History and trends of professional nursing

HISTORY & TRENDS
of Professional Nursing

GERALD JOSEPH GRIFFIN, B.S., M.A., Ed.D., R.N.

Director, Department of Associate Degree Program, National League for Nursing,
New York, New York

JOANNE KING GRIFFIN, B.S., M.A., R.N.

Former Instructor, Division of Nurse Education, New York University,
New York, New York

with a special unit on Legal Aspects by
Robert G. Bowers, B.A., J.D.
New Bern, North Carolina

SEVENTH EDITION

WITH 62 ILLUSTRATIONS

THE C. V. MOSBY COMPANY

SAINT LOUIS 1973

SEVENTH EDITION

Copyright © 1973 by The C. V. Mosby Company

All rights reserved. No part of this book may be reproduced
in any manner without written permission of the publisher.

Previous editions copyrighted 1943, 1950, 1955, 1959, 1965, 1969

Printed in the United States of America

Distributed in Great Britain by Henry Kimpton, London

Library of Congress Cataloging in Publication Data

Griffin, Gerald Joseph.
    History and trends of professional nursing.

    First published in 1943 under title: A history of
nursing, by D. M. Jensen.
    Includes bibliographies.
    1. Nurses and nursing—History. I. Griffin,
H. Joanne King, joint author. II. Jensen, Deborah
(MacLurg) 1900-   A history of nursing.
III. Title. [DNLM: 1. History of nursing. WY 11
G851h 1973]
RT31.G74   1973   610.73'09   73-4553
ISBN 0-8016-1977-7

CB/CB/B 9 8 7 6 5 4 3

To the **"Cinders"** *four*
Mary Hope, Jerilyn, Maura, *and* **Jennifer**

PREFACE

■ Updating of any written history about nursing in today's world is an all but impossible assignment, even for someone who is more than an onlooker in nursing's mainstream. Change, usually a slow and erosive process, has speeded up to a point where it is nearly visible.

In this edition we have attempted to consolidate the subject matter and combine many of the sections that previously were scattered throughout the text and that often overlapped. The bibliographies of some chapters have been combined to reduce duplication. Despite our attempts, there may be some areas where there is repetition and, unfortunately, of necessity, there are omissions.

We have made a serious effort to identify and describe all of the modern trends in some manner. The most constantly recurring theme throughout the book is the evolutionary role of women in our society today. We consider this a transitional edition be-cause the changes that are taking place in nursing and in the delivery of health services are as monumental as those that influence the lives of all men and women.

We wonder if the current turmoil in nursing, which concerns the extended role of the nurse, indicates that we probably should have followed the American system outlined by Lillian Wald in the early twentieth century. We also consider this edition as a nostalgic effort, especially the pictures of graduates of famous hospital schools that may no longer be in existence.

We sincerely thank the people who have contributed serious critical comments in the past to help make this edition more accurate and meaningful.

It seems imperative to acknowledge once again our admiration of Deborah MacLurg Jensen who still exemplifies some of the best attributes of the twentieth century nursing educator.

Gerald Joseph Griffin
Joanne King Griffin

CONTENTS

UNIT ONE
Pre-Florence Nightingale nursing and a current beginning

Nursing is not a product of modern medicine in the sense that socal service, dietetics, and occupational therapy are. It should be remembered that medicine and nursing had independent origins and existed as such for many centuries without much contact because the practice of medicine and surgery was relatively simply and undeveloped and required no technical skill. During the centuries known as the Middle Ages, nursing needs were met by a group of uneducated or untrained women, by members of the family, or by religious or military groups whose prime function was other than nursing. It was the evolution of medicine, surgery, and public health into complex technologies requiring specially trained persons with an understanding of scientific principles that brought the two professions more closely together. Fortunately, by the time the demand became urgent, nursing reform had been well started by motives arising within the nurses themselves, stimulated by changing social demands and conditions.

Today the two major health professions are becoming more distinct as a result of the promulgation by state legislatures of the legal definition of nursing as a profession. The New York State definition, a landmark achievement, was signed into law March 15, 1972. It clearly describes for the first time in the history of the profession the nursing function, and it establishes full legal authority for the implementation of the independent role of the nursing practitioner.

The New York State legal definition of nursing clearly establishes the professional status of nurses. Because of this status the public will expect, and rightly so, far more accountability on the part of all nurses. Therefore it is imperative that more nurses become involved in matters relating to nursing and health care.

Following is the legal definition of nursing practice as stated in the New York Education Law:

Section 6901:
Definitions. As used in Section 6902:
1. "Diagnosing" in the context of nursing practice means that identification of and discrimination between physical and psychosocial signs and symptoms essential to effective execution and management of the nursing regimen. Such diagnostic privilege is distinct from a medical diagnosis.
2. "Treating" means selection and performance of those therapeutic measures essential to the effective execution and management of the nursing regimen, and execution of any prescribed medical regimen.
3. "Human Responses" means those signs, symptoms and processes which denote the individual's interaction with an actual or potential health problem.

Section 6902:
Definition of the practice of nursing:
1. The practice of the profession of nursing as a registered professional nurse is defined as diagnosing and treating human responses to actual or potential health problems through such services as case-finding, health teaching, health counseling, and provision of care supportive to or restorative of life and well-being, and executing medical regimens prescribed by a licensed or otherwise legally authorized physician or dentist. A nursing regimen shall be consistent with and shall not vary any existing medical regimen.
2. The practice of nursing as a licensed practical nurse is defined as performing tasks and responsibilities within the framework of case-finding, health teaching, health counseling, and provision of supportive and restorative care under the direction of a registered professional nurse or licensed or otherwise legally authorized physician or dentist.

Section 6906:
2. Nothing in this article shall be construed to confer the authority to practice medicine or dentistry.*

---

*Amendments to Article 139 of the New York Education Law, effective March 15, 1972.

CHAPTER 1 WHY A HISTORICAL BACKGROUND?

■ History is the study of the trends of human thought and action as they influence the pattern of our lives. No longer are we much interested in the dates of births and deaths of kings or of great battles. They form the skeleton around which we build our story; our real interest lies in the principles for which great men and women fought and in the conflicts that lie behind the tests of armed strength. The strategy of war and the tactics of battle remain subjects for the student of military science; we wish to understand the outcome of the battle in terms of its effect on political thinking, economics, or religion.

As we study history in this manner we learn that great principles are the essential factors that determine human life. Great men are great only in part because of their inherent qualities; in part they owe their greatness to the setting of the stage upon which they enter. Without the conflicts that called them into action, George Washington and Abraham Lincoln might not have grown to the gigantic proportions that they now assume.

While studying history we must distinguish between conflicts of power politics and great movements that surge through Western Civilization as a whole. The conflicts that rage between nations at the present time are evidence of the significance of power politics. Although present events command our attention and claim the energies of all of us, in the eyes of the future historian they may seem like incidents when compared to the great social changes that in our time are sweeping through the entire world. These social changes are characterized by greater assumption on the part of government of responsibility for all citizens, limiting the individual's freedom of action, avowedly for the common good. Broad changes sweep so simultaneously through the entire world that any country in it resembles any other country more than it resembles itself as it was a century ago.

We are the products of our time; characteristics of any social group are conditioned by its greater movements. Therefore to understand the development of any group some time should be devoted to studying the movements on which it depends for its origin and growth. We speak of history in the sense of growth and change, not in the chronology of names and dates.

EVOLUTION OF PROFESSIONAL NURSING

To understand the evolution of nursing we should understand other important developments that have profoundly conditioned and influenced its growth. These are, fundamentally, the Crusades, the Renaissance, the Reformation, the Industrial Revolution, and the development of modern science and health facilities. Finally, the emancipation of women came to be part of the evolution of the nursing profession more than the other factors, because the newly gained freedom of women enabled them to develop and participate in community interests. The very fact that women demonstrated they could develop a profession greatly strengthened them in their fight for the further freedom that they desired.

Nursing is closely allied to medical progress and practice. In fact, just as one cannot understand nursing without some understanding of medicine and surgery, one cannot understand the evolution of nursing without knowing something about how medicine grew out of witchcraft, how the science was born through the clear thinking and observation of Hippocrates, and how it receded during the Dark Ages until the Hippocratian principles were rediscovered by the English clinicians of the seventeenth century. It is important to understand that modern medicine rests upon the physiological principles that Harvey discovered and the correlation of symptoms with organic changes as Morgagni taught it. When these great principles became integrated with clinical medicine, they gave to it the impetus under which we still progress in the understanding, cure, and prevention of disease.

The Industrial Revolution and the growth of medicine inevitably led to the need for hospitals. When poor people crowded together in tenements, it became necessary to segregate the sick in institutions designed for their care. Communities gradually began to assume some responsibility for the relief of their sick and unfortunate members. The growing medical science demanded working conditions and special facilities that the tenement did not afford. The aggregation of many patients under one roof favored specialization among the physicians. The outcome was the modern metropolitan hospital with its hundreds or thousands of beds separated into departments according to medical specialty.

As medical knowledge grew, the de-

mands on the individual doctor became greater and his training became more complicated. A need arose for an entirely new group of persons who could tend to the sick and carry out many procedures that they could master, often better than the doctor. This need was met by the modern nurse even before the doctors as a group realized how great it would become.

When medicine was passing into its modern phase, nursing was at a low ebb. Originally, nursing had developed to satisfy a fundamental need in all families. This impulse to care for the sick and weaker members of the group took different forms of expression among different peoples, influenced largely by the form of religion they practiced, their intelligence, and their humanitarian interests. Among all early peoples the dominating influence in nursing is the religious one. It is difficult at times to differentiate between ceremonials of worship and of purification and medical and nursing measures.

There is little evidence that any organized group of women nurses existed before the Christian Era. The ideals of brotherhood, service, charity, and self-sacrifice were preached by the early Christian church. Thus, groups of workers whose main function was to care for the sick and needy developed and became organized as deacons and deaconesses; often nursing of the poor was a way of atoning for sin.

Nursing as a function of the church, linked to this old ascetic idea, prevailed until after the development of nursing as a secular activity. The concept of nursing as an economic, independent, and secular vocation, an art requiring intelligence and technical skill as well as devotion and moral purpose, was developed first by Florence Nightingale.

Nurses in the early nineteenth century had much practical experience in looking after the sick, but they had no concept of scientific medicine and no social standing or responsibility. The doctor needed an assistant who could work scientifically and could observe and assist intelligently without relinquishing the old qualities of common sense and sympathy with those who suffered. The new nurse needed specialized training and, as the craft grew into a profession, began to require professional education.

A distinction must be drawn between "nursing" and "modern nursing." Nursing in the sense of caring for the sick dates back to prehistoric times and became a distinctive characteristic of the social structure as it rose above the level of the herd. It would also be natural that in any social grouping those who had proved themselves most adept in caring for the sick would be called upon to nurse friends or acquaintances or even would acquire the reputation to establish a practice of nursing. This is the usual state of affairs in primitive societies. The concern here is with the evolution of an organized group within a society who have received a recognized preparation for their work, devoting the major part of their time and effort to the systematic pursuit of a task— with recognition as a social group devoted to this task.

When viewed historically, the development of nursing seems to fall into three periods: (1) from the earliest times to the latter part of the eighteenth century, (2) from the latter part of the eighteenth century to the establishment of the first modern school for nurses at St. Thomas's Hospital, England, in 1860, and (3) from 1860 to the present.

The first period was a long preparatory one; there was no special training or education in nursing. The obvious and most pressing needs of the patient, a natural adaptation or liking for this work, and occasionally some sort of appointment by a religious group started the nurse in her work. The practical experience received at the patient's bedside constituted the training.

The second period was much shorter in time but is marked off from the long pre-

paratory period by definite attempts at reform and at beginning actual training for those wishing to equip themselves to care for the sick. Many far-reaching discoveries in the field of science and in social thought occurred during this period. The foundations for the tremendous activities of the nineteenth century were being laid in all fields as well as in nursing and nursing education. For example, in 1798 Dr. Valentine Seaman began a series of lectures for nurses in the New York Hospital. In 1833 Pastor Fliedner founded his noted Institute of Deaconesses, where Miss Nightingale received her only formal education in nursing.

The third period is characterized by the establishment of schools for nurses, college schools, both undergraduate and graduate; by the establishment of the associate degree nursing programs and their rapid growth; by the development of specialization in nursing; by the development of nursing organizations; by the beginning of study and research; by the expanding of opportunities for the graduate nurse; by legislation affecting nurses and nursing; and by the development in the community of interest in health and medical activities.

CONCLUSION

In studying the history of nursing it is obvious that the fight for professional advancement is entangled with the struggle for the political, economic, and educational freedom of women. In no other field has the emancipation of women been of greater or more practical importance. This struggle evolved from the philosophy of the eighteenth century, was nourished by the revolutions of 1789 and 1848, and culminated in the general reaction against the Victorian era. The result has been a newly won freedom that has enabled the modern woman to achieve that about which her mother hardly dreamed.

To further enhance the new freedom is the women's liberation movement, which is having revolutionary repercussions that affect us socially, economically, and politically.

There is an acceptance of newer life styles, which include pairings as well as marriage. Recent magazines dealing with newer concepts of mothering and child rearing continue in the vein of woman's new freedom.

Because of modern methods of contraception, for the first time in the history of civilization, women can, with almost absolute certainty, control what was once considered their primary function—child bearing and rearing. Also, the Supreme Court decision striking down existing abortion laws now permits the elimination of unwanted pregnancies legally.

This in itself has implications for nursing care and raises questions for large groups of nurses. It has made staffing difficult in some clinics because nurses have traditionally been educated and trained to preserve life, and it is simply physically and emotionally impossible for them to work in units where they feel life is being destroyed.

Medicine itself did not remain within the confines of the hospital or the sickroom. As it developed, its purpose spread beyond the cure to the very prevention of disease. To prevent disease requires work among the healthy in the community, schools, factories, and army camps. Laboratories that control the development and spread of disease need not be part of hospitals. Thus a new science arose—public health. It aims at protecting the population as a whole by instituting relatively simple measures. Once these measures have been devised and standardized, they can be executed by trained assistants to the doctors. Again the nurse became the ideal agent. Since its birth but a short time ago, public health nursing has grown into a field of unequaled opportunities.

The story of the evolution of modern nursing must be understood against the background of the Industrial Revolution, the evolution of modern science and health care, and the emancipation of women. When this background is comprehended, the history of nursing can be traced from antiquity through the Dark Ages to the rise of the great leaders in nursing of the last century. The results of their lifework may then be traced in Europe, America, and elsewhere. Finally, the more abstract but nonetheless real efforts of nursing in its work for international cooperation and understanding may be studied; this work may eventually prove to be its greatest achievement.

CHAPTER 2 NURSING IN ANTIQUITY

■ Very little mention is to be found in ancient history of nursing as a separate occupation. Certain activities must be performed, and specific needs must be met by society. Reference is made to the midwife and occasionally to women who looked after children. Of course, in the study of many ancient religions, priestesses are described who often performed functions now recognized as belonging to the nurse. The temple or place of worship in ancient days was also the health center; people who were ill went there for the treatment of disease as well as to worship. In fact, many of the health instructions were intermingled with concepts of religion and magic.

EGYPTIAN MEDICINE

Medicine originated in the practice of magic. In early Egypt certain empirical knowledge regarding sickness slowly accumulated from the witchcraft. The practice of medicine never entirely outgrew the superstitions that surrounded its origin. Today even the very educated patient looks toward his physician for something more than the logical application of a technical science. Medicine in Egypt reached a surprisingly advanced stage of knowledge. The custom of embalming enabled the Egyptians to become well acquainted with the organs of the human body. From clinical observations they learned to recognize some 250 different diseases; to treat these they developed a great number of drugs and procedures, including surgery. At the time of Herodotus, about 484-425 B.C., neurosurgery was advanced to a point beyond the imagination of the visiting Greeks. However, their ignorance of normal and pathological physiology and of experimental investigation limited their theories.

Egyptian medical practice was centered in the personage of Imhotep, chief physician to Pharaoh Zoser of the Third Dynasty about 3000 B.C.

Imhotep was not only chief physician but also by far the most trusted advisor to Pharaoh Zoser. One of his major contributions was in architecture, which affected the beauty of the projects of the dynasty for generations; another major contribution was in the care of the sick. This remarkable man also left behind much wisdom in the formulation of his wise proverbs. The common people sang these proverbs for centuries after his death. His fame was such that he became a demigod almost immediately upon death and was raised to the honor of full deity centuries later. On the Isle of Philae a temple was erected to Imhotep, and actual worship to him continued into the sixth century of the Christian Era.

With the decline of Egyptian civilization, medicine came under Greek influence. Although the Greeks brought their own ideas regarding medicine, they undoubtedly absorbed much of the knowledge found in Egypt, thus becoming bearers of some of the ancient truth to our own time.

7

GREEK MEDICINE AND HOSPITALS

Hippocrates (about 460 to 370 B.C.) stands out as a real person in the mythology surrounding early Greek medicine. The chief contribution of his school was to change the magic of medicine into the science of medicine. Hippocrates taught physicians to use their eyes and ears and to reason from facts rather than from gratuitous assumptions. His writings on fractures and dislocations remained unexcelled until the discovery of the x-ray. The Oath of Hippocrates possesses such a vitality that even today many are admitted to the practice of medicine with it, and the Hippocratian school has perhaps erroneously been given credit for the first ethical guide on medical conduct.

In ancient Greece we distinguish between two refuges for the sick: the secular and the religious. Physicians directed the secular, which corresponded roughly to spas or health resorts of today. Some were endowed and had outpatient departments, and some were used for the instruction of medical students. The secular places of healing and the sanctuaries of the gods, especially Aesculapius, were closely associated; of these, the one at Epidaurus, his birthplace, is the most famous. Most important here was the play upon the patient's emotions by a compli-

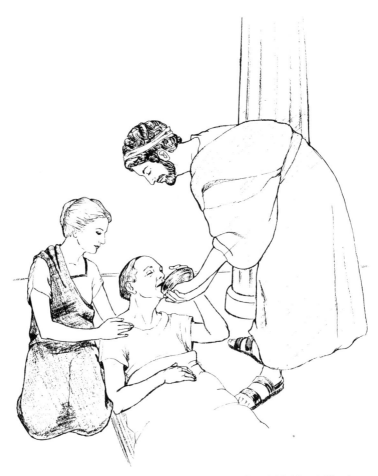

Specially trained care of the sick has been a characteristic of highly civilized peoples. The ancient Greeks had several centers for such care—among them the Temple of Hygeia, named for the goddess of Health, the daughter of Aesculapius.

cated ritual. Other practices that may have been more effective in bringing about cure were rest, wholesome food, physiotherapy, and fresh air and sunshine on porches overlooking the blue Mediterranean while the patient awaited the appearance of the god in his dreams. There were more than eighty such sanctuaries throughout ancient Greece. One of the most famous is the Temple of Cos, the birthplace and later seat of activity of Hippocrates.

The first suggestion of women being associated with the healing arts is found in Greek mythology. Aesculapius, who eventually became deified as the God of Healing, had five children; one daughter, Hygeia, became the Goddess of Health, and another, Panacea (our word for "cure-all"), the Restorer of Health. Aesculapius is represented by the familiar caduceus. Later most Greek healing centered around shrines in which many patients congregated. Among the attendants were the so-called "basket bearers" and those who were supposed to look after the sick somewhat in the manner of nurses. In the writings of Hippocrates there are many references to procedures that would be undertaken in modern hospitals by nurses but no reference to a nursing vocation as such. In ancient Greece and Rome the nursing of the sick and wounded was probably an incidental household duty, since there is no reference to any organized nursing group.

EARLY CHRISTIAN CHURCH

The great element of altruism contained in the Jewish religion later became further emphasized by Jesus Christ. Love is the fundamental element of His teaching. Its practical expression appeared in the early Christian church in the form of succor to the orphans, the poor, the travelers far from home, and above all, the sick. The deaconesses of the early church visited the sick, much like modern visiting nurses. They were lay women appointed by the bishops. These appointments were highly esteemed and were given to women of good social standing. The women were often sent on distant and varied missions to accomplish their appointed tasks. Gradually their work was assumed by the various orders, and their activities declined. One of the best known deaconesses of the early Christian church was Phoebe, a Greek lady who is also remembered as the bearer of St. Paul's epistle

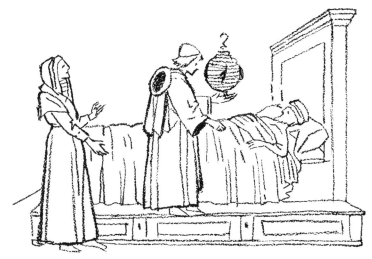

In ancient Greece "basket bearers" cared for the sick in a manner like nurses.

to the Romans. Visiting nursing soon became an important part of the work of these early deaconesses, and Phoebe is often referred to as the first visiting nurse as well as the first deaconess. During the fourth and fifth centuries the names of three Christian matrons of patrician Rome, Fabiola, Paula, and Marcella, were associated with charitable work. These matrons were particularly interested in the care of the sick.

In the early days of the Christian Era the Roman Empire was at its peak. At the height of its splendor Claudius Galen (A.D. 130-201) was physician to the Emperor Servetus. He worked with incredible industry observing, experimenting, and gathering information. Unfortunately, many of his conclusions were based on speculation. Although his anatomical and physiological observations were admirable, his later dominance over medieval and Renaissance medicine came about largely by the force of obscure and erroneous notions that retarded medical progress for centuries.

However, Galen's voluminous writings contained virtually all of the medical knowledge of his day—knowledge that only through his industry survived the destruction of the Roman Empire. The translation of his writings into the Arabic chiefly accounted for their preservation; therefore, until the time of the Crusades, Arabian physicians became the standard bearers of medical knowledge.

EARLY CHRISTIAN HOSPITALS

Although early Christendom at first encouraged women to visit the sick and to nurse them, refuges for the sick made an early appearance. Patients were sheltered in the bishop's houses, but when this proved impractical, special institutions were established by endowments throughout the Roman Empire. In Rome the first large hospital was established by Fabiola, a beautiful, worldly woman, who thereby did penance for her second marriage. She administered

this hospital so well that her death was mourned by all Rome.

In the eastern Roman Empire several large hospitals were established; the Emperor Constantine founded one at Constantinople, A.D. 330; but the largest of them all was the one that St. Basil of Athens built on land granted him by the Emperor Valerian near the city of Caesarea in Asia Minor. It was tremendous, constituting a town all of its own, with separate hospitals for lepers, children, the aged, and strangers. These hospitals, however much contemporaries may have been impressed by them, did not continue into the later centuries.

A few centuries later in the Western world the first hospitals immediately under the auspices of the Roman Catholic Church were founded; these still exist. In Lyons the Hôtel Dieu was established in A.D. 542 by Childebert; it is now the hospital with the longest record of continuous service. Detailed records were kept of the Hôtel Dieu in Paris, which was founded about A.D. 650-651 by St. Landry, bishop of Paris. It was greatly enlarged in the thirteenth century by St. Louis and was the prototype of the medieval hospital. The records of this hospital constitute a principal source of information regarding nursing in those days.

MOSLEM HOSPITALS

During the eighth to the tenth centuries magnificent hospitals were erected throughout the Moslem world. For the times they had excellent endowments. One in Bagdad received about $1,200 a month, and the physician-in-chief served gratuitously. In addition these hospitals had a great advantage over their European contemporaries, for they were staffed by physicians superior to any in the world. Greek knowledge had been preserved by the Moslems.

One large hospital in Bagdad had a staff of 24 physicians. In 869 its superintendent published the first known pharmacopeia. By 1160 there were some 60 medical institutions in that city. Best known to Western lands, however, were the big institutions in Damascus and Cairo. The hospital in Cairo was founded by the sultan of Egypt in 1276 as a thank offering for having been cured of the colic.

It was endowed with an income of 25,000 pounds, and contained four great Courts, each with a fountain in the centre, wards for each separate disease, a lecture room, and a department for attending patients at their own homes. Musicians and storytellers were provided for the amusement and benefit of those troubled with sleeplessness, and the convalescent patient received, at his departure, five pieces of gold, about 50 shillings, that he might not be obliged to return to work immediately.*

Such was one of the hospitals of the "infidels," whom the Crusaders tried so hard

*British Medical Journal, 1908, p. 1448.

to exterminate. These structures were in marked contrast to the rather gloomy Gothic Hôtels Dieu in France of a few centuries before.

MOHAMMEDAN MEDICINE

Physiology and hygiene were studied by the Arabian scientists, knowledge in materia medica was expanded, and surgeons used various drugs as anesthetics, but Moslem belief in the uncleanliness of the dead forbade dissection. The following names stand out: Rhazes (860-932), noted for his study of communicable disease, and Avicenna (980-1037), who wrote extensively —his *Canon of Medicine* was used long after his death.

CHAPTER 3 MEDIEVAL MEDICINE AND NURSING

■ During the Middle Ages medicine in Europe was under two influences—the lay medicine that followed what was left of the Roman traditions and the ecclesiastical medicine that existed in the monasteries, around which most of the existing hospitals were built.

For 1000 years after Christ, there were no attempts to organize nursing. As the Middle Ages advanced, three organizations developed that either have persisted in some form to the present day or that established certain principles still recognized as important. These organizations were the military, regular, and secular orders. All worked under the auspices of the church, which, as we know, profoundly influenced all activities of the Middle Ages.

The most spectacular product of the feudal system was the Crusader, a man who was supposed to combine a lofty spirit devoted to the service of God with a fierce, belligerent temper, ready to fight the infidel wherever he was to be found, that the holy ground upon which Christ trod might again belong to his followers. He carried the principles and the glory of knighthood to their fullest as he traveled over the continent of Europe and throughout the Mediterranean basin. When he traveled in the Near East, he learned much from the enemy; the idea of the organized hospital was originally borrowed from the Arabs. The natural places for the establishment of hospitals were the outposts, particularly Jerusalem itself, where those wounded in battle sought refuge while they recovered. The hospital had to be staffed by physicians and nurses who were members of the regular orders. The nurses went to battle and then retired to attend the sick. They were called "knight hospitalers." In later years they devoted themselves entirely to nursing. Two great influences shaped nursing practice in the Middle Ages—the religious and the military. Gradually the care of the sick was considered more and more to be a religious duty.

MILITARY ORDERS

Three nursing orders became preeminent: Knights of St. John, Teutonic Knights, and Knights of St. Lazarus. Corresponding with these were three orders for women who tended female patients in special hospitals.

Knights of St. John

About 1050, Italian merchants of Analgi founded two hostels in Jerusalem, one for men and the other for women. The former was dedicated to St. John the Almoner; the latter to St. Mary Magdalene. Some 50 years later the Order of St. John became prominent, and it is generally assumed that this order originated in the nursing staffs of these two hospitals. Peter Gerard, an intensely devout man, was active in the organization of the order on a high religious plane under the grand master. The members were divided into three classes: the priests, the knights, and the serving brothers. The women's branch of the order, organized under Agnes of Rome, devoted itself to religion and nursing; they gave up the latter pursuit, however, when the order was driven from Jerusalem.

The Order of St. John proved a huge success; branches were established everywhere, and its extraordinary vitality is shown by the fact that it has persisted to the present day and is active in England. St. John's Ambulance Association and the National Association for the Aid of the Sick and Wounded During War are activities of the order. The order was active in the organization of the International Red Cross, which carries its insignia as its mark.

The order had a long and varied career. At the reconquest of Jerusalem by the infidels it was driven to Cyprus and from there to Rhodes where it established a magnificent hospital that was used as recently as World War I. At this very moment some of the apartments once used by the knight nurses house refugees from other eastern Mediterranean countries.

The order became a prominent, affluent, and important factor in medieval Christendom. Many of the customs that it established have remained the heritage of nursing to the present day. Being military in character the discipline was strict, and modern nursing traces its tradition of obedience to superiors to the Order of St. John. The order also established the organization of rank and the principles of complete and unquestioned devotion to duty. Although extreme subservience does not belong to our day and age, it must still be remembered that in an organization in which exact execution of orders and minute attention to instruction may determine the difference between life and death of patients, strict attention to detail must continue.

Teutonic Knights

The Teutonic Knights made up the German equivalent of the Order of St. John.

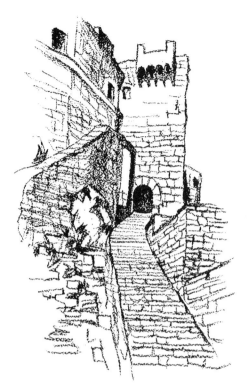

THE HOSPITAL OF THE
ORDER OF ST. JOHN AT RHODES

The Knights of St. John established branches throughout Europe, one of which still exists in England.

They date back to a hospital founded by Germans in Jerusalem soon after 1100. They took an active part in the subsequent wars in the Holy Land, especially the siege of Acre in 1190, when they established a tent hospital for wounded crusaders. In consequence they were established as Brothers of the Hospital of St. Mary of Jerusalem. Later they became a separate order under the rule of St. Augustine. Their organization was modeled on the Order of St. John, and they seem to have been, for a while, under the jurisdiction of that order. Like their model, they gradually came into possession of great property, especially in Sicily. They always remained under German leadership, however, and eventually their main seat was moved to Germany where they became primarily a military order. The nursing of this order was largely done by men; women were not admitted to full membership but retained a secondary position. Sisters of this order were, however, engaged in nursing as late as the end of the fifteenth century.

Knights of St. Lazarus

The Knights of St. Lazarus were established primarily for the nursing of lepers in Jerusalem after this city had been conquered by the Christians. Later, Boigny near Orleans became their main seat, but as leprosy became less prevalent by the end of the fifteenth century, the order was dissolved and its property was absorbed by the Order of St. John.

REGULAR ORDERS

As the early Christian church developed, those who devoted their lives to the service of God followed the example of Christ, and the very spirit of the church led it to care for the fatherless, the poor, and the sick. In antiquity, when the Pax Romana prevailed, people could safely travel. The deaconesses could go to people's homes and nurse their sick; later, because of the insecurity of the early Middle Ages, men sought protection behind moats and walls. The men and women of God established monasteries in which they organized hospices to house their charges. In the beginning, travelers, paupers, and patients were housed under the same roof; the modern words of hostel, hotel, and hospital, now with different meanings, all have the same origin—hospice or hospitium, a place of refuge. The early hospital was called a "Hôtel Dieu." Soon, however, it became advisable to care for the sick separately, and with the knowledge the crusaders gained from the Arabs, the hospital, as we now know it, had its origin. As society again became better organized, and with the growth of cities, hospitals tended to become separate institutions apart from monasteries

although many of them continued to be staffed by the regular orders.

Of these, the sisters who took charge of the Hôtel Dieu in Paris are the best known, because their records are the most complete. They began about A.D. 650 as a small group of volunteers who looked after the sick in the hospital. They remained primarily a nursing order called the Augustinian Sisters. For the first 600 years of their existence as a nursing order they were without severe restrictions, but about 1250, Innocent IV caused them to become cloistered under the rigid rules of St. Augustine. The Augustinian nun wore a white robe, and when she became a full sister, a hood was added to her habit. In Hôtel Dieu she worked very hard, both early and late, with no recreation, and apprenticeship the only method of instruction.

In spite of very inadequate medicine and nursing during the Middle Ages there began to be an increase in the institutions for the care of the sick. Sometimes this was stimulated by epidemics. The number of individuals, mainly volunteers, who devoted themselves to nursing also increased. During the fourteenth century one of the outstanding and devoted women whose activities were linked with the care of the sick was St. Catherine of Siena (1347-1380). At night her lamp represented to the sick of Siena what Miss Nightingale's lamp was to mean in the Crimea. Catherine was not of noble birth; she had been trained in what we would call a middle-class home to help with housework as was the custom of the day. A devout Catholic with a decided bent toward asceticism, she found great happiness in nursing, and in spite of the protest of her parents, she devoted a great deal of her time to working in the hospital in her native town. She taught herself to read and, some years later, to write. She became a tertiary of the Order of St. Dominic, an organization within the regular order to which she could not be admitted because of her youth. However, the members decided that, because of her great homeliness, it would be safe to allow her to nurse and visit in the homes of sick patients. In 1372 the plague came to Siena, and Catherine worked day and night at nursing. She became particularly well known about the hospital at La Scala; it stands as a memorial to her today.

St. Hildegarde (1099-1179), a Benedictine abbess in Germany, is associated more with medicine than with nursing, since she actually prescribed cures and was supposed to perform miracles. However, she trained young noblewomen in the care of the sick in her abbey.

In the sixteenth century the Ursulines, an order that emphasized the care of the sick and the education of girls, was founded. It is of great interest to nurses and teachers in the United States because some of the early schools and hospitals were staffed by Ursuline Sisters.

The nursing provided in the Middle Ages was simple. It consisted mostly of providing for the patient's physiological needs, giving medications and bathing and dressing wounds and ulcers. The ideas concerning cleanliness and ventilation differed considerably from ours: windows were often placed so high that they were difficult to reach, and bathing and the changing of bed linen would not measure up to modern standards. Heating, lighting, and plumbing arrangements were either very primitive or nonexistent. When the mother superior made her evening rounds, it was by the light of a torch that she was carrying. Nursing appliances were also primitive. Much equipment that we consider essential, such as thermometers and hypodermic syringes, were entirely missing; the use of rubber was unknown and accessories like bed rings were made of leather stuffed with hair; draw-sheets were made of leather and later of oiled cloth. At the Hôtel Dieu there were no washing machines; the nurses carried the dirty linen down to the river on washdays. Many of the activities of the sisters were limited by prejudices. Because the human body was considered inferior and unclean, it was thought improper for the nurses to undertake certain procedures, such as giving enemas to men or vaginal douches to women. An important duty of the sisters was to minister to the spiritual needs of the patients; in an age when religious considerations dominated every activity, this took a great deal of time.

The nursing order was definitely organized; the sisters advanced from the stage of probationer to wearing the white robe to receiving the hood. They were all under a "superintendent of nurses" or director of nursing; in those days she was called a prieure or maîtresse. In the beginning there was no uniformity of dress; nurses wore their regular clothes when on duty. Clothes became gaudy as the Middle Ages advanced; and because the church secluded itself from the more worldly aspects of life, there was a tendency to adopt a uniform dress that eventually became entirely standardized. We have thus studied the first organization devoted to nursing; now let us consider its strong and its weak points.

The strength of the nursing order was its organization into an institution under the immediate guidance of the strongest spiritual and secular power of the time, the church. Absolute devotion to the sick without mundane or selfish motive made the nursing order acceptable to all, and it was thus able to survive for many centuries. The Augustinian Sisters at Hôtel Dieu in Paris can look back upon its record of over 12 centuries of uninterrupted service. The nursing order was not firmly associated with the medical profession for two reasons: it was sponsored and dominated by the church, and the medical profession in the Middle Ages had not developed into a profession capable of exerting leadership over nursing.

However, the strength of the nursing orders was also their weakness. By being so closely attached to the church, they had to share the vicissitudes of that organization; and because it later suffered censure for practices that were at variance with its professed purpose and ideals, the nursing orders suffered with it. They were sent out of countries in which the Protestant Reformation had gained the upper hand, and their property was confiscated. Those countries then passed into what has been called the "dark age" of nursing. Their close attachment to the church also sometimes prevented them from enjoying the advantages of the medical progress that did occur. When the interests of church and medicine conflicted, the church prevailed, often to the detriment of the patient. As time passed, and as the Catholic church recovered from weaknesses occurring during the Middle Ages and adopted broader policies of modern days, these difficulties were largely solved. The Catholic nursing orders now seem perfectly capable of serving both

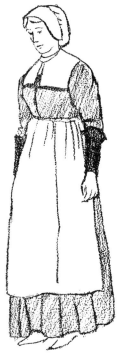

SIXTEENTH CENTURY NURSE

Secular nursing groups often had many characteristics in common with regular and religious orders, such as uniformity of dress.

church and patient without detriment to either.

SECULAR ORDERS

Some of the drawbacks of the nursing orders were apparent also to their contemporary observers. Demands for complete and perpetual devotion to God would not always attract those best suited or inclined to care for the sick. Consequently, organizations developed for the primary purpose of nursing. Many of them, it is true, prospered under the auspices of the church, often as lay branches of the regular holy orders, but some of them remained relatively independent. On the whole the tendency in the course of time was to make the secular orders approach the regular ones by requiring temporary vows, uniformity in dress, and religious observances. Many of these orders possessed extraordinary vigor and have persisted to the present time. They were very numerous but similar; this description will be limited to six of the more interesting ones.

Third Order of St. Francis

About the year 1200 St. Francis was a lively young man in Assisi in northern Italy. He had generally led a carefree life until illness and disagreement with his father brought out the more serious side of his character. At first he retired into the wilderness, but soon he decided to devote his life to the service of God and man. He began by rebuilding a local church, and he attempted to lead a life as similar as possible to that of Jesus. Soon he was joined by friends, all of whom devoted their lives to poverty and service to the poor. When the group numbered 12, they obtained papal sanction as an order and dressed in brown or gray woolen hooded robes ("Gray Friars") with ropes around their waists. They set forth traveling from place to place to spread the Gospel and to teach the better way of life they had learned to live. Eventually their number increased, and they became a great and powerful order with branches throughout the countries of Europe. They were the First Order of St. Francis.

Among those who watched the work of St. Francis was a young girl from his home town. Her name was Clarissa. She was so influenced by his work that one night she ran away from home and joined the small band of Francis and his friends. Francis consecrated her at the altar and cut off her beautiful hair as a sign that she had abandoned vanity and devoted herself to God; she dressed in a simple robe similar to that of the brethren. After having lived in a Benedictine convent for protection, she eventually established an abbey of her own; the sisters who gathered around her grew into a regular nursing order, "The Poor Clares." These were the Second Order of St. Francis.

The work of St. Francis greatly stirred the people of his time; there was a great surge to abandon the temporal for the life of God. St. Francis soon realized that to admit unlimited numbers to his order would not be practical, so he instituted the third or tertiary order, which was secular in the sense that the members did not give up their social relationships or take vows of chastity but devoted their lives to the order in their home town, without neglecting their duties as citizens. These people improved their communities as they served the order. One of their most important duties was nursing. For centuries male and female nurses belonging to the Third Order of St. Francis could be found in hospitals and homes.

Order of St. Vincent de Paul

Nearly 400 years later, about 1600, another inspired priest, St. Vincent de Paul, founded with prophetic vision another nursing order that has become very important. St. Vincent lived in Paris, France, where he joined in the care of the sick of a neighboring hospital. Here he discovered that charity was often poorly directed, being bestowed to excess on some, while others equally deserving went without aid; therefore, St. Vincent organized charity wherever he could. He devoted special attention to begging, which was rampant at the time, and whenever possible he tried to guide tramps and beggars into useful occupations. His greatest work, however, was done in companionship with Louise de Gras (Saint Louise de Marillac). She was a widow of a noble family who had devoted herself to visiting nursing, and directed a group of volunteer women devoted to this purpose. She was a rare woman, for along with her feeling of social responsibility she was highly educated, being conversant with the Scriptures, Latin, philosophy, and painting. Under the guidance of St. Vincent she studied closely the various lay organizations of charity devoted to the care of the poor and the sick all over France. Finally, on her return to Paris, she organized the "Dames de Charité" (the Ladies of Charity), an institution devoted to social work.

Soon she found that these ladies had difficulty in establishing the right kind of contact with the poor of the slums of Paris; their duties as ladies of charity conflicted too often with their domestic duties. Louise then decided to train her own social workers. In 1633 she opened her home to young peasant girls who as "The Community of the Sisters of Charity" became the foundation of one of the most important of nursing orders. To be accepted the girls must be of good family and of good character; they enter with the consent of a male relative. Each year on March 25 they dedicate and rededicate themselves to their work, but if they do not wish to do so, they are free to resign from the order to marry or to take up some other occupation.

In their training and practice they have made every endeavor to overcome the difficulties that were noted in the discussion of the regular orders, and by working closely with physicians and by assuming all nursing duties they have spread all over the world and set a fine example of what a nursing order should be. One of their greatest services was in the Crimean War, for here they not only nursed the French wounded but also, by their example, indirectly stimulated the discontent in the British army that eventually resulted in Florence Nightingale's great work.

The Beguines

The Beguines are a most interesting group of lay nurses originally organized in Liege, Flanders, about 1170 by the priest Lambert le Begue. The concept of their organization was that it should be liberal but devoted to the service of suffering mankind. Groups of women lived together in little houses, four or five in each. If they occupied a number of houses, these might be surrounded by a wall; however, in small communities this was not the case. These women were available for all kinds of household aid, especially nursing of the sick, but they also sewed, made lace, or taught. They did not beg but supported themselves by their wages and fees for services to those who could pay, as well as by special funds provided for them by the community. They made no vows but accepted certain standards as long as they belonged to the order. For instance, they could not marry and remain Beguines. The adoption of a uniform was optional; when a group designed one for themselves, it was generally in accordance with contemporary dress. They became immensely popular, and the order spread from Flanders into the Netherlands, France, and Germany. At its height about the middle of the fourteenth century it numbered approximately 200,000 members. They staffed hospitals where necessary but generally devoted themselves to work throughout the community; some were found in every community, their number depending upon the need for their services. They always endeavored to live within walking distance of their work. At all times, even to World War II, they served their communities, often in a manner comparable to that of the Red Cross.

Similar groups have from time to time come under the domination of the regular orders as tertiaries. Such a fate overcame the entire Order of the Visitation of Mary that was established in Dijon, France, by St. Jane de Chantal with the help of St. Francis de Sales. They began as an order of visiting nurses, with activities like those of the Beguines, but because the church insisted upon cloistered seclusion, they had to change their activities and to restrict themselves to offering succor to those who could come to them.

The Oblates

The Oblates, founded in the twelfth century in Florence, Italy, are another order similar to the Beguines. They gained distinction by the manner in which they staffed the hospitals of Florence and by the broad training that they received for this task. They still remain an established order.

Order of the Holy Ghost (Santo Spirito)

The Order of the Holy Ghost originally had branches for both men and women, although this order is remembered chiefly as a male nursing order. It was founded in Montpellier, France, in the twelfth century by Guy de Montpellier. The numerous "Holy Ghost" hospitals, churches, and streets may be traced back to the activities of this order.

THE MEDIEVAL HOSPITAL

Moslem ideas about hospital construction and administration were adopted by the Crusaders and influenced the great hospitals of the military nursing orders in Jerusalem. Later, as these orders were driven west, the Moslem influence appeared in the hospitals that they constructed in Rhodes and Malta. Inspired by what he had learned in the East, Pope Innocent III about A.D. 1200 decided to build a modern hospital in Rome.

He called on Guy de Montpellier of the growing Order of the Holy Ghost to establish this hospital on the bank of the Tiber. Because of its architecture, efficient management, and nursing care, it remained in operation until destroyed by fire in 1922.

When this hospital was finished, the pope begged the bishops from foreign lands to come and to inspect it and then to go back and to construct similar hospitals in their home dioceses. During the next 100 years literally thousands of such hospitals under the Order of Santo Spirito, Heiligen Geist, or Holy Ghost were spread all over Europe. Street names bear witness to their locations down to the present day. The best of these hospitals were magnificent places, architecturally beautiful with painted Gothic doors, and with window and wall coverings of precious hangings in the manner of the times. The high, wooden ceilings were beautifully carved; privacy of the beds was secured by partitions that could be removed when mass was said. The greatest artists contributed to these decorations, which made the hospitals beautiful and attractive.

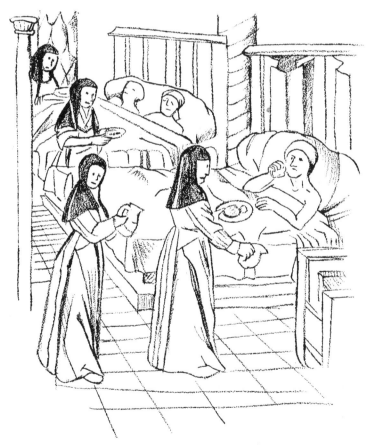

SIXTEENTH CENTURY HOSPITAL

Most early hospital architecture was profoundly influenced by Moslem ideas which were adapted by the Crusaders and military nursing orders. Often these hospitals were quite beautiful from an aesthetic point of view.

Not until the present day has the wholesome effect that pleasant architectural designs and attractive furnishings have on the patient's morale been appreciated. In fact, some medieval hospitals were so attractive that even well-to-do citizens who were left alone in the world would move into them bag and baggage and turn over all their property to the hospital in return for carefree old age.

In this period a distinction must be made between the two types of hospitals in the medieval towns. There were the city hospitals proper, built within or actually in the walls of the city. There were also the isolation hospitals placed outside the city called "plague" or "leper houses" that served as refuges for those unfortunate outcasts of society. Nursing in them was largely provided by the Order of St. Lazarus. When the Black Death swept Europe in the fourteenth century, it seemed like a fire to consume all who were weak and ailing; following it, leprosy almost disappeared, with consequent neglect and decay of the leper houses.

The better hospitals had resident and visiting physicians who were also often professors of medicine. If they had known a little more medicine, the hospitals would have been a setup for fine medical services, for nursing by religious orders was then at its height, its devotees being enthusiastic servants of Christ.

MEDICAL SCHOOLS AND MEDICINE IN THE LATER MIDDLE AGES

The establishment of the famous medical school in Salerno, Italy, was a great medical event of the ninth century. Until the fourteenth century this school was the center for all medical teaching and was not primarily dominated by the church. It was abolished by a Neapolitan decree in 1811, but had been in a decline for a long period before that. In the twelfth and thirteenth centuries, many famous universities were established in Europe. The growth of medieval cities with the corresponding increase in wealth and power influenced this development. The medical school at the University of Montpellier established in the twelfth century was the most famous medical school for several centuries, probably because it was practically independent. The University of Paris had a medical faculty at the same time, but within the department of philosophy. In Italy the medical school at the University of Padua was gaining a favorable reputation, as was the University of Bologna. By the end of the fifteenth century there were well-organized medical schools in many European countries and in Great Britain. Laws governing the practice of medicine were in effect in these same countries. It was to these centers of medical learning that the great medical men of the Renaissance turned for information and inspiration.

Physicians or doctors of medicine at that time considered the practice of surgery inferior and beneath the dignity of scholars. In the fourteenth century the student of medicine in Paris had to swear that he would not do any surgical operations. Surgeons of that period often traveled from place to place performing operations for the stone, hernia, and cataract, as well as blood-letting, pulling teeth, applying cups, and giving enemas. In England the Union of Surgeons and Barbers lasted until 1745, and in 1800 the present Royal College of Surgeons was founded.

By the end of the fifteenth century the newly invented technic of printing resulted in the rapid increase in both the number and variety of medical books that before then could only be reproduced painstakingly by copyists.

Although names such as Paracelsus (1493-1541) are recorded as outstanding in their time, they do not represent any fundamental advance of physicians of their era generally. What little practice of medicine there was, was so involved in superstitions and erroneous assumptions that it must have done little good. Patients who recovered often did so because their desire to live overcame not only the disease but also the treatment to which they were subjected.

THE RENAISSANCE IN MEDICINE

The well-known name of the forerunner in the great medical developments of this period is that of Leonardo da Vinci, whose anatomical studies and sketches remain classic. Vesalius (1514-1564) is remembered as the founder of anatomy as a science and, with Harvey, of a medical science based on fact rather than on tradition. The work of these sixteenth century anatomists enabled the surgeons to work on a more solid basis. Ambroise Paré (1510-1590), a military surgeon, wrote a great book on natural history in general and on surgery in particular in which he emphasized that it was not necessary to dress wounds with boiling oil and that bleeding could be controlled with ligatures as well as by red-hot cautery. He also devised artificial

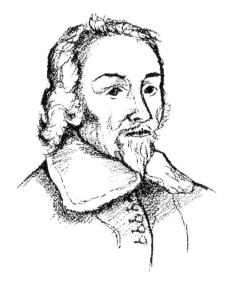

WILLIAM HARVEY

William Harvey is often called the father of modern medicine because he established the principle of the physiological experiment.

limbs for the victims of war. During this period nursing reached a high level of organization and efficiency in the religious and military orders.

Harvey and his time (1578-1657)

We ordinarily associate William Harvey's name with the discovery of the circulation of the blood, but his contribution to medicine is much greater than the discovery of a single physiological fact, however important, for he established the principle of the physiological experiment. He received his anatomical training at Padua and returned to the St. Bartholomew's Hospital in London where he served as demonstrator of anatomy at the Physicians' College in Amen Street. Here he completed his great discovery, which he communicated in a lecture in 1616. His book was not published until 12 years later. In due course he became attached to the court of King Charles I, left London with that monarch, and was in Oxford during the siege of that city. While there, his home in London was searched, and all of his manuscripts and notes were destroyed. What loss medicine thereby suffered can only be surmised, for some of the titles were of great promise, including "The Practice of Medicine Conformable to the Thesis of the Circulation of the Blood" and "Anatomy in Its Application to Medicine."

Following these disturbances, Harvey returned to London and became one of the scientific leaders of his day. He donated his library to the College of Physicians and established a lectureship that has continued to this day and to which we owe, among others, Osler's marvelous oration of 1905* on the founder himself. Harvey exhorted the fellows and members of the college to study the ways of nature by means of experi-

---

*Osler, William: The harveian oration on the growth of truth as illustrated in the discovery of the circulation of the blood, Lancet, October, 1906.

ment; and, most important, they were urged to continue in love and affection among themselves. These traditions are still highly regarded in the old college.

Thomas Sydenham, 1624-1689

The simple methods taught by Hippocrates were all but forgotten when they were suddenly resurrected by a man who later was called the English Hippocrates, Thomas Sydenham. Sydenham was Puritan by birth and outlook. He took part in both the Cromwellian wars.

Sydenham's great contribution to medicine was that he first set the example of true clinical method. His independent and unprejudiced spirit, combined with great powers of observation, made him the prototype of the clinical investigator. It was he who resurrected the great principles of Hippocrates: to observe phenomena and to let observations logically lead to conclusions. He expounded, "We should not imagine or think out, but find out, what nature does or produces." That this sounds obvious to us is only because Sydenham succeeded to such an extent that his teaching has become commonplace. In his time medical science carried a superstructure of wanton speculations and theories so complicated and cumbersome that it became deprived of real value. In fact, Sydenham was attacked because he made the practice of medicine too simple and easy. In modern times his name is most commonly associated with his description of chorea, although his description of gout was much more of a masterpiece.

Undoubtedly Sydenham received great support from his friendship with his colleague, the physician-philosopher John Locke, the private physician to Lord Shaftesbury. Locke was a proponent of common sense and straight thinking and the forerunner of Hume and Kant. The essence of his philosophy was to consider the reasonableness of taking probability as our guide in life. In thus eliminating the fantasies and vagaries of the mind, Sydenham met on common ground with Locke; the two must have been great mutual supporters.

It has been stated that Sydenham was considered little better than a quack by his contemporaries. It is true that his views met with great opposition and that he did not participate in the activities of the Royal Society of Medicine. But during his lifetime he was considered one of the great physicians of the age, although the true magnitude of his accomplishments was not appreciated for several generations.

CONCLUSION

During the seventeenth century London abounded in quackery of all kinds. Quacks, mountebanks, chemists, apothecaries, and even surgeons, who in those days were not supposed to treat internal diseases but nevertheless did, joined in exploiting the healing crafts. Druggists copied prescriptions they were supposed to fill and sold the drugs privately over the counter. One was said to have profited a hundred times as much out of a single prescription as did the doctor who wrote it. Consequently, five sixths of the physicians went with their hands in their pockets all day, the greatest part of the business passing through only a few men's hands (although some of them were more ignorant than others). It was considered that medicine was overstocked with students graduating from the universities. He who began practice must have had to resolve to be a perpetual slave and servant to the meanest and basest all the days of his life. Upon the physician were imposed taxes, polls, large fees for houses, servants, and entertainment—more in this age than formerly. The main requirements for beginning a practice were to have a good understanding with the druggist and to be seen regularly at church.*

---

*Payne, Joseph Frank: Thomas Sydenham, New York, 1900, Longmans, Green & Co., pp. 165 ff.

CHAPTER 4 THE DARK PERIOD IN NURSING AND SOCIAL SETTING FOR REFORM

■ The dark period in nursing and the social setting for reform dates roughly from the end of the seventeenth to the middle of the nineteenth century. The dark period was characterized by nursing conditions so terrible that some time must be spent on an analysis of how such conditions could come about. It should be noted that during the same period the principles upon which modern medicine was built were established and that remarkable progress in other fields of human endeavor is evident. Medicine developed rapidly during these years. One great man after another made important contributions, not only to detailed medical knowledge but also to its basic principles. There has always been a lag between medical discoveries and their practical adoption. In present times, this is a very short span. One notes, for example, the rapid adoption of insulin or the sulfonamides, but in the old days when postgraduate communication was slow and medical instruction proceeded along primitive lines, physicians persisted tenaciously in old habits.

The general practitioner and most specialists practiced as did their medical predecessors until well into the eighteenth century. During the years that followed, the changes were not great. The doctor of those days simply was not in a position to demand good nursing, for he did not know what comprised good nursing. Good nursing is predicated upon a knowledge of anatomy, physiology, hygiene, and bacteriology; a knowledge that in those days was nonexistent. Assumed knowledge and superstition, the details of which are now practically forgotten because they are worthless, occupied the place of scientific knowledge. Therefore, in the practice of medicine, in spite of the growth of medical knowledge, nothing existed to stimulate the evolution of nursing as a profession. The new knowledge was not to bear practical fruits for many years to come.

The guiding principle of ecclesiastic nursing was charity; there was no concept of medical progress or of medical efficiency. Nursing services, therefore, were as good as the organization within the church that supported them; some orders continued nursing efficiently until the present time and experienced no "dark age." For the most part, in Catholic countries, nursing remained more or less on the same level, ready to take advantage of progress when it appeared.

The emergence of an organized group such as the nursing profession can be understood only if we understand its background. Nursing as we know it today was greatly influenced in its professional development by the social and economic change called the Industrial Revolution. By referring to this change as an industrial revolution we do not mean to focus our attention on one element, the mechanical change that occurred in Western Civilization, for it must be realized that the entire process was fostered by economic change. Economy originally meant the rules governing housekeeping; here we use it in the sense of the producing or procuring of the essentials of life. As this activity changed, it altered the entire lives of men, including their environment, their thinking, and their political philosophy and conduct. Out of this setting emerged the world as we know it today. We must look upon the present world as the outcome of the past and the beginning of the future. There is nothing static about it, nor anything hard and fast. Yet to understand nursing we must understand its most important elements of the past as well as those that are likely to dominate its future. In other words, we must think of nursing as a social function.

INFLUENCE OF THE REFORMATION

Nursing sank to its lowest levels in the countries in which the Catholic organizations were upset by the Reformation. The state closed churches, monasteries, and hos-pitals. In England alone it was said that over 100 hospitals were closed, and for a while there was little or no provision for the institutional care of the indigent sick. When the demand became too great to be ignored, lay persons were appointed to run the hospitals. For example, this was done in the case of St. Bartholomew's Hospital in London and in St. Giles in the Fields and St. Katherine's Hospitals. These hospitals were not run because of the principle of charity but because of a social necessity. There was no honor attached to running a hospital or to being on its staff. At St. George's Hospital a man and his wife were engaged at salaries of £8 and £10 per annum to be messenger and matron, respectively. The matron remained there in charge of the nurses, and a nurse in charge of a ward or a division was called a "sister," possibly because it was thought that by retaining the title, some of the devotion and dignity of the old days might be retained also. This, however, was not the case, for when deprived of the dignity of the church, nursing somehow lost its social standing. Nurses were no longer recruited from the respect-

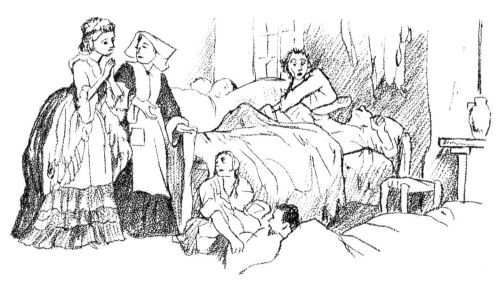

EIGHTEENTH CENTURY HOSPITAL

Nursing care during the eighteenth century was guided by charity, not by knowledge or principles of safety and hygiene.

able classes of the community but from the distinctly lower classes. The new Protestant church abhorred cloisters and religious institutions and did not feel the same responsibility to the sick that had characterized the early Catholic church. Nurses were drawn from among the discharged patients or from the lower strata of society—women who could no longer eke out a living from gambling or vice often turned to nursing.

Another factor in this situation was the status of women in the social structure of 200 or 300 years ago. From the antiquity of Rome to the Middle Ages the Catholic church had assigned to woman a place in society that afforded her much freedom and opportunity to move about in the world. Thus women of ability could carve out careers for themselves, and the lay nursing orders especially offered them great opportunities to contribute to the life of the times.

The Protestant church, although it stood for religious freedom and freedom of thought, did not think much of freedom for women. In the seventeenth and eighteenth centuries and into the Victorian era the place of the average respectable woman was in the home—a "career woman" would have been next to unthinkable around the year 1700. All teaching, secretarial work, and literary endeavors were confined to men, and work then unsuitable for men, such as nursing, was entirely out of the reach of the average woman, even if she had wanted to do it. Housework demanded infinitely more effort than nowadays, and those women who had enough servants to free themselves from domestic tasks gave their efforts entirely to the shallow and superficial life of society. The only profession open to women was acting, and that was not very respectable. So women faced with the necessity of earning their own living were practically forced to enter domestic service; nursing was considered a type, although not a very desirable type, of domestic service. After all, the chief duties of a nurse in those days were to take care of the physical needs of the patient, and to make sure that he was reasonably clean, although this was not considered very essential in the early municipal hospitals. Dressings were applied by dressers or by surgeons; the dispensing of medicines was the responsibility of the doctors and the apothecary.

It is possible to understand the low and dismal state of nursing. It existed without organization and without social standing. No one who could possibly earn a living in some other way performed this service; and those who did lost caste thereby, for, as you are judged partly by the company you keep, a woman who began to practice nursing was almost certain to become corrupted if she was not so already. Most nurses were venal, drunken, and given to even worse vices than these. They expected and took bribes wherever they could be obtained, and liquor was their chief solace.

There were reasons why the nurse should fall a victim to these vices. Her pay was poor; if she had to provide only for herself, she could perhaps eke out a miserable living; but if she had children or other dependents to support, her pay was entirely insufficient, and she was forced to supplement it by any means available in order to survive. Her hours were so long and her work so strenuous that she had no opportunity to supplement her income by additional work. Her work was cheerless and depressing if she thought about it. If she worked in the hospitals, she was dealing with riffraff and the scum of creation; if she were lucky enough to be admitted to nurse respectable persons, she was considered the most menial of servants. As well as the long hours (sometimes nurses worked 24 or 48 hours at a stretch) they received poor food and sometimes none at all during the long night shift. There was no future toward which these women could look; this was the end of the road. They should, therefore, not be judged too harshly if they turned to the only source of comfort that was open to them—the bottle.

Seen with our eyes, nursing was a blotch on seventeenth and eighteenth century society, but the contemporary attitude was one of inertia and complacency. The high ideals of the Middle Ages were gone, and a demand for adequate nursing had not yet risen. However, when men with the inquisitive spirit of the eighteenth century began to look into social evils, nursing was examined along with the rest of them. Hogarth's cartoons and later Dickens' description of Sairey Gamp were caricatures that had their effect. In a more serious vein the writings of John Howard (1727-1789) have become famous.

INDUSTRIAL REVOLUTION

The Industrial Revolution emerged from a social state called feudalism. Feudalism was stationary, and if it had not been for the Reformation, which really was a product of the Renaissance, and the great scientific discoveries, it might have gone on for centuries. In almost every respect it differed from our world; it was essentially static with fixed concepts of class relationships defined by insurmountable barriers. Life was strictly localized; it centered around the manor, which offered a measure of protection and exercised a crude but effective form of law and justice in return for hard work by the individual to obtain the bare necessities of life. So much work was required to obtain food, clothes, and shelter for the present that there was very little chance of obtaining reserves for the future or for barter. There was little time for education or for leisure, and freedom to pursue them became, of necessity, restricted; and limitations became further imposed by the social order on the right of movement as well as upon political and religious thinking. It was a conservative, patriarchal state of society, offering few of what we today consider the amenities of life; the individual lived in continuous fear of famine, pestilence, and the figments of his own imagination, such as witchcraft and other superstitions.

The Crusades, acting as a catalyst, began to change all this. Knights returning from the Middle East yearned for the knowledge, pleasures, gracious living, and comforts they had enjoyed so briefly. Out of the ferment came the sixteenth century with its great changes. New, rich lands were discovered beyond the seas, and men began to emigrate and to bring back treasures to the old centers of population. The immediate effects of this were tremendous: the treasures from the new lands made for a richer life, a "surplus economy" was being created, transportation was encouraged, and the center of gravity was shifted from the Mediterranean to the Atlantic seaboard, a change that was to chiefly benefit England. During the time that followed, there was progress in domestic agriculture. Under the feudal system it had been, to a certain extent, communal; it now became more individualistic, and methods were improved. This led to a better yield, fewer men were required to till the ground, and with better food more men survived to a productive age. This agricultural surplus population moved to the cities in which industries had begun to develop in response to the growing wealth. These industries did not offer attractive careers; at first, they had few, if any, machines and it was long before they utilized power other than that of man and beast. There were the guilds, but their range was narrow, and the early industrial worker was limited by fixed wages, inability to move, and many social customs. Essentially the feudal outlook was carried into the early industrial community.

It is questionable whether this Industrial Revolution would have extended very far had it not been stimulated by the new thought.

NEW THOUGHT

The origin of the new thought may immediately be traced to the Reformation. Although the religious aspects of this movement are most spectacular, more important than these fundamental elements is the new stimulus to thought provided by the freedom that generated from the Reformation and eventually transformed our ideas of government, politics, business, and philosophy. The right of private judgment was established, which later led to individualism in politics and business and to the concept of the free contract and the right of property. In the feudal order the right of property, by custom, was vested in the sovereign who could, in all ways, abrogate the rights of the individual to hold and to utilize the individual's property. The thinking of Locke, especially, established individual prerogative: the individual's right of property antedates that of the state, and he cannot be deprived of it without his consent (or "due process of law"). With the right of free contract it follows inevitably that the individual is also privileged to acquire and to hold as much property as he can within the limits of the law. This is the fundamental philosophy of capitalism, and it is essential that we grasp it, for without it the Machine Age of the nineteenth century would be unthinkable. Unless we understand it we cannot understand the modifications that it later undergoes and that have profoundly influenced the development of nursing.

Natural sciences

Free thought extended also into the realm of natural science; men began to ask questions to which they expected to find rational answers based on facts alone. The scientific method of inquiry was born. This method of reasoning led to objective observation and to the physical and physiological experiments that form the basis for the modern natural sciences. The writings of Locke, Bacon, and Hobbs guided men's thoughts. Suffice it to mention that Gilbert of Rochester assembled all knowledge pertaining to magnetism and introduced the word electricity; Newton invented calculus and discovered laws governing optics and the law of gravity; Boyle introduced the atomic theory. Thus, through hundreds of observa-

tions and discoveries, which often in the most unexpected way gained practical importance, the foundations for sciences were established. It was the scientific attitude that led to the discovery of steam power and the construction of the steam engine and somewhat later to the discovery of electromagnetism and the construction of the electric motor. Without it the modern engines would hardly have come into being, and the Industrial Revolution would have remained unborn. In the course of time, the scientific attitude also laid the foundations for modern medicine, for, as we have seen in Chapter 3, Harvey's and Sydenham's fundamental work was its direct outgrowth. Thus, clearing the air for straight thinking eventually led to the construction of the engine by which our entire lives were to be altered.

Political philosophy—mercantilism

Along with studying the laws of nature the philosophers of 200 and 300 years ago began to ask questions regarding the conduct and the rights of man. The right of contract to which we have referred was but one of their conclusions. They studied the laws that seemed to govern the growth of population: thus, Petty founded the science of vital statistics, and Graunt showed that the population increased in a geometric ratio but that this increase was checked by various factors which in turn were studied by Davenant and de Mandeville; these studies eventually led to the sciences concerning trends in population that are now so essential in grasping the fundamentals of public health. Although purely scientific in their beginning, they were to lead to knowledge of the greatest importance to the modern public health nurse.

The study of the laws of population growth is but a short step to the study of economics, and soon this field was under scrutiny. Gresham founded the science of public finance, and soon the men who guided the new thinking arrived at certain conclusions that by their general acceptance were to exert a fundamental influence on the growth of the state. Their views on the right of property and on national ambition led them to an economic and political philosophy that has been called mercantilism. Property was the watchword, especially property represented by holdings of precious metals or bullion. To obtain these metals foreign trade had to be encouraged, even at the cost of domestic trade. Because trade flourishes when a country has a product to sell, preferably a manufactured product, the importance of manufacturing was stressed. To be able to produce finished goods came to be considered preferable to producing the raw materials from which these goods were manufactured, because the profit was greater.

This was in the days when machines had to be tended laboriously by men and were not the labor-saving devices of today. The chief motor power was man power; therefore the men of mercantilism began to welcome increases in population, because these increases in man power would eventually mean increases in wealth. We had, at the same time, retained from feudalism the concept of the sovereignty of the head of the state—"L'état, c'est moi," proclaimed Louis XIV—and that was the view to which most persons acquiesced. It was therefore the monarch or his representative who personified more than anyone else the practical aspects of this philosophy. The common man is the principal asset of the state, and the personification of the state is the monarch —this is the absolute monarchy. The state became a dynamic entity that, depending chiefly upon the industrial centers of the cities, competed with other states for trade monopolies and far-flung colonies. This was the era in which colonial empires were built.

This political philosophy had one interesting result: since it was realized that the power of the monarch ultimately depended on the number and opulence of his subjects, the monarch became concerned for their welfare. This led to the enlightened monarchy, which was one of the most efficient forms of government ever devised by man. Its defect was the lack of checks and balances that would become effective when the monarch ceased to be benevolent, and that was the cause of its ultimate doom. However, while the enlightened monarchy lasted, the concern of the state for the health and welfare of its citizens resulted in formulation of our first notions of public health. Although factory towns of the eighteenth century may have appeared dingy to us, they were, nevertheless, far in advance of the dirty, smelly cities of the century before. Wealth accumulated, and many strata of the population improved their living conditions. It was also this outlook, which, together with the rapid growth of the cities, was responsible for the rapid increase in hospital construction of this era. Here we have the beginning of public health in the setting of the society that produced it.

Beginnings of revolutionary thought

There were other currents of thought that were to influence men in the future. The philosophers of the seventeenth century who had accepted the right of property and of free contract soon began to ask by what right the sovereign owned the state and by what right he collected tax moneys to be spent on his own personal ambitions rather than on the common good. The answer soon was found to be—by the acquiescence of his subjects. This doctrine of consent of the governed led directly to the political philosophy of the eighteenth century engendered by Rousseau, Voltaire, and Hume.

These political philosophies led to a revaluation of human rights and to the new concept of political liberty. Once the people understood that concept, the Boston tea party was inevitable, leading as it must to the American Revolution and then to the French Revolution. The citizen is no longer the chattel of the sovereign; he is the state, and "citizen" became in France an appellation of honor. The French Revolution and the American Revolution were not revolutions in the sense that the proletariat was placed in power, as occurred in the Russian Revolution a century later; the absolute power of the head of the state was abolished and replaced with a constitutional form of government—immediately in America and eventually in Europe—in which the real power was placed in the hands of the bourgeoisie, the propertied classes.

MACHINE AGE—THE RISE OF ENGLAND

During this same eighteenth century, industrialism, which so far had been very primitive, developed into the Machine Age; the steam engine had now been invented, it multiplied man's power in the factory, and eventually the railroad and the steamship revolutionized transportation. Now factories could be placed near the chief source of their raw materials. All during the eighteenth century and at an accentuated pace during the nineteenth century, England forged ahead of the industrial states. There were many reasons for this: her capitalists had apparently been more awakened by the new philosophies than had been her continental confreres; she understood first what production for the masses really implied; her isolated position had largely protected her against the devastation of wars; she was traditionally a nation of sailors; and when it came to getting colonies, she got the lion's share, including the plum of them all— India. The greatness of the British Empire was to a large extent built upon the riches of India. So we come to look to England as the leader of the Machine Age and consequently as the source of many of the movements that were direct products of this age.

Evils of the Machine Age

England became the first great nation of factories, but certain elements that were part of that development later had to be discarded. We learned that the value of a cer-

tain measure of public health was appreciated by the proponents of mercantilism, but these concepts of public health were limited by restricted medical knowledge and furthermore were partly ignored when the absolute monarch disappeared; in fact, they were largely squeezed out by the aggressiveness of the new capitalist. As a type he was so impressed with the right of free contract and the right to acquire and hold property that he forgot that when a man has only the choice between absolute starvation and starvation wages he is not really a free agent. The result was the early dark years of the Machine Age when the capitalist was protected by law in his exploitation of the worker under the guise of free contract. The result was child labor, sweatshops, unhygienic factories, and hours of labor fixed only by the limits of human endurance. This led to the gin shop and all the social evils that soon were to be so graphically described by their reformers. Not the least of these evils were the hospitals. The advances in medicine were so far largely theoretical and had not yet borne practical fruits, so that while medicine definitely was advancing, it was still proceeding slowly and without the dramatic developments that were to mark the end of the nineteenth century. The hospitals were large and crowded, and the conditions of nursing, which were brought about by the Reformation when the Catholic institutions had been closed, had been steadily aggravated until they now reached an all-time low.

HOSPITAL REFORM AND CONSTRUCTION

A new development in our social structure in the eighteenth century, and more so in the nineteenth century, influenced the construction and administration of hospitals: the rise and evolution of capitalism and industrialism. Wealth was created by the manufacture of natural resources brought to the industrial countries from faraway colonies. Manufacture demanded factories, factories required workers, and the profits from individual enterprises went into relatively few pockets; therefore large numbers of people congregated in the new cities, and the gulf between the new-rich industrial employers, on the one hand, and the laborers, on the other, grew even wider. The result was that extensive sections in industrial cities were inhabited almost entirely by laborers. In sickness these individuals required ever larger hospitals, and as a direct result of the Industrial Revolution the demand grew for bigger, but not always better, hospitals. So we see during this period the foundation of the great city hospitals. The London Hospital in the East End of London, the Grosse Charitee in Berlin, and the Allgemeines Krankenhaus of Vienna all originated during the eighteenth century, and the development continued through the nineteenth century with the growth of the great cities.

The following notes, taken from the catalogue of the London Hospital, give an interesting account of its progress.

The first course of lectures on surgery was delivered in 1749. In 1772 iron bedsteads were first introduced. In 1780 surgeons were henceforth to be members of the company of surgeons in London. In 1781, Mr. Blizard was granted permission to deliver courses of lectures on anatomy and surgery. In 1791 a thermometer was purchased. In 1820 feather beds were bought for special cases. In 1833 gas was installed in the corridors, though not in the wards. In 1838 an ordinance was passed that medicine was to be administered only by nurses who could read and write. In 1842 special wards were set aside for Jewish patients. In 1849 a microscope was bought. In 1852 the committee held that the apothecary was not the fit person to administer chloroform. In 1856 Miss Florence Nightingale was elected life governor. In 1896 x-rays were introduced.

The evolution during these two centuries cannot compare with the developments of the last 50 years, neither in regard to number of beds nor in regard to technical improvements. Some changes of the nineteenth century must, however, be recorded.

The pavilion system of hospital construction was introduced in the French Academy of Sciences in 1788. It became generally accepted both in Europe and in this country. Its outstanding expression is in the beautiful Bispebjerg Hospital in Copenhagen, which probably is the most expensive hospital to heat yet designed, and also the one which, in proportion to its size, provides the most extensive walking exercises for all who work there, because of the distances between its divisions. As implied in the name, the hospital consists of pavilions and is not built in large blocks as was hitherto the case. In this country the first buildings of the Johns Hopkins Hospital were built by the pavilion system.

Originally as a result of the writings of John Howard, who had severely criticized the hospitals of the eighteenth century, this period also saw the introduction of better hygiene throughout the hospitals, from the nursing service to the plumbing and heating, because the old hospitals had been very cold and unsanitary places. Florence Nightingale, although she failed to appreciate the significance of bacteriology, thoroughly understood the value of fresh air, soap and water, and sunshine. This all preceded the antiseptic and aseptic operating room. We shall learn more later on about the nursing reforms.

During the nineteenth century there was also a tendency to develop hospitals for various specialties. This reached its height in London where the start was made with the Royal London Ophthalmic Hospital, which was founded in 1804 and which was followed by many others: the Royal Free Hospital run for women by women doctors, St. John's Hospital for diseases of the skin, the Royal Victoria Hospital for diseases of the chest, and many, many others. For a while this tendency also appeared in this country, until the disadvantages of thus emphasizing specialties appeared. The tendency has now been modified so that separate departments are developed within the same hospital, easily accessible to each other.

Outpatient department

With the development of the hospital idea it also became apparent that the hospital's responsibility toward the patient did not always end with his discharge. He may require aftercare while he is ambulatory, or poor patients may wish to avail themselves of the experience of the hospital staff although they are not sick enough to gain admittance to the wards. It thus became logical to establish outpatient departments in connection with the hospitals. Although dispensaries, that is, clinics in which poor patients could be seen gratis and could obtain medicine at cost or free, had been organized in the beginning of the eighteenth century, the outpatient department idea was not thoroughly developed until near the end of the nineteenth century, but when it was developed, the possibilities for medical teaching that it offered were first grasped and best developed in England. In the United States we have been rather slow at appreciating the excellent source of clinical material for nurses as well as for doctors, which is found in the outpatient department.

Early English hospitals

The early movement to construct fine hospitals also reached England. The first one was built at York in 937. This one, however, did not influence further development. For hospitals of enduring importance, we must turn to London, where following the Conquest, three important hospitals were founded—St. Bartholomew's Hospital by Prior Rahere in 1123, St. Thomas's Hospital in 1213, and the Hospital of St. Mary of Bethlehem in 1247. All three of these have so importantly influenced British hospital history that a brief sketch of each is in order.

At the beginning of the twelfth century a cleric of humble birth became ill while on a pilgrimage to the Holy Land. In his misery he vowed that, should he be spared, he would on his return to London build there a hospital dedicated to the glorification of God. In answer to his prayer, St. Bartholomew appeared to him in a vision and instructed him to erect a church in Smithfields, London, and name it after him, the Saint. In obedience to his vow, Rahere, who was a courtier as well as a cleric, obtained a grant of land from the king and erected a church and hospital on the chosen site, where it has since remained. The church could still be seen before World War II, but the original hospital had long since been replaced by more recent, if far from modern, structures. St. Bartholomew's Hospital was closed by Henry VIII along with other similar institutions from the Reformation that had ushered in the dark period of hospitals and nursing, but after a few years it was reopened at the request of the Lord Mayor of London. It had then a capacity of 100 beds. During the next century it expanded, and medical teaching was organized there. Since that time "St. Bart's" has been in the heart of British medicine, and some of the most prominent medical men of English history have been on its staff. Outstanding among them is Dr. William Harvey, whose work was discussed in Chapter 3. Although the medical practice, past and present, of St. Bartholomew's Hospital has always been outstanding, it shared in the general decay of nursing during the post-Reformation period, and much of our information on how bad nursing became was obtained from the records of that hospital.

St. Thomas's Hospital was founded, south of the Thames, by the prior of Bermondsey in 1213. It was rebuilt on various sites before it was finally moved to its present location on the south side of the river overlooking the Houses of Parliament. This hospital is of special interest to us, because at the time of this last reorganization, Miss Nightingale established her school of nursing there. St. Thomas's Hospital has, throughout the years, remained among the leading London hospitals. It was badly bombed during the blitz of 1940.

Finally there is the Hospital of St. Mary

of Bethlehem. In 1247 on the feast for the Translation of Edward the Confessor, Simon Fitzmary gave a tract of land for the erection of a monastery for the brethren of Bethlehem, the second monastic order created in 330 in Bethlehem by Constantine. This land was situated in the eastern part of the city of London, around what is now Liverpool Street Station, and is extremely valuable. In those days it was covered with marshes, fields, and gardens; on this the original Hospital of St. Mary of Bethlehem was erected. It was more of a monastery than a hospital at this time. However, it, too, suffered in the Reformation when Henry VIII expropriated it and handed it over to his political friends who managed it badly. The character thus changed from a monastery, doing charity work, to a regular hospital, and gradually it became purely a lunacy asylum. As such it became a place of horror to the patients and of amusement to the visitors. In those days there was no understanding of mental diseases. The patients were treated with cruel restraint, and it was thought proper to exhibit them to spectators for a small fee. So a visit to see the sights of London included a visit to "Bedlam" as the place eventually was called in common parlance. Later the building was wrecked, and in 1676 a new and magnificent structure took its place. It lasted until 1812 when the last and final structure was commenced.

For many years Bedlam played an important part in London life. Fiction writers sent their characters to languish within its walls, and artists painted its terrors; probably Hogarth's final stage of *A Rake's Progress* was as pictorial a representation of lunacy as was ever accomplished. Awe was inspired by a public exhibition, the horrors of which exceeded the imagination. Although Bedlam presented the horrors of maltreatment of mental disease, it was also responsible for the first rays of the new dawn. It was in connection with the tortures sustained by one American, James

Norris, that William Tuke, a York tea merchant in 1792, suggested that mental disease be treated along humane lines. His plea was without immediate effect, but it was the next year that the Frenchman, Pinel, introduced the famous reform of the treatment of mental patients. When reform did occur, the Bethlehem Hospital was again in the vanguard and has taken its place among modern hospitals devoted to the treatment of mental disease. Tuke's work did have an important effect in the United States, for when the Bloomingdale Asylum was opened in 1821 in connection with the New York Hospital, it was modeled after Tuke's "York Retreat" and emphasized the mild and humane treatment of the patients.

THE STATE OF MEDICINE

It has been noticed that, while nursing was in a very bad condition during this period, medicine was advancing rapidly. During the first part of the eighteenth century Hermann Boerhaave (1668-1738) of Leyden, Netherlands, was easily the most famous physician of Europe. Princes and statesmen alike crowded his waiting room. When he appeared after a sickness, the whole town was illuminated, rejoicing in his recovery. A letter from a Chinese mandarin, addressed "To the illustrious Dr. Boerhaave, Physician in Europe," found him without difficulty. His greatest contribution was his pupils. There was hardly a prominent physician in Europe and North America who had not at some time studied under him. He occupied several university chairs at the same time and excelled in wisdom and classical knowledge. He was one of the first great physicians who appreciated music. When he died in 1738, he left a large fortune of about 2 million florins.

The seventeenth century had seen two great principles established: (1) disease is to be observed like any other natural phenomenon, and (2) the functions of the human body can be investigated by means of physiological experiments. A third great principle was to be added: symptoms and disturbances of function are associated with changes in the organs of the body and this relation is frequently very specific. It is to Giovanni Morgagni (1682-1771) that we owe this contribution.

His principal work, *On the Seats and Causes of Disease,* appeared in 1761 when he was 79 years old. It is in the form of a series of letters to an unidentified young man. Morgagni excelled in his infinite capacity for working diligently and carefully. He insisted on examining every organ, as well as the one that he suspected of being chiefly affected. He marshalled with the utmost care from his own experience and that of his predecessors all instances in which the disease had existed apart from the symptoms of the lesion or the lesion apart from the symptoms. He discussed each of these incidents with severe exactness, and only after exhaustive investigation would he allow the inference that the organ referred to either was or was not the seat of the disease. Thus he created a work of classic importance and beauty, which even today delights the mind of the scholar.

Thus Morgagni came to reap the highest honors bestowed on living men. He was a friend of popes and princes, honored by all the scientific groups of importance in Europe, sought by every student of medicine; he died beloved by his family in his eighty-ninth year. Twice when hostile armies invaded his town, their commanders gave strict orders that no harm come to Morgagni and that his work be not hampered. His wife, who could not have been surpassed in judgment or affection, bore him 11 children—eight daughters who all became nuns, one son who died young, one son who became a Jesuit priest, and one son who married and reared a family.

In Delft, Holland, an unlettered man had the honor of first using the microscope systematically and of perfecting its construction. Anton van Leeuwenhoek (1632-1723) lived quietly, pursuing his microscopic studies and communicating most of his observations to the Royal Society.

In spite of the great leaders who had risen in the seventeenth century, British practice and the teaching of medicine and surgery fell to a low ebb by the middle of the eighteenth century. Obstetrics as a science was just being founded through the efforts of William Smellie (1697-1763). But that was about all. Then suddenly anatomy, surgery, and obstetrics received a great impetus through the efforts of the brothers John and William Hunter. Alike in their zeal and industry for the advancement of science, they otherwise differed most strikingly.

William (1718-1783), the elder, was born in 1718 near Glasgow, where he received his early classical and professional education. Still in his youth he, like so many celebrated Scots, gravitated to London. He became associated with Dr. Smellie, the first male-midwife, founder of obstetrics. He was one of those fortunate few who early in life were placed exactly in the situation for which they were best suited by nature and by education. Given the opportunity to teach anatomy, he soon found himself in charge of the most famous school in the country, and turning to obstetrics he advanced rapidly and eventually became obstetrician to the queen. In spite of his success, he never let financial considerations crowd out his professional ideals. He realized that a man may do infinitely more good for the public by teaching his art than by practicing it, because the influence of the teacher extends over a whole nation and descends to posterity. So Hunter continued to combine in himself the qualities of a polite scholar, an accomplished gentleman, a complete anatomist, and a most perfect demonstrator as well as lecturer. *The Pregnant Uterus* is his main work, which for all time will stand as a landmark in medical literature. About his teaching, he said that he aimed at showing not what he knew but what he thought his students ought to know.

Through his professional efforts he accumulated much wealth, most of which he spent on a magnificent collection now in Glasgow. It contains famous paintings, valuable books, a large number of coins, besides medical and zoological specimens all gathered with great taste and discernment. Thus he combined in himself the qualities of a great teacher, investigator, patron of the arts, and scholar. Besides, he earned additional credit as the man who brought his younger brother to London.

In contrast to the polished William, John Hunter (1728-1793), ten years younger, was considered a misfit for the first 20 years of his life. Not until his brother had introduced him to the art and science of anatomy did his native ability assert itself, but from that day John developed into one of the greatest geniuses of all time. His great intellectual powers triumphed over his early defective training, and he marched onward step by step despite vast obstacles to the highest achievements. After serving a term in the army, he became surgeon to St. George's Hospital, and he gradually acquired the leading surgical practice in London of his day. In contrast to his brother, his progress was slow, for he did not possess the charming manners of William but had to advance by sheer ability. In fact, to the end of his days he remained crude in his expressions and highly undiplomatic; for instance, he generally gave precedence to his poorer patients, saying they had no time to spare, whereas the wealthy ones, having nothing to do, could afford to wait.

Although he had never read Bacon, his mode of studying was as strictly Baconian as if he had. Characteristic is his answer to Edward Jenner (1749-1823), his student: "But why think? Why not try the experiment?" Yet he himself was so busy in his search for knowledge and so cautious in his estimate of it that he always delayed to publish what he knew. He was 43 years old when he published his first work, and at his death he left many valuable manuscripts and notes, which, to the inestimable loss to the world, were destroyed by his brother-in-law.

A wave of enthusiasm was apparent in France after the French Revolution. Young men now advanced by ability and no longer by privilege and nepotism. This also applied to medicine, and in that century medical science advanced as never before. Beginning with Napoleon's own physician, Jean Nicolas Corvisart (1755-1821), the list runs through François Xavier Bichat (1771-1802), the pathologist, who unfortunately died young; Réné Laennec (1781-1826), to whom we owe the stethoscope and our knowledge of diseases of the chest; to Pierre Louis (1787-1872), who first introduced statistical methods into medicine and who, more than the others, attracted young American students, especially the pathetic figure of James Jackson, Jr., whom he considered almost like a son. The famous school of Dublin, which soon was to shine with the names of Robert Graves (1796-1853), William Stokes (1804-1878), Robert Adams (1791-1875), and Dominic Corrigan (1802-1880), had not yet reached its climax; and on the continent Karl Rokitansky (1804-1878) and Rudolf Virchow (1821-1902) were not yet famous. By the middle of the eighteenth century interest in real clinical medicine was being stimulated; for example, decisions were based on examination of the patient and the diseased organs rather than on the study of classic texts and the use of metaphysical discussion.

One of the most successful clinicians of the century was William Heberden (1710-1801). Among other things for which he is remembered is the description of angina pectoris, which has been made available to modern students in reprints. He also described the rheumatic nodules on the fingers called "Heberden's nodes."

William Withering (1741-1799) is remembered for the discovery of the use of foxglove (digitalis) in the case of dropsy.

CONCLUSION

Thus we see the stage being set for the social reforms of the late nineteenth and early twentieth centuries. These reforms included nursing which was soon to be looked upon not only as a skilled technic necessary in scientific medicine, but also as a community service essential to the health and welfare of every community.

CHAPTER 5 EARLY REFORMS

■ The torch of liberation was carried largely by the intellectuals who continued to follow the views on the human right to happiness that had been championed by the humanitarian liberals of the eighteenth century. Recognizing the deplorable conditions that existed in the eleemosynary institutions, Parliament reformed the Poor Laws in England in 1832, but even this left much to be desired, and when Dickens, Carlyle, and others of their school revealed the social evils of their time, they met with a ready response among their readers. A sense of social responsibility and a desire to give this feeling a practical response developed among the well-to-do classes. Owen's sociological experiments are an example of this movement, but of greatest interest is its expression in the life work of Miss Nightingale, which was entirely devoted to the relief of the classes in society that could not help themselves. One of the most important accomplishments of this era was the entire reform of nursing education, which is the main topic of this book.

The beginning of the evolution of the nursing profession was primarily the private work of philanthropic persons; it was not sponsored by the state. In time the women who had done nursing in religious or military orders and those untrained and uneducated women who did nursing for money were replaced by the new profession. The government sponsorship of causes that so greatly increase the fields and scope of nursing is of still more recent origin and has developed out of trends that we have yet to explain.

EMANCIPATION OF WOMEN

The emancipation of women may be traced ultimately to the trend toward personal freedom, which was one of the factors in the Industrial Revolution. It is part of the fight for human rights, which was first audibly expressed in the eighteenth century and which became one of the principles of the French Revolution. It is a step without which nursing might have developed as a craft but never into the profession as we know it today. Therefore the emancipation of women forms part of the background that we must know to understand the evolution of nursing. Many attitudes of Florence Nightingale appear peculiar to us if we do not appreciate the difference between the social position of women 100 years ago and now. Furthermore the emancipation of women can no more be considered a completed process than can the Industrial Revolution, the evolution of modern medicine, or even the very evolution of nursing with which we are principally concerned.

The word "moral" comes from the Latin *mos, moris,* custom, and if we use the word in its original sense, we may say that the emancipation of women is fundamentally a moral process, its various practical manifestations—suffrage for women, legal rights, and educational and occupational opportunities—are secondary to the moral aspect.

The customary social attitude toward women a few hundred years ago was one that was almost as old as Christendom and that, in fact, had been dictated by the church—not by Christ, for his attitude toward women was, as far as can be judged, quite liberal—but by the early church, especially as influenced by Paul. During the sixth to eighth century the stern attitude toward women was relaxed somewhat, but it was generally believed that woman's place was in the home only.

There were practical reasons for this: the work of housekeeping, like that of producing the necessities of life, was so complicated that it left little time for other pursuits. One part of housekeeping was the rearing of children, which because of the high rate of infant mortality was a most inefficient process. It was not uncommon that out of ten or twelve pregnancies, labors, and months spent taking care of infants there resulted but two or three effective citizens for the community. The energy lost in this manner of procreation was appalling, especially when compared with modern marriages. Young couples today are often limited to two to four pregnancies, but nearly all result in effective citizens. By an effective citizen we mean one who grows to productive manhood or womanhood. Thus there was a good physical reason which would have restrained all but a small privileged class of women from enjoying any measure of freedom even if it had been granted them, and even if the Machine Age had reduced the time required for domestic work, the professional woman as a social class still would not have been possible.

Society's attitude toward women

Another fundamental factor in the emancipation of women was the changing attitude of society toward her. When, during the period of the French Revolution, Condorcet upheld the rights of women and Mary Wollstonecraft wrote her *Vindication of the Rights of Women,* it is doubtful if many understood that these were the germs of a movement that eventually was to transform society. Few realized that women needed any "rights." In fact the rights that women already had (such as the franchise, which women had in the United States under the first constitution of New Jersey from 1776 to 1807 and in England prior to the Reform Act of 1832) were not used and consequently were abrogated without contest.

Until the middle of the nineteenth century there was no place for women in the professions or in public life; whatever they wished to do had to be accomplished behind the scenes, hence "the little war office" at Burlington Hotel where Florence Nightingale worked out the army reforms with Sir Sidney Herbert and Dr. John Sutherland. As we shall see later, this failure to recognize women in public life may have been the real reason for Miss Nightingale's illness. Those few who bravely broke the bonds of tradition, such as Elizabeth Blackwell, the first woman doctor, and Miss Dorothea Dix, faced a great resistance, purely because they were women.

The real difficulty in securing for women a place of equality with men was the negative attitude of society; its members took refuge in all types of rationalizations. The meeting of the argument, therefore, did not change the fundamental attitude of the opponents. The passing of laws or the exercise of previously unused constitutional privileges or rights does not accomplish much as long as these efforts are not in accord with the emotional attitude of the dominant citizenry, for our moral or customary attitudes are fundamentally determined by emotions. This has best been illustrated in our own country by the failure of the Eighteenth Amendment and the partial failure of the Fifteenth Amendment in the South, attributable to this cause. The relative inertia of our emotional attitudes, together with our social structure, is still effective in maintaining certain social handicaps for women long after they have legally and politically been given rights practically equal to those of men.

In spite of the fact that the professions are open to women, very few enter the medical, legal, and, especially theological schools or attain high executive positions. On the other hand, society expects some professions to be staffed preponderantly by women, for example, those of nursing, elementary school teaching, and social work. In our evaluation of the progress of the movement for the equalization of women with men, these two distinct aspects must be borne in mind. Nevertheless, the fact that women can now enter almost any career open to men on more or less equal terms is an indication of the trend of the times even though the lag is still markedly felt.

The emancipation of women is characterized in four main areas: judicial, political, educational, and occupational.

Judicial emancipation of women

Before women can hope to advance as a group they must be equal with men before the law. The original concept of the family was that of a unit ruled by a head; the change in legal concept has been to recognize the members of the family as equivalent members of society. This change has been wrought by many individual laws, some of which pertain to franchise or occupation, others again to the civil standing of women in the community. Some of these changes may be mentioned: a married woman is now capable of acquiring and holding property, something that she could not do before; prior to 1925 a mother in England did not possess the same rights as the father did of guardianship of her children; divorce laws have all been changed in favor of the wife. In some cases custom has changed ahead of the law.

Thus, although laws placing women at a disadvantage have gradually been displaced by others giving women the same equality as men, the increasing participation of women in trade and industry has led to the introduction of many laws protecting but at the same time limiting the activities of women. These laws are justified insofar as they take into account the physical difference of women, but not if they limit their rights and privileges, as, for instance, the many laws that allow lower wages or salaries for women performing the same service as men. There are, in this respect, still many inequalities that should be corrected.

Enfranchisement of women

In recent history the vote has proved to be a most powerful weapon when used by an organized group. This was appreciated by the early champions of women's rights. If a woman could vote, she could enforce the correction of many injustices. In spite of Condorcet's efforts, suffrage was not extended to women through the French Revolution; and because this movement soon became unpopular in the Anglo-Saxon countries, the cause did not gain impetus until about the middle of the last century.

The agitation for women's vote was more intense in America than in England. This was brought about especially by the antislavery movement in which women took a very active part. It was led by Lucretia Mott and Elizabeth Cady Stanton and supported by the Quakers. As a result of their activity the first Women's Rights Convention met in Seneca Falls, New York, in 1848. During the next few years the movement continued to gain strength. It received wide publicity in the press, and soon other leaders joined in. Most famous among these was Susan B. Anthony who remained actively interested until her death in 1906.

In England the early efforts were made between 1840 and 1850 when suffrage for women was advocated by such men as Cobden, Disraeli, and Hume. The most potent protagonist, however, was John Stuart Mill, who entered Parliament in 1865, having placed women's suffrage in his election address. Later he published his *Subjection of Women,* which had a tremendous influence. Women now began to organize themselves and to present petitions to Parliament. When a reform bill was to be introduced in 1884, they thought that they stood a good chance of achieving their goal; however, Gladstone killed the bill through the treason of 104 liberal members. The movement became greatly discouraged although at this time women gained electoral rights in local government.

The women in America had no better luck in obtaining suffrage. Working through state legislatures was found to be futile; therefore they turned to national organizations. In 1869 the National Women's Suffrage Association was formed in New York under the leadership of Mrs. Stanton and Miss Anthony, and in the fall of the same year the American Women's Suffrage Association was formed in Cleveland under Lucy Stone; in 1890 the two were joined. By annual conventions and by repeated appearances before the legislature in Washington, D. C., they pressed their claim. The movement grew, and in 1888 it assumed an international character. When the older leaders died, new ones took up their tasks, and eventually the states began to yield. By 1920 general suffrage had been obtained by ratification of the Nineteenth Amendment.

The movement had to pass through more troubled waters in England. After the setback in 1884 it grew without any dramatic events until 1897 when a national union was formed of the various smaller societies. This step strengthened the effort. In 1903 the Women's Social and Political Union was formed; this was the famous organization that for the next decade, under the leadership of Mrs. Pankhurst, was to obtain such notoriety. Offhand the new union changed tactics. Formerly each candidate for office had been questioned on his views, but this method had achieved nothing. Now the union applied directly to the government, and as the liberal party came into power in 1906 it was hoped that it would be more

favorable than the previous conservative rule. Instead the new government handled the suffragettes roughly, and when they attempted to hold a meeting, they were brutally thrown into the street and eventually into prison. The ensuing notoriety gave a tremendous impetus to the movement; they now began to adopt "militant" tactics with parades, heckling of ministers when they appeared on public platforms, and general disturbances all in the name of propaganda. Their efforts showed the world what determined propaganda could do: everybody all over the world was talking about them, and the papers carried pictures of their activities, with the result that the movement became tremendously popular. New societies sprang up everywhere, and the membership grew by leaps and bounds. In 1907 they organized their first public demonstration, and on a rainy afternoon 3,000 women marched through London; soon one mass meeting followed another, and no one could move anywhere in England without encountering their propaganda.

After a while the suffragettes became so violent that they had to be arrested; in prison they went on hunger strikes and had to be released, and immediately they resumed their tactics. To combat hunger strikes the "cat and mouse" act was passed, whereby prisoners who refused to eat could be rearrested when they had recovered their health. A few efforts on the part of private members to introduce bills failed, and finally in 1910 a committee was organized under Lord Lytton for the purpose of drafing an acceptable bill. Even this effort came up against the unyielding resistance of the government under H. H. Asquith. The struggle reached its climax when the government, in 1911, proposed to introduce a new franchise bill, "for male persons only." New and violent protests followed, but in decisive matters Parliament supported the government, and seemingly the suffragettes made no progress.

The suffragettes now decided to support

the party that would further their course. This happened to be the labor party. By 1913 they believed that they had public opinion behind them, and they had. The government's cause was virtually lost and British women would probably have been enfranchised if World War I had not begun in 1914, when all efforts were turned toward winning the war. The Women's Social and Political Union was dissolved, and the National Union undertook war relief work; the women thus gained even greater favor in public opinion. Finally in 1917 a conference called by the Speaker of the House of Commons (that is, the government) recommended that the vote be given to householders and wives of householders. A bill drafted along these lines was passed in the House of Commons by a majority of 7 to 1 and soon became law. The next year women became eligible to run for Parliament, and in 1919 Viscountess Astor was elected. The experience with women's franchise was so entirely favorable during the next ten years that by 1928 women were given voting rights similar to those of men, and the movement came to a successful close.

Women's suffrage apparently has not materially altered the course of Anglo-Saxon civilization, but it has given to women a potential power with which they can support any movement in which they choose to take interest, and although it may never be given any bias as a whole (the women's vote has in general been divided along party lines similar to those of the male vote), protecting the rights of women before the law in the professions and in the labor market is always extant. A movement such as the state (or national) registration of nurses would always receive a more favorable treatment in the hands of legislators if it were to be backed by nurses as voters rather than by a disfranchised profession. This whole movement, therefore, now successfully completed, has been of the greatest value and may be of still greater potential value in the progress of American nursing.

Education of women

The placing of women on an equal footing with men, before the law, had politically enabled them to seek careers comparable to those of men. Thus it became further necessary to give them educational facilities equal to those that were offered to men. Early in the nineteenth century it was very difficult for a young woman to obtain an education except through private tutoring, which was very expensive and therefore limited to a privileged few. Thus, Miss Nightingale received much of her education from her father and by travel and social contact. There was no "college" to which she could have been sent. If there had been, the evolution of nursing might have developed quite differently. As it is, the growth of colleges and universities for women has profoundly affected nursing education; therefore a short review of this is in order.

Before 1800, occasional schools in America had been open to girls, but educational opportunities for women were practically nonexistent until 1821, when Emma Willard opened a Female Seminary at Troy, New York. "Academies" and "seminaries" soon followed in various parts of the East, and about the middle of the century the public high schools, which were coeducational, had been extensively established. Higher education for women, however, lagged somewhat behind; the first colleges open to women were Oberlin in Ohio (1833) and Wheaton at Norton, Massachusetts (1835). Mount Holyoke also dates from this early period, having been established in 1857. A number of other colleges were established during the next 30 or 40 years. Outstanding among them was Vassar, which opened in Poughkeepsie, New York, in 1865; it is remarkable for its high educational standards, which have been maintained from the first.

During the latter part of the century, when higher education for women became more generally recognized, large numbers of institutions all over the country admitted women. Some of them were separate colleges for women; others were established within already existing universities, some of these being coeducational. Among colleges for women established during this period, Smith, Wellesley, and Bryn Mawr became outstanding. Mount Holyoke also obtained a college charter (1888). Simmons College in Boston was established in 1899 for the specific purpose of preparing women for independent professional careers. Tulane University in New Orleans and Western Reserve in Cleveland were the first universities to open their doors to women (1887 and 1888) and soon others followed their example. The University of Chicago was established in 1893 on the basis that it should be open in equal measure to men and women. To mention them all would be tedious; in general, not only did the number of women admitted to college increase but the educational standards of institutions admitting them advanced rapidly during this period.

These schools and colleges have maintained very high standards. All the good ones have had their pick of students, with the result that their material to start with was superior; they have been led by educators of vision who have emphasized the liberal arts education as applied to the individual, with the result that more and more of their graduates have sought and qualified for distinguished professional careers. The American Association of University Women has been active in creating opportunities, often by establishing fellowships for the advanced education of women, with the result that an increasing number of women have obtained the degree of doctor of philosophy. Most of these women enter advanced teaching or research in the physical sciences, where they are beginning to occupy more of the important posts.

The participation of the nursing profession as a whole in the development of the education of women will be extensively discussed later; in addition we may note that an increasing number of women seeking professional education go into nursing.

Thus it will be clear that the advances made in the education of women form an important integral part of the professional evolution of nursing.

Occupational emancipation of women

Perhaps some of the early emancipators of women visualized a world in which woman took a place in society in all respects similar to that of man. Obviously that dream has not been and is not likely to be realized. As long as the family remains the unit of Western Civilization, the larger proportion of women's efforts will be concerned with homemaking and child rearing. Therefore, although the growing freedom of women has resulted in their admission to most occupations, this movement has encountered certain countercurrents of considerable power.

Experience has shown that, physically and temperamentally, women are less suited than men for certain pursuits although they are eminently fitted for others. In certain professions women still constitute a small percentage, and it is of great significance that this percentage in some instances tends to decrease; thus there are fewer women doctors, both absolutely and proportionately, than there were a few decades ago. It has also been found necessary to protect women in the labor market by limiting their participation in certain activities by law; for instance in England women may not be employed in mines below ground, and they are protected by special hour and wage regulations. On the other hand, in some professions, preeminently nursing, the superiority of women has been generally recognized; this profession is unique in that all its positions, even to the highest national offices, are occupied by women.

Thus, as far as the participation of women in occupations and professions is concerned, the movement is finding a level consistent with the compatibility of women for the various tasks.

Another important countercurrent is survival of the old attitude toward women—

"prejudice" it is often called—although it is not strictly so, but rather survival of a view that formerly was both justifiable and proper. This, however, is waning steadily, and it is slowly being realized that women should be admitted to any place or career in society for which they are constitutionally and educationally fitted without the handicap of old custom.

RISE OF SOCIALISM

The social reformers of the early part of the nineteenth century were promoting ideas of philanthropic enterprises on the part of those who were privileged to be in a position in which they could carry them out. The power of the organized lower classes was not prominent in the reforms that they suggested, although an awareness of the powers of the French Revolution existed, as is evidenced in the writings of both Carlyle and Dickens. The impulse that eventually was to stimulate action by the workers themselves was to come from another source. About the middle of the century Karl Marx wrote *Das Kapital,* and he and Engels founded the socialistic movement that was directly or indirectly to influence so much political thinking and action. The socialistic way of thinking shifted the center of gravity in society. The industrial system, so far, had acknowledged individual freedom to act and to extract from one's fellowmen whatever one could within the law. The state was for the protection of the individual, but it had no obligation to him. According to the socialistic doctrine it is the duty of the individual to give his work to the state; in return this state will see that he receives his full share of the proceeds of his labors. In the socialistic state all are politically equal. As this aimed at abolition of political and economic privilege, the masses had but one means to enforce their demands: to organize.

Organized labor movements began to develop in Europe during the second half of the nineteenth century, slowly at first, but gradually gaining momentum. Organized labor advanced in Europe much more quickly than in America, where the labor unions are of relatively recent origin. Consequently the by-products of labor organization, with which we are particularly concerned, developed more gradually in America than in Europe. The chief enemies of the laboring man are old age, sickness, exploitation, and unemployment from the shutdown of factories. It is, therefore, reasonable that requests for protection from these enemies should soon be added to the demands for improved working conditions and that they should become important objects of social legislation.

Social legislation

The first moves for sickness and unemployment legislation were not initiated by the labor movement itself but by Bismarck in Germany, who thought that by anticipating the demands of labor he could control its development. The passing of legislation in Germany protecting labor against sickness and unemployment has progressed even during the more recent periods when the electorate was relatively impotent. Another effect of Bismarck's reform, one that he perhaps did not anticipate, was that it established a precedent and acknowledgment of the obligation of the state to the underprivileged. From this time the revaluation of the rights of man, which had been going on throughout the century, became rapidly accentuated. The right to life, liberty, and the pursuit of happiness was given an even more liberal interpretation, except perhaps as far as liberty was concerned. The modern era has seen industry increasingly regulated: hours have been shortened, health and safety requirements regarding workshops have been steadily improved and better enforced, and there has been a steady trend in wage increase. Altogether the present age has been one of social and industrial reform foreshadowed in the preceding century; these reforms are still far from completed.

Extension of medical care

The general trend had embodied an ever-increasing demand for hospitals and medical and nursing services. This demand has had an economic aspect: there has been an increasing interest in the cost of medical care in its broadest sense. Studies have been and are being made of means by which it could be distributed in such a manner that families would not be crippled financially in case of severe sickness and whereby those in society who cannot afford medical care can receive it in a properly organized manner and not as a more or less accidental charity. The attempts to distribute the cost of medical care have led to the development of numerous schemes; the Krankenkasse system in Germany, the panel system in England, and group hospitalization and sickness insurance by private insurance companies in the United States are but examples of a field so vast that it requires a special study to be understood in its entirety.

These developments have been met with resistance, the chief and general argument being that they had led to "socialization" of medicine, by which in general was meant that they would interfere with the professional freedom and initiative of those engaged in the healing art. This social conflict has many aspects that, however, are beyond our scope. We can merely note that in Western Civilization as a whole such schemes have progressed at an accelerated pace. For our purpose, suffice it to say that this evolution of the healing arts is of the greatest significance for nursing, for it continuously widens its scope: we continue to build new and larger hospitals, public health activities continue to expand, and new industrial positions continue to become available. We shall consider all these developments in their proper places, but when we do, we should remember to study them against the background we have just described.

Benefits of industry

Social reforms within the society of the United States are premised upon the ability

of the industrial system to carry its share of the burden. Now let us consider how industrialism has become so prosperous. When we described feudalism, we noted that most people were occupied fulltime simply in obtaining food and other basic commodities. When we described the advent of the machine, we pointed out how it essentially led to the saving of time that could be used for other work or for leisure (by "leisure" we mean here any activity other than productive labor, such as education, and engagement in the luxury trade). As our machines became increasingly efficient this saving of time became increased at an almost incredible rate. As an example of this we quote A. J. Todd:

It has been calculated that to copy by hand a volume of 100,000 words would require 14 days and cost approximately $54.40; to write 1,000 copies would require 44 years, 45 weeks and 2 days and cost $54,400. To do the same work with a modern power press would require some preliminary work which the author estimates would occupy 96 days and cost some $1,780, but once that was done, 1,000, and as many additional thousands of copies could be run off at less than a cent a copy in less than 10 hours. This example could be amplified by thousands more all showing how the machines increase our efficiency and save us time.*

This tremendous advance applies not only to the production of goods but also to their transportation. For example, modern transport renders it more profitable to carry letters at eight cents apiece than it was to carry them at a dollar apiece when mail service was first established.

A further study of this subject will make it clear that there is a striking difference between poverty of feudalism and poverty of the modern Machine Age. Feudal poverty was inevitable, for the work of all the people could produce commodities barely above subsistence level, while the productive power of the modern industrial structure is such that it can produce ample commodities for

*Todd, A. J.: Industry and society, New York, 1933, Henry Holt & Co., Inc., p. 109.

all the people living under Western Civilization if they will turn it to productive purposes at full capacity. In modern society there are two causes of poverty: either society fails to provide an adequate distribution of its commodities or the citizens at the bottom of the economic scale lack the capacity or education to acquire a reasonable share of the communal wealth.

Public health

Defective distribution of commodities, however intriguing, is too complicated a subject to fall within our scope, but the second cause of poverty is definitely our concern. There is now general agreement that failure to achieve a reasonable standard of living can be traced in many cases to an unhygienic environment with resulting disease that is preventable or curable. The whole subject of hookworm anemia and the deficiency diseases as causes of chronic illness is pertinent. The prevalence of venereal diseases and tuberculosis among the less-favored classes is another illustration. For generations these social evils have been brought to public knowledge by social reformers, and gradually, although slowly, society has accepted an ever-increasing responsibility for their existence. The acceptance has been furthered by enlightened self-interest, for we are to an increasing extent realizing the truth of the mercantilistic axiom that the wealth of a state depends primarily on the number and opulence (including health) of its citizens. This became particularly evident in the examinations of recruits for World War II. The practical realization of this truth has led the state, be it local or federal government, to assume a greater share in the prevention and treatment of preventable diseases. Consequently, governmental medical care in city institutions, veterans' hospitals, or other institutions has greatly increased and is still increasing both in the number of beds being made available and in the quality of services offered.

The field of public health sponsored by public or semipublic bodies is ever expanding. As this view is being accepted the great corporations are following suit either because of pressure of public opinion, ever the severest taskmaster, or because they find that it is to their advantage to maintain a high standard of health and safety measures on their premises and thus avoid damages and compensations that had to be paid in the past. As public goodwill becomes more important, many corporations and governmental bodies take pride in making known the health measures they sponsor. Organized health measures require more and better nursing; it will now be seen how the Industrial Revolution and its collateral economic, political, and philosophical developments may be considered the soil that nurtured the growth of all the healing arts.

MEDICINE DURING THE NINETEENTH CENTURY

The vigorous intellectual, political, and social activity of the nineteenth century affected medicine and resulted in a remarkable development in America as well as in all the European countries. Some of the outstanding men and their contributions will be outlined briefly, but the reader is referred to books on the history of medicine for the complete discussion of this fascinating period. During this period the tendency to specialize in a single clinical field had its beginning. General physicians practicing in all branches of medicine became proportionately fewer in number; this trend was encouraged.

Ignatz Philipp Semmelweis, 1818-1865

One of the most tragic figures of medicine —Semmelweis—was the genius who banished childbirth fever from maternity hospitals. Hungarian by birth, he was assistant at the second Vienna clinic about 1845 when the death rate from puerperal sepsis had reached the appalling figure of 10% of all those delivered. At the same time it was only about 3% at the first clinic. Medical students were taught at the second clinic, pupil midwives at the first. Semmelweis proved that the high rate of death at the second clinic was caused by the filthy habits of the students. They were dissecting and doing postmortem work at the same time that they took their obstetrical work. Often they walked directly from the postmortem room and proceeded to examine a woman in labor without washing their hands. Rubber gloves were not used in those days. Semmelweis showed that this practice was the cause of the appalling mortality; the fever was caused by decomposing organic matter that had gained access to the mother's system through the wounded generative organs. He also showed that other sources could cause it—the examining hand could carry the infection from woman to woman and from infections occurring elsewhere in the body of other patients. Most important, he demonstrated that the infection could be prevented by cleaning the hands with a solution of chlorinated lime before examinations. This work was done before Pasteur began his great task.

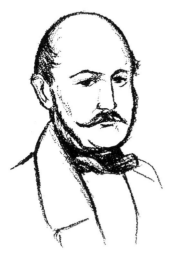

IGNATZ SEMMELWEIS

Ignatz Semmelweis had a share in the "emancipation of women" by helping to free them from the spectre of puerperal fever.

Semmelweis died young, at the age of 47 years. His biography is the story of the fight to gain recognition of an idea. In having to wait long years for the victory of his discovery, Semmelweis shared the fate of Harvey, Jenner, and many others. Semmelweis was met by his contemporaries not only with antagonism but also with derision—he was called "the fool from Pesth."

In America, Oliver Wendell Holmes (father of the chief justice of the Supreme Court) has been extolled as the hero who with Semmelweis conquered the scourge. In fact, the contagiousness of puerperal fever had been suggested by him, before Semmelweis published his papers, in a paper *On the Contagiousness of Puerperal Fever* (1843). Holmes was agreeable to his friends and clever with his pen, whereas Semmelweis was difficult to get along with and an awkward writer. Although Holmes held the professorship of anatomy at Harvard and Dartmouth, he is now remembered mainly for his wit and clever pen. His work on puerperal sepsis was his most important contribution to medicine.

Another person with whom it is tempting to compare Semmelweis is Lord Lister (1827-1912), who in 1883 visited Pesth where he learned of the fate of this unfortunate man. Studying the lives of these two men offers a good opportunity to learn the effect of circumstance on the association of fame and genius. Why should Semmelweis's life have been such a tragedy while Lister's was a triumph? The work of Semmelweis was advanced for his time; he died in 1865 before Pasteur's great work was accepted, the year Lister began his researches. Semmelweis had a small and unimportant promoter. Lister's promoter was his father-in-law, the master surgeon of his day in Great Britain, Mr. James Syme (1799-1870). "There are few things more encouraging to aspiring youth than a strong and triumphant master; few things more discouraging than an unpretentious or timorous one." Semmelweis died at the age of 47 years; Lister did not experience his final triumph until 1879 when he was 52 years old. Semmelweis had difficulty with his environment; Lister was never known to speak a sharp word to a house surgeon, dresser, or anyone in his employ. Lister was fortunate in finding prompt support. If circumstances had been different, Semmelweis might have attained a fame as great as that of Lister.

Joseph Lister, 1827-1912

Joseph Lister, the father of modern surgery, was born in 1827, the son of a well-to-do Quaker merchant. He received his early medical training in London, after which he went to Edinburgh and became the house surgeon of Syme, whose daughter he afterward married. In due course, partly through Syme's influence, he became professor of surgery in Edinburgh. In 1877 he came to London where he worked until his retirement.

When Lister entered the surgical wards he found a condition as bad as that found by Semmelweis in the obstetrical wards. Particularly, he was impressed by the huge

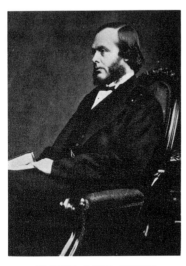

JOSEPH, LORD LISTER

This photograph was taken about the time Lister discovered antisepsis. (From Smith, Alice Lorraine: Principles of microbiology, ed. 6, St. Louis, 1969, The C. V. Mosby Co.)

mortality from sepsis following compound fracture and amputation. After much thought and experimentation, he discovered that if wounds were cleansed with carbolic acid and were kept clean, sepsis did not occur. Out of these observations he developed his antiseptic surgical technique. Although his results were conclusive, his methods were accepted slowly, for it not only takes a great man to make an important discovery but it also takes a great man to be the next to adopt it. Saxtorph of Copenhagen was, in this case, the first to adopt Lister's method, and soon it spread to Germany, France, and elsewhere. England and America were very slow to appreciate Lister's methods. However, by 1879 the evidence in Lister's favor was so overwhelming that it enforced the acceptance of Lister's principles, which since then have guided all surgical work.

Lister, on every occasion, recognized his debt to the genius of Louis Pasteur (1822-1895), whose germ theory supplied the missing link in his reasoning. The assumption of pathogenic bacteria made everything clear. If this effect of great minds upon each other could have happened a few years earlier, another of the greatest catastrophes of history could have been avoided, that is, the casualties from wound infections during the Franco-German war when for the first time the modern war machine was unleashed.

Rudolf Virchow, 1821-1902

In 1881 an international medical congress was held in London under the presidency of Sir James Paget. Among the many thousands attending were some already famous and many destined to become so later. Among them were these four, each of a different national heritage: the Latin Pasteur, the Teuton Virchow, the Anglo-Saxon Lister, and the young and relatively unknown Celt, Osler, who had come from Montreal with his chief, Palmer Howard.

Eldest of these was Virchow. Born in 1821, he soon displayed an interest in natural history which, as so often happens, became supplanted by the love of medicine. He combined a brilliant mind with great industry, and in his twenties the young professor occupied the chair of pathology at the University of Berlin. With the exception of a few years spent at Würzburg, largely for political reasons, he remained in this position until his death at the age of 81. The mind of this intellectual giant was enormous. His fame is founded in his many different contributions to medicine, but he is famous in his own right in many different sciences. He is possibly the greatest pathologist who ever lived. His conception of the cellular changes of disease transformed the entire outlook of the scientific world. Besides his fundamental contribution, he founded or contributed to our knowledge of leukemia, thrombus formation, tumors, septicemia, and much else. Under his direction about 50,000 postmortem examinations were performed. He founded and personally edited the first 170 volumes of his *Archives*. He was also active in politics; he became

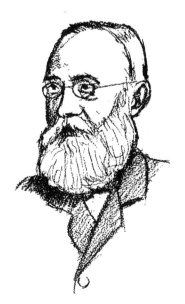

RUDOLF VIRCHOW

Rudolf Virchow is justly famed for his many contributions to medical knowledge. His greatest work was probably as a pathologist.

associated with the liberal movement of 1848 and suffered for his views.

After the age of 50, at the time when most men willingly slow down, Virchow became active and famous in the fields of anthropology and archeology. His knowledge and contributions were so great that people wondered how he could do this work and still remain a leader in pathology. He contributed to the science of public health; he studied the epidemics of typhus and did much to stamp them out. He helped plan the system of sewage disposal of Berlin. It was partly a result of his efforts that Germany for a while was leading the world in public health research. Virchow was active in the sanitation program of the German army in the war of 1870, in the heating and lighting of schools, in the organizing of the duties of school physicians, in the training of nurses, and in the organization of the medical profession into national and local associations. In short, his mind was encyclopedic.

Louis Pasteur, 1822-1895

Then there was Pasteur. The son of a country tanner in moderate circumstances, he did not show any promise of genius at first. His father was one of Napoleon's veterans and instilled into his son a wholesome respect for truth and industry, love of family, and appreciation of the glory of his beloved France. Pasteur traveled one road from his youth to his death, but it was a mountainous one leading him, like the youth in "Excelsior," to ever-greater achievements. He began by solving the molecular structure of racemic acid. He then discovered the true nature of the fermentation of wine and of vinegar and of the production of beer. The relation of these substances to infectious processes and certain fortuitous circumstances led him to the study and eventual conquest of silkworm disease, anthrax, "swine fever," chicken cholera, and finally to the greatest of all his achievements—the preventive treatment of hydrophobia. Any-

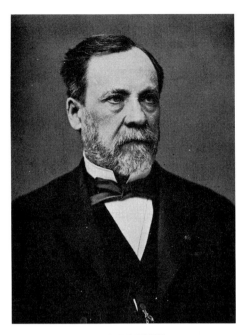

LOUIS PASTEUR

The genius of Pasteur, first evidenced by his discovery that polarization of light could be related to the structure of crystals, carried him to the solution of many problems: the spoilage of beers and wines with accompanying pasteurization process; the discovery of anaerobic bacteria, virus vaccines, and attenuation of virulence; and studies of spontaneous generation. His studies in immunology have rightly earned him a position as father of the science. (From Carpenter, P. L.: Microbiology, ed. 3, Philadelphia, 1972, W. B. Saunders Co.)

one of these conquests would have assured him immortal fame.

He gave all his attention to his work; thus his wife wrote: "Your father is absorbed in his thoughts, he talks little, sleeps little, rises at dawn, and in one word continues the life I began with him 35 years ago." But with it all, Pasteur upheld the highest ideals. As he himself expressed it: "Blessed is he who carries within himself a God, an ideal, and who obeys this ideal of art, ideal of science, or ideal of gospel virtues; therein lie the springs of great thoughts and great actions. They all reflect light from the infinite." This was the man who established the science of bacteriology

—and yet he never possessed a physician's diploma.

Other medical advances in Europe

In 1847 James Simpson in Scotland discovered the use of chloroform, which was the leading anesthetic for many years until its place was taken by newer and safer drugs.

Psychiatry was first considered a separate branch of medicine toward the end of the eighteenth century. The most famous doctor associated with modern reform in the treatment of patients with mental illness was Philippe Pinel (1745-1826).

Concern for community hygiene and public health began to emerge during the eighteenth century. At that time there were no city sanitation departments, and open sewers ran through the streets into which people dumped all their garbage and waste. English doctors and medical societies became interested in trying to control communicable diseases as well as in treating them.

The discovery by Edward Jenner (1749-1823) of vaccination against smallpox not only was an important scientific discovery but also was one of the first steps in scientific prevention of disease and has been followed by many other more modern discoveries.

At about the same time that Dr. Jenner was working in England, Johann Peter Frank (1745-1821), an Austrian physician, was outlining the whole structure of modern systematic hygiene. He described the principles of state hygiene and maintained that the government should be responsible for the public health not only during periods when threatened by serious epidemics or disaster but at all times. The theory of Frank was supported in the writings and activities of many nineteenth century social reformers.

Antituberculosis legislation was begun in Italy toward the end of the seventeenth century. Important in the dissemination of medical knowledge among practitioners was the development of medical journals, which began to appear in all countries during the eighteenth and nineteenth centuries. No longer were physicians attached only to the courts of princes, they also began to practice in towns and to appear in localities all over the civilized world.

EARLY REFORMS IN NURSING

Partly as a result of Howard's writings and partly as a manifestation of the general change in attitude toward the penal and eleemosynary institutions, it was realized that nursing, in and out of hospitals, was thoroughly unsatisfactory both in England and on the Protestant continent. At the same time, as we have seen, development for the social liberation of women moved slowly. Because of the great loss of men in the frequent wars, many women could not find husbands and were naturally looking for careers for themselves.

Mrs. Elizabeth Gurney Fry (1780-1845) was an outstanding social reformer in England, particularly concerning conditions in prisons. While she was engaged in this work, she was visited by Fliedner, the father of the deaconess movement. Later she became interested in nursing and established the order that inspired the Fliedners.

Nursing Sisters

In the British Isles, the first efforts at systematic lay nursing institutions were made in Ireland by the Irish Sisters of Charity and the Sisters of Mercy. They antedate the modern deaconesses and orders sponsored by the Anglican church by a number of years and are more closely related to the Sisters of Charity of de Paul than to the later English orders.

The Irish Sisters of Charity were started by Mary Aikenhead (Sister Mary Augustine). In 1812 she and a friend went to the Convent of the Blessed Virgin Mary at York where they studied the work of nuns who practiced visiting among the poor, and in 1815 they began similar work in Dublin. Some years later they sent three sisters to study nursing at the Hôpital de la Pitié in

Paris, and when they came back, the sisters got their own house and hospital in Dublin. This hospital, which was begun with 12 beds, later expanded into St. Vincent's Hospital, the name of which suggests its relationship to the French order of Sisters of Charity.

The Sisters of Mercy was a similar order founded by Catherine M'Auley. It began as a home for destitute girls but soon included visitation of the sick. In 1830 it was made a presentation order with increasing emphasis on nursing. This order also sent branches to different parts of the world, and from the branch in Bermondsey near London some sisters went with Miss Nightingale to the Crimea. The order came to the United States in 1843 when Mother Warde brought some sisters across the ocean. Among their outstanding hospitals in this country are the Mercy Hospitals in Chicago and in Pittsburgh.

These orders are important as being the first modern nursing orders in the British Isles; they are, however, Catholic and derived from the French orders. They did not in their original conception embody the modern training school for nurses. This idea was first propounded by Dr. Robert Gooch, who around 1825 suggested that lay nursing orders should be established for women. The applicants should first be entered as pupil nurses in the big hospitals in London and Edinburgh, should be supplied with regular textbooks adapted to their needs, and should be regularly examined so that their progress could be checked. After graduation they should, after the manner of the Beguines go into the country or districts where they should live together in small houses. This plan, excellent as it was, did not materialize for many years. But Dr. Gooch was a friend of Mrs. Fry's, and it is not impossible that some of these ideas were conveyed to Mr. Fliedner and thus first materialized in Germany.

Deaconesses at Kaiserswerth

The need for better nursing was also acknowledged in Germany. In Hamburg,

Amelie Sieveking had organized "The Friends of the Poor," who did home visiting and nursing. Efforts were being made in many towns to improve nursing in the hospitals. Nursing manuals were being written. Still, it all lacked the spark of genius that was eventually to overshadow all similar efforts in Europe.

This spark was contributed by Theodor Fliedner and his wife, Fredericke (nee Münster). As a young minister Mr. Fliedner was called to Kaiserswerth near Düsseldorf. He found a community in the throes of an economic depression and little prospect of earning even a modest livelihood. However, in spite of tempting offers elsewhere, he decided to remain at his post and to travel abroad to raise the funds necessary to work where he was.

In 1822 he traveled through Holland and England, and because he had introductions to all sorts of influential people, he was soon able to solve his financial problem. He also had the opportunity to study firsthand many efforts at relieving shame and suffering; in Holland he observed the work of the deaconesses, and in England he formed a close friendship with Elizabeth Fry, who allowed him to study her work in the prisons. He investigated schools, hospitals, almshouses, and other eleemosynary institutions, so that he returned to Kaiserswerth one of the best-informed men in his field.

It took his wife and him many years to materialize their plans, and not until 1833 were they able to open their first refuge for discharged prisoners. However, the problem of the deaconesses lay closest to their hearts. They had seen what the Sisters of Mercy were able to do, and they appreciated the intrinsic value of the deaconesses. They also realized that a nursing organization, such as they had in mind, must be modernized to meet the demands of the times. The training had to be more systematic than it had been in the past, and the organization had to be more closely knit, although elastic enough to meet the most varied demands.

In 1836 they bought the biggest house they could find in Kaiserswerth, hoping somehow to pay for it later—which they did. Soon afterward their first patient, a servant girl, arrived, and Mrs. Fliedner persuaded her friend, Gertrude Reichardt, to enter as the first deaconess. Mrs. Reichardt was a doctor's daughter, middle-aged, who had already had extensive experience dealing with sick people in assisting her father with his practice. She arrived at the Kaiserswerth Hospital expecting little in the way of equipment, but even that was not there. Four bare walls and a patient were about all the new institution had to offer, and Gertrude Reichardt was just about ready to give up and go home when the first load of equipment unexpectedly arrived, and somehow the young hospital got started. By the end of that year there were six more deaconesses; eventually there were 120 deaconesses, and by 1842 the hospital had 200 beds.

Fredericke Fliedner had a marvelous talent for organizing, and soon each girl found herself in charge of her own department with no one else's interfering. Furthermore, to complete their training, the deaconesses rotated from service to service, all the while receiving systematic instruction. Mr. Fliedner instructed them in ethics and religious principles, and Mrs. Fliedner instructed them in the principles of practical nursing. A physician gave them theoretical training and bedside instruction in the care of the sick, and they learned enough pharmacology to pass the state examinations for pharmacists.

Thus the fully trained deaconess could nurse sick and convalescent patients, manage children, and dispense medicines; she was familiar with occupational therapy, parish or district visiting, and religious theory and instructions.

The organization that accomplished so much was managed very strictly. No student could assume a privileged position; all were equal before their instructors. In this way they differed markedly from the later English and American orders. To be admitted to the course a girl had to be at least 18 years of age and had to present letters from a clergyman and a physician certifying both her moral standing and her health. She would then be admitted for three months' probation; later this probation was replaced by required attendance at a preparatory school, sometimes for as long as a year. She received a regular, small allowance of pocket money. Rotating through the various services, she in turn became a junior, senior, and finally head sister. Through the course she received, besides practical instruction, regular theoretical classroom instruction. The course took three years, and she was required to wear a uniform. For the first time in history we observe, complete with all the essentials, the modern training school for nurses.

The modern training school was a huge success, and it grew rapidly. The Fliedners already had a normal school for the preparation of deaconesses, and soon there was added to the hospital a lunatic asylum for female patients and in 1842 an orphanage for Protestant girls. They also organized an infant school and a day school for girls. Finally they organized an asylum for released female prisoners and for wayward girls, in an attempt to readjust them to society.

When the hospital was fully developed, its facilities included, besides wards for male and female patients and children, a unit for communicable diseases, one for convalescents (this is remarkable, for many modern hospitals still have no such department), and one for sick deaconesses. There were also an apothecary shop, the administrative offices, the chapel that took care of burials, and the garden that furnished vegetables.

Not only did the institution prosper in Kaiserswerth but there were also calls for branches from all over Europe and from America. As early as 1846 Fliedner went to London with four deaconesses to begin the nursing in the German Hospital there. In 1850 he took a group to Pastor Passavant in Pittsburgh, and at the same time a deaconess home and hospital were founded in Milwaukee. Branches were established throughout the Near East in such cities as Jerusalem, Smyrna, Constantinople, and Alexandria, and by the time Fliedner died in 1846 there were about 1,600 deaconesses working in 400 different fields, and they had 30 motherhouses. Since that time the organization has continued to grow, so that there is now hardly a community, excluding the strictly Catholic countries, without its group of deaconesses.

The growth of the organization was a result of the urgent need for such an organization and the incessant industry of the Fliedners. Along with her enormous task Fredericke Fliedner found time to bring into the world five children before she died in 1842. Theodor Fliedner was fortunate in marrying Caroline Bertheau, a former pupil of Amelie Sieveking, one year later. She had been in charge of the nursing of the female surgical department of the Hamburg Hospital. She was able to carry the mantle of Fredericke, and she did not neglect the domestic side of life, for she made her husband a good wife—they had eight children before he died in 1864. After his death she continued to direct Kaiserswerth until 1882.

There remains but a brief evaluation of the order. It was primarily religious, it was modern, and it was practical and democratic. If the directions and the spirit of Theodor Fliedner had always been followed, there would have been no difficulties. However, not all clergymen possessed his wide vision, and sometimes interference by the clergy would hamper its efficiency in spite of the principle that doctor's orders should prevail. Exaggerated idealism on the part of the girls would occasionally lead to excessive self-negation, and sometimes they were exploited by unscrupulous leaders. Some opposition to the order resulted, manifest in the appearance of "free sisters" who later became organized, but, on the whole, deaconesses have weathered all storms and are now the outstanding Protestant religious nursing organization. The security of the motherhouse, which means so much to the European girl, has been somewhat modified in America. They have offered and still offer a unique opportunity for serious-minded young women to do good in the world. They require no vows; a deaconess may retire or marry, but in return for a life of faithful service a deaconess can look forward to an old age secure from want.

BRITISH NURSING ORDERS
Protestant Sisters of Mercy
(the Nursing Sisters)

Fliedner's work made a great impression on interested persons especially in England and on the European continent. As we shall see, Florence Nightingale received much inspiration from his work, visited the institution repeatedly, and for a while even participated in the Fliedner's activities. Mrs. Fry also followed the work closely, and finally in 1840, largely under the inducement of Dr. Gooch and the poet Robert Southey, she organized the first Protestant nursing order in England, the Protestant Sisters of Mercy or the Nursing Sisters, as they were later called. These women received some training in their preparation for the care of the sick; they visited Guy's Hospital in London for several hours each day where they received some instruction from the doctors and the ward nurses. However, these doctors and nurses were uneducated and could not be expected to be very valuable instructors. These pupils received neither classroom nor theoretical instruction; they were trained entirely for practical home nursing. The order is still in existence.

Anglican nursing orders

The Church of England sponsored the most important early nursing organizations in England. As a result these organizations were dominated by the clergyman's conception of nursing as primarily an act of mercy and of religious devotion. It was thought that such service must be free to the patient.

It took a considerable amount of time before the idea could be accepted that nursing by good, devoted women could be a profession with services rendered for remuneration and that these women should be trained as carefully and thoroughly for this as for any other profession. There was an obvious need for a profession for women, and consequently refined and capable women were attracted to this work. More and more nursing activities were sponsored by the upper classes and more nurses were recruited from the middle classes of the country.

The Park Village Community, established in 1845 by Pusey, was the first of the Anglican nursing orders. The emphasis here was largely upon friendly visiting of the sick in their homes; there was no emphasis on systematic training or care of patients. About the same time, Miss Sellon organized a similar group, the "Sisters of Mercy" in Devonport. These orders were established for the purpose of home nursing and did not participate in the reform of hospital nursing that took place in the next few years.

A primary factor in this reform was St. John's House, established by the Church of England in 1848. Its purpose was to establish systematic training of nurses in the hospitals and to attract young ladies of the middle classes into nursing. Like the nurses of the Hôtel Dieu they were to advance through three stages. For the first two years they were to be probationers, after which they were to qualify as "nurses," when they would receive board, lodging, and a salary besides. After having worked for five years as nurses, they could advance to become "sisters," who had the privilege of living at home with their families. Women of the better classes could enter as "nurses." Training in obstetrics was not included until 1861. St. John's House became identified with nursing activities in most of the important London hospitals at one time or another. At first the probationers were trained at Middlesex and Westminster Hospitals, and then, from 1849, at Kings College Hospital where in 1856 they took over the entire nursing service until the hospital established a school of nursing of its own in 1885. The order also nursed in Charing Cross Hospital and was finally taken over in 1919 by St. Thomas's Hospital. The order is now known as the St. John's and St. Thomas's House and is maintained on a cooperative basis as an institution for private nurses. The order contributed 26 nurses to Miss Nightingale's expedition.

A similar order, the Sisterhood of All Saints, was founded in 1851 by Miss Byron. This order also concerned itself with the training of nurses in hospitals. It was especially connected with University College Hospital; from 1857 it was responsible for the nursing of a few wards, and from 1862 to 1899, for nursing in the entire hospital. The order assumed direction also of St. John's House from 1883 to 1893.

Finally, St. Margaret's order, established by the Reverend Dr. Neele in East Grimstead in 1854, should be mentioned, Although this order emphasized nursing, the training that it offered its members was not outstanding.

In the United States the Protestant Episcopal church established similar nursing orders, patterned after the English. A branch of the English order, the Sisterhood of St.

Margaret, nursed at the Children's Hospital in Boston from 1872 to 1912. The Sisterhood of the Holy Communion has nursed in St. Luke's Hospital in New York since 1854, and the Sisterhood of St. Mary has nursed in St. Mary's Free Hospital for Children in New York since 1870.

ON THE CONTINENT
La Source

One continental development should also be mentioned. In 1859 Comtesse Agenor de Gasperin and her husband established L'école normale evangelique de gardes-malades independents, briefly called "La Source," in Lausanne, Switzerland. They endowed this school of nursing and provided it with a building. The students received instruction for six months during a preliminary course, after which they nursed in the homes of the poor. Since 1891 the institution has had its own hospital. The order, if it may be called that, is based upon the principle of personal liberty. The nurses are salaried and make no vows. The quality of the nurses issuing from this institution has sometimes been questioned, but about its importance as a new departure in the form of an endowed school for nursing, there can be no argument.

CHAPTER 6 PIONEER DAYS IN AMERICA

■ The time of the great discoveries in medicine and the early immigration to America was also the time of the Reformation, which split the European nations into either Catholic or Protestant states. The early Spanish explorers and the French were Catholic and brought with them as missionaries Dominicans, Franciscans, and Jesuits and, later, the nursing orders. The care of the sick and the wounded among friend and foe in the missions and in the wilderness was largely their task. The old term for quinine, "Jesuits' bark," is reminiscent of those days when medical knowledge was in the hands of the clergy. In the Spanish civilization nursing continued to be the responsibility of the monks, and any high degree of efficiency was never reached. During the eighteenth century, when the great European hospitals began to develop, American hospitals were also beginning to be established. Mexico City can justly claim the first American hospital to be built by the white man—established by Cortez in 1524;—and the early French immigrants built hospitals in Quebec, New Orleans, and St. Louis.

BEGINNINGS OF HOSPITALS AND ORGANIZED NURSING SERVICE

The Charity Hospital of New Orleans established in 1737 is considered by many authorities to be the oldest hospital still existing in America for the care of the sick. In 1737 a sailor, Jean Louis, died in New Orleans and left a bequest of 10,000 liras "to serve in perpetuity and the founding of a hospital for the sick of the City of New Orleans and to secure the things necessary to succor of the sick."* The contract for this hospital gives the following description: "A hall measuring 45 feet in length, by 24 feet in breadth, and 14 feet in height including the foundation, the whole in walls of well conditioned brick."*

This building was completed in 1737 and named St. John's Hospital. In official records it is mentioned as "L'hôpital des pauvres de la charité," and it is considered the original Charity Hospital of New Orleans. The institution served both as a hospital and as an asylum, but most of the early hospitals performed both functions. The school for nurses, however, was not established until 1894.

The Ursuline Sisters came to Canada from France in 1639 to teach. They were accompanied by three Augustinian nuns who were to nurse in a hospital in the new land. However, nursing care was needed so badly that they all did nursing at first until the new Hôtel Dieu was built in 1658. These early settlements of New Orleans and farther up the Mississippi were to have great influence on American nursing. The early Ursuline Sisters in France had done nursing as well as teaching, and in 1727 a small group of them came to New Orleans where even then colonial life had achieved

*Sister Henrietta: A famous New Orleans hospital, American Journal of Nursing 39:249, March, 1939.

certain standards of luxury in a civilization based on slavery. However, the people living in the settlement were ravished by epidemic diseases, most important of which were yellow fever and smallpox; all the scourges of a seaport town were encountered. During the nineteenth century the Ursuline Sisters were active throughout the entire territory of Louisiana. They opened many hospitals and performed many heroic deeds, which were climaxed in the nursing done during the Battle of New Orleans. Soon after this they practically gave up nursing and restricted themselves to teaching.

As the growth of settlements in the new country proceeded, the need for nursing became urgent; the various Catholic nursing orders responded to the call. The Sisters of Charity were among the first; in 1809 Mother Elizabeth Bayley Seton in Emmitsburg, Maryland, established the Sisterhood of St. Joseph as a branch of the Sisters of Charity. In 1849 the Sisters of Charity be-

came affiliated with the Order of St. Vincent de Paul. In 1830 the Sisters of Charity established the first hospital west of the Mississippi River—a log cabin in St. Louis. Almost at once it proved insufficient for the demands made upon it, and in 1831 a larger hospital was built on Spruce and Fourth Streets. This came to be known as the Mullanphy Hospital; in 1874 it moved to bigger quarters, and in 1930, during its centenary, it was replaced by the DePaul Hospital, then one of the most modern and certainly one of the most beautiful hospitals in St. Louis at that time. The Sisters contributed some of the best nursing during the Civil War. Sister Anthony O'Connell, a Sister of Charity from Cincinnati, is remembered in the history of this period as the "Angel of the Battlefield."

The Sisters of Mercy, the Sisters of the Holy Cross, and also the Irish Sisters of Mercy who came to America in 1843 extended their orders throughout the new country, establishing hospitals everywhere and practicing the highest standards of nursing of the times.

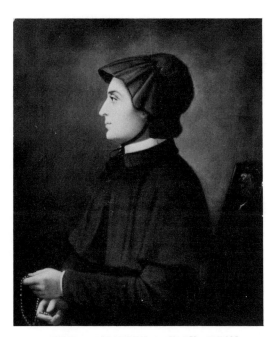

MOTHER ELIZABETH BAYLEY SETON

Mother Seton founded the American branch of the Sisters of Charity of St. Vincent de Paul.

EARLY NURSING IN PROTESTANT HOSPITALS

Protestant settlements did not fare as well. We have previously seen the havoc that was wrought during the Reformation to the Catholic nursing orders and to all for which they stood. The result was that wherever Protestant pioneers advanced, there was no organized effort to take care of the sick and wounded. The task was done by persons who felt inclined thereto; although these persons apparently performed their task with kindness, their skill was limited by their inherent ability. As the colonies grew and as settlements became better established, they followed the pattern of their homeland and organized institutions for the care of the sick and the poor, not so much out of Christian charity as for social convenience —something had to be done with the unfortunate ones. The result, according to the

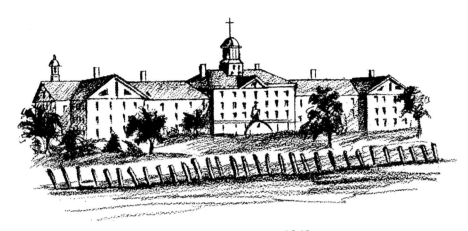

BELLEVUE HOSPITAL, 1848

Originally Bellevue Hospital was established as the New York Public Workhouse. The name was taken from its second site, Belle View on Kip's Farm, where it still stands.

descriptions that have reached us of these early refuges of poverty, sickness, and immortality, was a fair match for what Mrs. Fry found in British workhouses and hospitals during the same era. For in those early days the poorhouse and hospital were under a common roof, and no one who could possibly be nursed elsewhere would go to a hospital. Consequently the public developed a fear of hospitals, remnants of which survive even today, long after hospitals have ceased to be dens of horror and torment.

The most accurate information about nursing in American hospitals before the reform movement is found in the records of the investigation of 1837 and later of the Bellevue Hospital Visiting Committee. This was an agency of the New York State Charities Aid Association.

Dirt and squalor were predominant factors; no money was available with which to accomplish anything; and everybody lived, or died, close to a subsistence level. There was neither ventilation nor hygiene; plumbing was defective. The "nurses" were ill-paid individuals from the lower strata of the community; they were venal to a degree and were tempted to supplement their meager pay with bribes and extortions from the patients. They could be trusted with nothing—neither with administration of medicine nor with gifts of food for the patients. Often they were so deficient in number or health that the sicker patients had to receive most of their nursing from other patients who could move about or from prisoners or inmates of the workhouse. No proper provisions were made for the maintenance of the nurses. Their food was poor, and there is record that they even had to sleep in the barns on bundles of straw. Now we realize that "hospital" and "nursing" had a different connotation in those days than they have today. Only the utterly destitute went to the hospital. Any others who had a home or place to stay remained there when they were sick, and nursing was provided by the mother of the home, or the grandmother, or in well-to-do homes by trusted servants. The "Mrs. Gamp" of English life does not seem to be quite as prevalent in early American days. In many neighborhoods certain women gained reputation in being especially good in nursing and were sought out for cases of sickness and confinement. These were called monthly nurses. Most of them were respectable women; many had a great deal of experience and, considering the limitation of medical experience of the period, were fully a match for the family doctors. Thus, considering the general state of medical knowledge and practice a hundred or more years ago, nursing of the sick in the middle and upper classes was not bad.

In order to present a few definite landmarks, we may remember that the Pennsylvania General Hospital was established in 1751, the New York Hospital in 1781, and the Massachusetts General Hospital in 1821. Two other institutions, the Philadelphia General Hospital and the Bellevue Hospital in New York, had their early beginnings before these came into being.

In 1713 the Quakers of Philadelphia established an almshouse for Quakers only. It demonstrated the value of such an institution as well as the need for one that was not restricted to Quakers. Accordingly, in 1731, the town established a general almshouse and, in connection with this, a hospital ward. After this institution had repeatedly outgrown its quarters, new buildings were constructed outside of the city in Blockley Township, and in 1834 it was transferred and, henceforth, assumed the name Blockley, later "Old Blockley." During this period it had become less and less of an almshouse and more and more of a hospital, and an increasing amount of instruction of medical students took place within its walls. Many famous medical teachers, the best known of whom is Dr. Osler, walked its wards. But all that did not prevent the standards of medical and nursing care at Old Blockley from sinking to a very low level until attempts were made to improve conditions during the early period of nursing reforms. Eventually Old Blockley developed into what is now known as Philadelphia General Hospital, one of the leading hospitals in the country. Its early origin can probably be traced back farther than any of the other early American hospitals.

About the same time as Philadelphia General Hospital emerged, Bellevue Hospital originated as the New York Public Workhouse. When the New York Workhouse was erected in 1736, where the city hall now stands, one large room in the west end of the building was set aside to be used as an infirmary, and a medical officer, Dr. John Van Buren, was employed at a salary of £100 a year to look after the sick inmates. By the end of the century the institution had outgrown its quarters and was moved to Belle Vue on Kip farm. Its name was taken from the place, and it has remained there since then, gradually changing its character from that of a workhouse and almshouse to that of a hospital. By 1825 a fever hospital was added, and from 1836 to 1838 the prisoners were moved to Blackwell's Island, after which it continued as one of the leading American hospitals. The leading part that it took in the development of American schools of nursing will later be discussed.

The first hospital to be organized as such was the Pennsylvania Hospital. It was built in response to a petition presented in 1751 before the Colonial Assembly by a committee of Philadelphia citizens. Prominent men on the committee included Dr. Thomas Bond and Benjamin Franklin. The governor granted a charter for the hospital and provided £2,000 to be paid in two annual installments toward its construction, provided a like amount be raised by private contributions. This was rapidly done, and after some negotiations, a site was acquired and the cornerstone was laid in 1755. The first patients were admitted by the end of the following year. The first president of the organization, Joshua Crosby, died within a month of the laying of the cornerstone. His place was taken by Benjamin Franklin, who remained in the post until he was appointed provincial agent at London in 1757. Among his many other accomplishments, Franklin was thus our first hospital administrator, and his views and organization here as in his other projects were quite progressive. The hospital has since continued its outstanding development.

When the Pennsylvania Hospital was being organized, New York City was still for many years to remain without a regular hospital for its citizens—during a time when all the great cities in Europe were building large institutions for their sick. That the defect was keenly felt was evidenced in the commencement address made by Samuel Bard to medical graduates at King's College in 1769: "It is truly a reproach, that a city like this should want a public hospital." This address immediately stimulated a movement that was heavily backed by Sir Henry Moore, governor of the colony. It resulted, in 1771, in the granting of a royal charter to the Society of the Hospital, in the City of New York. A site was acquired on the west side of Broadway, opposite Pearl Street. The necessary funds were procured, and construction was begun on a fine hospital. It was almost finished in 1775 when, accidentally, a fire destroyed the entire inside of the building. However, the men behind the movement, including the new governor, renewed their efforts; new funds were raised, partly by a grant of £4,000 from the Colonial Assembly, and the rebuilding was completed within a year, when the Revolutionary War broke out. With the occupancy of New York City by the British, the hospital was used as a barracks and occasionally as a military hospital. There followed, after the war, a prolonged period of reconstruction, and not until the year 1791 was the hospital finally opened for regular medical service.

The Philadelphia Dispensary established in 1786 was the forerunner of our modern outpatient department and clinic for ambulatory patients. It was independent of any hospital and supported by civic-minded citizens in Philadelphia. The Philadelphia Dispensary for Out-Patients was so successful that the idea soon spread to other early American cities.

CONCLUSION

Because of the growth of medical knowledge and of the hospital as a social institution, the deficiencies of nursing became glaringly apparent. As we have pointed out, the growth of modern medicine really began to gain momentum about the year 1800; there were doctors, then, who realized that properly trained nurses would be a great asset. In 1798 Dr. Valentine Seaman, attending surgeon to the New York Hospital, gave regular courses to nurses in anatomy, physiology, obstetrics, and pediatrics. He did not restrict instruction to lectures; he gave practical demonstrations also. He published a synopsis of these lectures, probably one of the earliest attempts at preparing nursing texts.

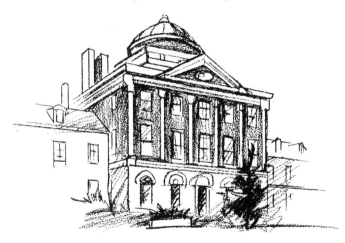

PENNSYLVANIA HOSPITAL

The first hospital to be organized as such in America was Pennsylvania Hospital, whose first administrator was Benjamin Franklin.

QUESTIONS AND STUDY PROJECTS FOR UNIT ONE

1. What were the nursing activities of the following orders?
   a. Third Order of St. Francis
   b. Order of St. Vincent de Paul
   c. The Beguines
   d. The Poor Clares
   e. The Community of the Sisters of Charity
2. Discuss the nursing done by the sisters of the Hôtel Dieu in Paris during the Middle Ages. Include the real contributions made by them to nursing.
3. Discuss the "dark age of nursing" under the following heads:
   a. General social conditions in Europe
   b. Status of medicine
   c. Status of hospitals
   d. Status and regulations affecting religious orders
   e. Status of women
4. Write short sketches of the following persons and show their contributions to nursing and to its development as a profession: Dr. Valentine Seaman, Pastor and Mrs. Fliedner, Mrs. Elizabeth Gurney Fry, Mother Catherine M'Auley.
5. What lasting contributions to medicine were made by Hippocrates, Harvey, Sydenham, Boerhaave, and Morgagni?
6. Write a short paper on early American medicine.
7. Discuss the contributions of Pasteur and Lister to medicine. Show how these discoveries radically changed the nursing care of patients.
8. Show the relation between medical discoveries and the progress of professional nursing.
9. What were the effects of the Crusades on nursing and medicine?
10. What were the contributions of John Howard to the improvement of hospitals?
11. Describe the origin and early history of your hospital.
12. Discuss medieval hospitals and the nursing care given in them.
13. How and why have city, state, and federal governments in this country become interested in health, medical, and nursing activities.
14. Discuss the development of social legislation and its effects on public health during the nineteenth century.
15. Discuss the progress of the emancipation of women during the nineteenth and twentieth centuries.
16. Discuss the work of religious orders in hospitals during this period.
17. Describe the development of hospitals and nursing service in pioneer days in America.
18. Make an annotated bibliography of recent articles appearing in *The American Journal of Nursing, Nursing Outlook, Nursing Record,* and any other journals available in your library containing articles relating to the discussion in this unit.

REFERENCES FOR UNIT ONE

Austin, A. L., and Stewart, Isabelle, M.: History of nursing, ed. 5, New York, 1962, G. P. Putnam's Sons. pp. 23-64.

Deutsch, Albert: Dorothea Lynde Dix: apostle of the insane, American Journal of Nursing **36:** 987-997, October, 1936.

Doyle, Ann: Nursing by religious orders in the United States, American Journal of Nursing **29:**775, 1929 (Part I, 1809-1840); **29:**959, 1929 (Part II, 1841-1870); **29:**1085, 1929 (Part III, 1871-1928); **29:**1197, 1929 (Part IV, Lutheran deaconesses, 1849-1928); **29:**1466, 1929 (Part VI, Episcopal sisterhoods, 1845-1928).

Ferguson, E. D.: The evolution of the trained nurse, American Journal of Nursing **1:**463-468, April, 1901; **1:**535-538, May, 1901; **1:**620-626, June, 1901.

Fishbein, Morris: History of the American Medical Association, Philadelphia, 1947, W. B. Saunders Co.

Frank, Sister Charles Marie: Foundations of nursing, ed. 2, Philadelphia, 1959, W. B. Saunders Co.

Gallison, Marie: The ministry of women: one hundred years of women's work at Kaiserswerth, 1836-1936, London, 1954, The Butterworth Press.

Hamilton, Samuel W.: The history of American mental hospitals. One hundred years of American psychiatry, New York, 1944, Columbia University Press.

Hume, Edgar Erskine: Medical work of the Knights Hospitallers of Saint John of Jeru-salem, Baltimore, 1940, The Johns Hopkins Press.

Jones, Mary Cadwalader: The training of a nurse, November, 1890, Scribner's.

Lady nurses, Godey's Lady's Book and Magazine 32:188, 1871.

Levine, Edwin B., and Levine, Myra E.: Hippocrates, father of nursing, too? American Journal of Nursing 65:86, December, 1965.

Robb, Isabel Hampton: Educational standards for nurses, Cleveland, Ohio, 1907, E. C. Koechart.

Sharp, Ella E.: Nursing during the pre-Christian era, American Journal of Nursing 19:675-678, June, 1919.

UNIT TWO
Florence Nightingale—her life and influence on nursing

The Nightingale pledge*

I solemnly pledge myself before God, and in the presence of this assembly,

To pass my life in purity and to practice my profession faithfully
I will abstain from whatever is deleterious and mischievous, and will not take or knowingly administer any harmful drug.

I will do all in my power to maintain and elevate the standard of my profession, and will hold in confidence all personal matters committed to my keeping and all family affairs coming to my knowledge in the practice of my profession.

With loyalty will I endeavor to aid the physician in his work, and devote myself to the welfare of those committed to my care.

---

*This pledge was formulated in 1893 by a committee of which Mrs. Lystra E. Gretter, R.N., was the chairman. It was first administered to the 1893 graduating class of the Farrand Training School, now the Harper Hospital, Detroit, Mich.

CHAPTER 7 EARLY LIFE AND EDUCATION

■ The dominant figure in the development of organized nursing is Florence Nightingale. We have seen in the introductory chapters (1) how medicine was evolving into a scientific practice in which doctors, whether they knew it or not, would soon require more than menial labor from nurses, (2) how the general state of society and the improvement of hospital facilities were amenable to the new profession, and (3) how the Protestant ministers in various countries had begun to realize that in Protestant countries an organization was needed similar to the Catholic nursing orders, but perhaps freer, and how they in various ways had attempted to meet this need.

The training and organization of lay Protestant nurses had begun before Florence Nightingale made her contribution to nursing, but with her powerful personality, her vision, and her practical organizing ability she took the lead in the movement, placed it on a powerful foundation of organization, sound educational principles, and high ethics, and inspired it with an enthusiasm that gave to it an impetus under which it is still progressing. A few years before Miss Nightingale's time there was no such thing as professional nursing. At the time of her death nursing was a profession, administered by women and offering them nursing and educational opportunities, formerly unthinkable.

However, Florence Nightingale devoted only a part of her life to the advancement of nursing; she also contributed greatly to reforms in the army, the Indian Public Health Service, and public health in Great Britain. Her full stature cannot be comprehended unless attention is given also to these accomplishments.

EDUCATION AT HOME AND ABROAD

On May 12, 1820, a daughter was born to Mr. and Mrs. William Edward Nightingale. She was their second girl, and because the family was then staying in Florence, Italy, she was named after the city of

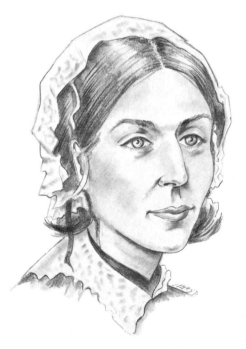

FLORENCE NIGHTINGALE

her birth. Her family was of considerable wealth, of good social standing, and highly cultured; therefore they could afford to give their children the best education available. Florence was brought up with a broad outlook and knowledge of French, German, and Italian. Her father took a very active part in her education by personally instructing her in mathematics and the classics.

When the Nightingale family returned to England, they built a new house at Embley Park, Hampshire, and most of their time was spent there or at the old family home at Lea Hurst, Derbyshire. Each year during the season an extended visit was made to London, and the young ladies grew up with opportunities to make the best social contacts, which later were to be of the greatest value to Florence.

In 1837 the family again went abroad, touring France, Italy, and Switzerland. In the winter of 1838 they traveled to Paris where Florence was introduced to the salons, in which she made acquaintances that she was to treasure throughout her life. When she returned to London, she was a young lady and was supposed to take her place in society. However, Florence was too serious to be satisfied with such a life. She felt a calling for something greater, although it took some years before her yearnings became articulate. From time to time she made inquiries into the possibilities of becoming a nurse, but knowing what we do of the social status and morals of those creatures, we cannot wonder that Mrs. Nightingale fought such ideas. Nevertheless, Florence had definite plans to become a nurse at the Salisbury Hospital not far from her home. Although these did not materialize, her purpose became even firmer.

In 1844 Miss Nightingale met the American philanthropist and his wife, Dr. and Mrs. Ward Howe (Julia Ward Howe later became known as the author of "The Battle Hymn of the Republic"). They stayed at Embley, the Nightingale home. Miss Nightingale was very much impressed with an institution for the blind that Dr. Ward had founded in New York in which he had worked out a plan to make medical care and nursing available without payment to elderly or ill American citizens. During their stay Miss Nightingale discussed with them the feasibility of working in English hospitals as Catholic sisters did. At that time no English women of any social standing would have sought a vocation outside the home, except to enter the church as a Catholic sister. During this year she felt she had reached the turning point of her life, and it was clear to her that her vocation was to be the care of the sick in hospitals. However, her family would not even discuss the possibility of her entering the hospital, so far was it removed from any of their thinking.

Until 1845 she had believed that qualities such as tenderness, sympathy, goodness, and patience were all that a nurse required. After experience in caring for some members of her own family during their illnesses, she recognized that knowledge and skill were also necessary and that acquisition of these required education and training.

It is not surprising that her family was shocked whenever she mentioned going to a hospital, either for training or to nurse, because in the middle of the nineteenth century, hospitals were at a low level of degradation and squalor. Dirt and lack of sanitation were common. They were crowded, and the patients who were dirty when they came to the hospital were likely to remain that way during their stay.

In 1847 after a busy "social summer" she set out for Rome with Mr. and Mrs. Bracebridge, close friends of the family—a visit that was to result in two important experiences. She went into retreat for ten days in the Convent of the Trinita dei Monti, where she absorbed much of the spirit of the church and where her religious belief greatly matured. Although she was much impressed with the practical endeavors of the Catholic church, she did not become converted to Catholicism; in fact it could never be said that she strongly preferred any particular branch of the church, although she remained deeply religious throughout her life. By tradition she remained within the Church of England.

Her second important experience was the meeting of Mr. and Mrs. Sidney Herbert. Mr.—later Sir—Sidney Herbert was to have the greatest influence on her life; it was through him that she was to go to the Crimea, and with him (and Dr. Sutherland) that she was to form "the little war office." For the present their contact was largely social, consisting of parties and visits to the galleries. There was some talk of nursing, for there were plans to establish a nursing home when they returned to England. It is interesting to note at this time that Mr. and Mrs. Sidney Herbert and many of their friends were beginning to be interested in hospital reform. Public opinion was being awakened, and Miss Nightingale, who had been collecting facts on public health and hospitals for several years, was able to give this group a great deal of information. Gradually she became known as an expert in hospital reform.

When Miss Nightingale returned to England, she was about 28 years of age, and it was about time for her to marry. In fact, marriage was seriously considered repeatedly but did not materialize. The next year she once more accompanied the Bracebridges abroad to Egypt and Greece. In the meantime she had grown considerably, both emotionally and intellectually, so she studied intently all that she saw; she paid much attention to institutions for the sick and poor. She had learned about the institution at Kaiserswerth. Through some friends she had received the Yearbook of the Institution of Deaconesses at Kaiserswerth in 1846. She studied it very carefully and realized that here she could receive the training she so keenly wanted. Because the institution was under religious auspices and the character of the deaconesses and pastors above re-

proach, she could go there without the stigma attached to the English hospitals.

On the return journey she paid it a visit. She was greatly impressed and became very eager to return to participate in the training. Miss Nightingale was so impressed with Kaiserswerth that on her return she issued anonymously a pamphlet called *The Institution of Kaiserswerth on the Rhine for the Practical Training of Deaconesses Under the Direction of the Rev. Pastor Fliedner, Embracing the Support and Care of a Hospital, Infant and Industrial Schools and a Female Penitentiary.* This was a 32-page pamphlet and was printed by the Inmates of the London Ragged Colonial Training School at Westminster where Miss Nightingale had taught and in which she had a great deal of interest.

She was well aware that to become a good nurse a thorough training was essential, and when in 1851 her mother and sister went to Carlsbad to "take the cure," she finally contrived to accompany them with the intention of paying an extended visit to Kaiserswerth. She spent three months at the Fliedners' institution and derived from it a great deal of instruction. She participated in the nurses' instruction even to the point of scrubbing floors and left much impressed with the organization and high purpose of the place. Her opinion of the actual training of the nurses was not so high. The experience at Kaiserswerth strengthened her purpose, but as yet she failed to give it practical expression.

In 1851 she met the famous woman doctor, Dr. Elizabeth Blackwell, through the Herberts. Dr. Blackwell visited Miss Nightingale at Embley, and although Miss Nightingale did not approve of women doctors in general, they had many discussions about hospitals and medical care. In the spring of 1853 she was in Paris again inspecting hospitals and infirmaries; finally she arranged to enter the Maison de la Providence for a course of training with the Sisters of Charity. An attack of the measles, however, promptly

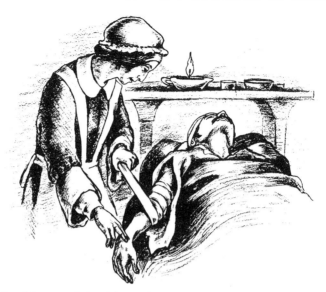

Florence Nightingale's care of the sick at all hours of the day and night during the Crimean War earned for her the grateful title, "Lady with the lamp."

forced her to receive nursing care instead of dispensing it. Her illness more or less put an end to this undertaking.

In the meantime she had entered into negotiations with the committee supervising an "Establishment for Gentlewomen During Illness." This was a type of nursing home in London for governesses who became ill, and after appearing before the committee she was appointed superintendent. In 1853 the establishment moved into an empty house at No. 1 Upper Harley Street, and here for the next few years Florence Nightingale found a limited expression for her desire to nurse. She had a number of difficulties with her committee, all of which she negotiated with tact, and she soon had the nursing home running smoothly.

As soon as Miss Nightingale had reorganized the institution, she again began visiting hospitals and collecting facts for reforming conditions for nurses. In the middle of the nineteenth century, social reform was becoming increasingly popular, and people like the Herberts and many of their friends became interested in the reform of medical and social institutions. Miss Nightingale realized that before any nursing reform

could be launched, some type of school for the training of reliable and qualified nurses must be organized. At this time, she realized that her first task was to help produce a new type of nurse. Because of her knowledge of hospitals, she was being consulted by social reformers and by many doctors who were beginning to recognize the need for the trained nurse. For example, Dr. Bowman, a well-known surgeon of that day, had performed a difficult operation on a patient anesthetized with chloroform, which was just beginning to be used as an anesthetic, and Miss Nightingale had assisted as his nurse. He was very eager for her to accept the position of superintendent of nurses in the King's College Hospital. However, when rumors of this reached her family, the objections they had always had to Miss Nightingale's going into large hospitals were again brought forward.

She remained in charge of the nursing home at No. 1 Upper Harley Street until her departure for Scutari, with the exception of a vacation to her home and a short leave of absence for the purpose of nursing at the Middlesex Hospital during an epidemic of cholera.

CHAPTER 8 THE CRIMEAN WAR

■ In the meantime the Crimean War broke out. The British, the French, and the Turks were fighting the Russians, chiefly near the Black Sea and the Crimean Peninsula. As the war dragged on, it became apparent that there were some serious defects in the organization of the British army, particularly in the handling of the sick and wounded soldiers. The letters of the war correspondent W. H. Russell to the *Times* stirred up emotion at home. His comparison of nursing in the French army to that in the British brought things to a climax, which resulted in the letter to the *Times* containing the famous question: "Why have we no Sisters of Charity?"

Many inquiries were made about town in a similar vein, and Miss Nightingale's name was mentioned repeatedly in this connection. Miss Nightingale herself was turning the matter over in her mind and finally wrote to Sir Sidney Herbert, who now was secretary of war, offering to take a group of nurses into the Crimea. Curiously enough, a letter from Sir Sidney requesting that she do so crossed hers. Her family consented, and she was soon hard at work enlisting 38 nurses. Among these were ten Roman Catholic sisters, partly from Bermondsey, eight of Miss Sellon's sisters from Devonport, and six from St. John's House. These were the best she could obtain at short notice, but several were inadequately trained and later had to be returned.

MISS NIGHTINGALE'S ACHIEVEMENTS

On October 21, 1854, the party set out for Scutari on the steamer Vectis. The problems that awaited Miss Nightingale were prodigious. The equipment for the hospital was defective or nonexistent, and the staff already there looked upon the expedition as a slur upon their own capabilities and were not kindly disposed to this arrangement of admitting female nurses into a military hospital. So her job required both organizing ability and tact.

The interested reader may refer to Miss Nightingale's biography for detailed descriptions of the conditions at Scutari. We are concerned with her contribution to organized nursing and may therefore treat the subject in a cursory manner. Plumbing and sewage disposal were next to nonexistent. The simplest means of hygiene and civilized living were lacking. There were no knives and forks, no bedclothes, no scrubbing brushes, no operating room—in fact, hardly anything but a crowded space full of suffering, dying, verminous, undernourished soldiers, attended by inexperienced orderlies and supervised by men who were largely inefficient and who considered the intruders with hostility.

At first Miss Nightingale and her nurses were ignored by the doctors. Although the patients were in great need and Miss Nightingale could get supplies for them, only one doctor would use her nurses and her supplies. She realized that before she could accomplish anything, she must obtain the cooperation and confidence of the medical staff. She was determined to stand by and wait until she was asked to help. This required a great deal of self-control because the need for nursing care and for the supplies that she could get was evident. She was determined that the doctors would ask for her help and was equally determined that no nurse would take care of patients unless she was reliable.

At last, as the fighting increased and the sick and wounded came in ever-increasing numbers, everyone—even visiting representatives from the British government—was pressed into service. At last the doctors turned to Miss Nightingale and her nurses. It gradually dawned on the medical staff and the hospital officials that Miss Nightingale was the one person who had money at her disposal and who had contacts with influential people who could help in critical situations.

Miss Nightingale and her nurses set to work at once. They had the authority from the war office, and they began by requisitioning several hundred scrubbing brushes. Before the war was over, there was a reasonable measure of cleanliness, special diet kitchens had been established, and the rats had been brought under some control. In brief, out of a shambles Miss Nightingale had established a hospital.

The manner in which she handled her staff is also interesting. They were there to cooperate, not to take charge. Miss Nightingale's nurses were strictly instructed not to undertake nursing except when requested by medical officers and to take orders regarding patients from the doctors only. Furthermore she established herself in the hearts of the men, dividing her time between administration and personal attention to patients. Famous are her nightly rounds when the day's work supposedly was done. Then with her lantern she made her tour of inspection past the long lines of cots, with a friendly word for some, a smile for others, but in all she inspired a feeling of comfort that someone was sympathizing with them and striving to make their hard lot a little less hard. Of all her activities in Scutari

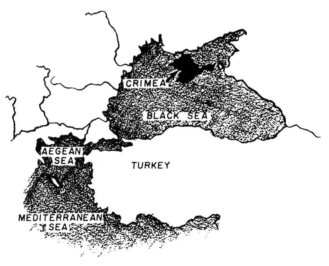

CRIMEAN WAR

The Crimean War dragged on for many years while the English, French, and Turkish fought the Russians. The English lacked the organization and personnel to care for their wounded until Miss Nightingale came to Scutari.

these nightly rounds are perhaps the most famous; they have been immortalized by Longfellow in his poem *The Lady With the Lamp*.

All this was not achieved without difficulties. One of the worst was that she was informed one day that 46 nurses were on their way to Scutari under the direction of Miss Mary Stanley. It has never been explained who initiated this move or how it was made without consulting Miss Nightingale. They were not sent to assist her but were instructed to report to the inspector general. Considering the importance of the experiment that Miss Nightingale was performing, her alarm at such an attempt at dual control can easily be imagined. She protested vigorously to Sir Sidney Herbert, and eventually the nurses came into her organization. Other nurses were added from time to time, and at the end of the war she had a staff of 125 nurses.

Miss Nightingale's interest extended beyond nursing. She was in the best sense a social worker. The army in those days had no recreational facilities for the soldiers when they were off duty. The only choice was such entertainment as they might find outside the camp. This entertainment was not of the best and was usually designed to part them from their hard-earned pay with the least possible effort. Many soldiers had brought their wives; these women were painfully neglected, especially during sickness or childbirth. Miss Nightingale did much to relieve the lot of these poor women. She established reading rooms, games, and other entertainments for the soldiers in an attempt to direct their attention away from the dramshop and loose living. She also established in her own office a type of savings bank through which the soldiers might transmit money to relatives in England. She was eminently successful in all these pursuits.

She gained the sympathy of the medical staff by furnishing them out of her own pocket with a dissecting room and the necessary instruments. In addition to all this she spent the better part of her nights writing: she wrote long official reports and private communications to Sir Sidney Herbert and did much of the work now incumbent upon the army chaplain by writing to the families of sick and dying soldiers.

She had hardly begun to get things into shape when a new and formidable task loomed before her. Her work so far had all been done at Scutari, across the Straits of Bosporus from Constantinople. The war itself was fought across the Black Sea at the Crimean Peninsula, and she felt it incumbent upon her to investigate conditions at the actual theater of war. So in the spring of 1855 she went to Balaklava in the Crimea and worked on the reorganization of the few hospitals there. Here she encountered great obstacles: the roads were dreadful, often nonexistent, and the official attitude of jealous superior officers caused her much grief. However, the commander of the British forces supported her, and she had done much toward achieving her purpose when she was taken sick with the Crimean fever (probably typhoid or typhus). For a few days her life was in danger. However, her convalescence was slow and she never recovered entirely. She refused a leave of absence to recuperate and returned to work too soon. She stayed until the very end of the war and left with the last contingent of nurses from Scutari.

At the end of the Crimean War two figures are prominent: the common British soldier and the nurse. At the beginning of the war most British soldiers were the drunken, immoral dregs of society. The status of the women doing nursing was not much better. Miss Nightingale, because of her experiment in the Crimea, did much to set the pattern for the improvement of conditions for these two groups.

NIGHTINGALE FUND

The significance of Miss Nightingale's work in Scutari became known and understood far and wide in England: in the future, nurses must be properly trained, and the nursing care of the sick must take its place beside the surgical and medical care. Accordingly a public meeting was held in London on November 25, 1855, under the presidency of the commander-in-chief, the duke of Cambridge, and it was decided to establish a fund, to be called the "Nightingale Fund," for the purpose of furthering nursing education. Some $220,000, of which $35,000 was subscribed by the army, was collected within a short time in England and in the Dominions. The medical profession, which ultimately was to benefit so greatly from this undertaking, did not enter it wholeheartedly but remained critical.

When Miss Nightingale heard of this fund, she accepted it with the proviso that it would be some time before she could utilize it, and she expressed fear that her health might not suffice for the task. In fact, several years elapsed before she established the first school of nursing.

MISS NIGHTINGALE'S ILLNESS

In August, 1856, she returned from Scutari, six months after the end of the war and began the strangest period of her life. It seem as if she had spent the strength of her body but not that of her mind. Although there is no record that she was suffering from any organic disease, she was never very well. During the first few months after her return to England she was so weak that she was not expected to live; but when new problems arose in 1857, she rallied to the occasion. For many years she displayed the greatest vigor of mind and undertook the most sustained mental efforts—and yet she was never well enough to see anyone who came to call out of curiosity or on trivial errands. By thus excluding herself from the superficialities of society, she managed to concentrate her energies on the truly great tasks of her life. Much has been written about her "illness." It cannot simply be dismissed as neurasthenia. It could possibly be considered an exhaustion neurosis from which she never recovered because she never afforded herself sufficient rest. It may also be considered an escape through which she, unconsciously perhaps, avoided certain conflicts that would have been inevitable if she had moved about in society hale and hearty. In mid-Victorian England it would have been unthinkable for her to obtain the official position in public life to which she might have legitimately aspired. As it was, she was an invalid. Those who wished her advice had to come to her; and by practically living the life of a hermit, she found time and opportunity to gather the tremendous amount of data and information with which she filled the reports that emanated from her rooms.

CHAPTER 9 MISS NIGHTINGALE'S POSTWAR ACTIVITIES

■ Miss Nightingale's first aim was the permanent rectification of the defects that had become glaringly apparent during the Crimean War. This was to be achieved through extensive reforms of the army. She accomplished this by working through a committee, the principal members of which were Sir Sidney Herbert and Dr. Sutherland. This committee, often called "the little war office," sat usually in her rooms, at first at the Burlington Hotel, later in various rented houses. This work was progressing when it was severely upset by the death of Sir Sidney (then Lord Lea) in 1861 and by changes in the government. The reforms were being made slowly; the origins of many reforms carried out years later can still be traced to the activities of Miss Nightingale.

In 1856 the result of Miss Nightingale's conferences and deliberations was published as *Notes in Matters Affecting the Health, Efficiency and Hospital Administration of the British Army.* This was a volume of nearly 1000 printed pages. In 1859 she published a small book called *Notes on Hospitals.* This was so successful that a second edition was published in 1860 and a third, rewritten and with many additions, in 1863. After the publication of this book she was constantly being asked for advice on hospital administration and construction. The plans for many hospitals were submitted to her.

In 1858 she was elected a member of the Statistical Society, and at the Statistical Congress of 1860 she presented a paper for discussion called "Miss Nightingale's Scheme for Uniform Hospital Statistics." Until this time each hospital had used its own method for naming and classifying diseases and keeping other statistics.

Although Miss Nightingale's interest in nursing and nursing reform had never diminished, her activities for reforms in the army had pushed it into the background.

In 1859 her book, *Notes on Nursing,* was published and caused quite a sensation for that day. Habits of personal hygiene taken for granted today were completely foreign to the mid-Victorian days. This book was very widely use, and thousands of copies were distributed to factories and schools. It was also translated into French, German, and Italian.

About 1860 she found time to devote herself to the establishment of a school of nursing to be financed by the Nightingale Fund. St. Thomas's Hospital was finally selected, and for many years Miss Nightingale took a most active part in all details concerning her school. This interest was slackened only by the feebleness of old age.

For the remainder of her life Miss Nightingale's interests were divided among "the Nightingale nurses," the construction of hospitals, reforms in workhouses, public health measures throughout England (and other countries), and the promotion of public health reforms in India. Because of her powerful personality and her vast knowledge, her advice was sought on most subjects in which she was expert, but she never stood out in an official capacity. Somewhat later she became interested in the development of district nursing, and during the Franco-German war she was frequently consulted by both belligerents regarding the care of sick and wounded.

In only two respects was she judged wrong by history. First, she did not appreciate the significance of the bacteriological discoveries that occurred during that period. In spite of her interest in public health and her good judgment regarding hygienic measures, wherever bacteriological facts conflicted with her ideas regarding hygiene, the facts were ignored. Second, she did not appreciate the importance of a central registry for nurses, similar to that for medical men. She thought that the reputation of nurses could be established better through their schools and that a central registry would lead to standardization that would have a detrimental effect on the profession as a whole. Experience, of course, has shown that this was not the case, but she did manage to delay this reform for many years.

In her writings Miss Nightingale dealt with many aspects of the fields in which she was interested. She wrote about the care of the sick in hospitals, workhouses, army camps, city tenements, and rural districts. She also discussed problems in the public health field, such as housing and sanitation, and was interested in health teaching. She wrote extensively on sanitary problems in India, of racial questions, and of the uses of statistics. Her writings appear in books, pamphlets, papers, addresses, articles, and many letters. The Adelaide Nutting Historical Nursing Collection at Teachers College, Columbia University, New York, probably contains the finest collection of her writings to be found anywhere. Following is a list of some of the writings of Miss Nightingale:

1. The Institution of Kaiserswerth on the Rhine for the Practical Training of Deaconesses under the Direction of the Rev. Pastor Fliedner, Embracing the Support and Care of a Hospital, Infant and Industrial Schools, and a Female Penitentiary. Printed by the Inmates of the London Ragged Colonial Training School, 1851.

2. Letters from Egypt. Privately printed, 1854.

3. Statements Exhibiting the Voluntary Contributions Received by Miss Nightingale for the Use of the British Hospitals in the East, with the Mode of Their Distribution, in 1854, 1855, 1856. Harrison and Sons, 1857.

4. Notes on Matters Affecting the Health, Efficiency, and Hospital Administration of the British Army. Founded Chiefly on the Experience of the Late War. Presented by Request to the Secretary of State for War. Privately printed for Miss Nightingale. Harrison and Sons, 1858.

5. Subsidiary Notes as to the Introduction of Female Nursing into Military Hospitals in Peace and in War. Presented by Request to the Secretary of State for War. Privately printed for Miss Nightingale. Harrison and Sons, 1858.

6. A Contribution to the Sanitary History of the British Army During the Late War With Russia. Harrison and Sons, 1859.

7. Notes on Hospitals. John W. Parker and Sons, 1859. 3rd edition, almost completely rewritten, 1863. Longmans, Green and Co.

8. Suggestions for Thought to the Searchers after Truth Among the Artisans of England. Privately printed for Miss Nightingale. 3 vols. Eyre and Spottiswoode, 1860.

9. Notes on Nursing: What It Is, and What It Is Not. By Florence Nightingale, Harrison and Sons, 1859.

10. Army Sanitary Administration and Its Reform Under the Late Lord Herbert. M'Corquodale and Co., 1862.

11. Observations on the Evidence Contained in the Stational Reports Submitted to the Royal Commission on the Sanitary State of the Army in India. By Florence Nightingale. (Reprinted from the Report of the Royal Commission.) Edward Stanford, 1863. "The Observations."

12. Introductory Notes on Lying-In Institutions. Together With a Proposal for Organising an Institution for Training Midwives and Midwifery Nurses. By Florence Nightingale. Longmans, Green and Co., 1871.

13. Life or Death in India. A paper read at the meeting of the National Association for the Promotion of Social Science, Norwich, 1873. With an Appendix on life or death by irrigation, 1874.

14. The Zemindar, the Sun, and the Watering Pot as Affecting Life or Death in India. Unpublished, proof copies among the Nightingale papers, 1873-1876.
15. On Trained Nursing for the Sick Poor. By Florence Nightingale. The Metropolitan and National Nursing Association, 1876.
16. Miss Florence Nightingale's Addresses to Probationer-Nurses in the "Nightingale Fund" School at St. Thomas's Hospital and Nurses Who Were Formerly Trained There, 1872-1900. Printed for private circulation.
17. Florence Nightingale's Indian Letters. A glimpse into the agitation for tenancy reform. Bengal, 1878-82. Edited by Priyaranja Sen. Calcutta, 1937.*

Thus for about 40 years Miss Nightingale was actively interested in some of the most important reforms of the times, but about the turn of the century her powers waned—she was then nearly 80—and the last ten years of her life she spent in a state of decline until she died quietly in her sleep on August 13, 1910. It was proposed that she be buried in Westminster Abbey, but in accordance with her wish she was interred in the family burying place at Willow, Hampshire.

MISS NIGHTINGALE'S INFLUENCE ON NURSING

Notwithstanding her great contribution in other fields, Miss Nightingale's greatest and most enduring work was done in nursing.

From her youth she believed that her calling was to nurse the sick, and as her purpose in life gradually evolved, she increasingly concentrated her efforts upon the organization of hospitals and the training of nurses. She availed herself of the training that was then available and always deplored that it had not been better. Although she accepted most of the good aspects of Kaiserswerth, she was keenly aware of the defects in the nurses' training. When she was sick in Paris, she criticized the nursing care

*Woodham-Smith, Cecil: Florence Nightingale, New York, 1951, McGraw-Hill Book Co., Inc., pp. 368-369.

that she received. When she was placed in charge of a nursing home, its greatest defect in her opinion was that it gave her no opportunity to train nurses. Again, the lack of trained nurses was at the root of the evils of Scutari and Balaklava, and her greatest single contribution in the Crimean War was the organization of nursing care and such training of nurses as she could effect. The next logical step in her career would have been the administration of the Nightingale Fund, and it was only because of the pressure of the army reforms and her poor state of health that the establishment of a school of nursing under her direction was delayed. However, the time was not wasted, for in 1859 she published two books, *Notes on Hospitals,* which advocated better construction of hospitals and better nursing care, and *Notes on Nursing; What It Is, and What It Is Not.* In the latter book she set forth the fundamental principles of nursing, and it became widely read; it was followed by a "popular edition" in 1861, called *Notes on Nursing for the Laboring Classes,* which include a chapter on infant care. Her *Notes on Nursing* was really one of the first nursing texts and was widely used as such by nurses. It was first published in 1859 and translated into several languages. The first American edition was published in 1860.

Finally, in 1859 a committee was appointed to select a hospital for Miss Nightingale's training school, and, as we noted, St. Thomas's Hospital was selected. The medical officer, Mr. R. G. Whitfield, was sympathetic to the plan, and the matron, Mrs. Wardroper, was a most capable woman. In 1860, fifteen probationers were admitted for a year's training. Miss Nightingale was consulted on all details of selection of pupil nurses, instruction, and organization. Throughout this chapter emphasis has been placed upon Miss Nightingale's appreciation of the necessity for training of nurses. This is so obvious to us that it is hard to understand that she had to fight to establish this principle. Most people, including many medical men, thought that nursing could be done "by intuition." If that attitude is understood, the magnitude of Miss Nightingale's contribution is better appreciated. Furthermore, she made it clear that she did not advocate a new "nursing order." She wanted to establish a secular career for women, similar to law and medicine for men. And she succeeded. If it had not been for Miss Nightingale, the elevation of nursing from a lowly craft to a respected profession might have been delayed many years, to the detriment of the progress of medicine and hospital administration.

As it was, Miss Nightingale placed the emphasis on the education of women in an endowed school; in fact she was less concerned with the production, in the first place, of practical nurses than with a group of educated women who could go abroad in the land and establish similar centers of training elsewhere, acting as leaders who would help raise the level of nursing everywhere. Again she succeeded. More nursing pupils were admitted, more instruction was instituted, and gradually the old type nurses were replaced by younger women to whom nursing was a career and not a last resort.

Along with all this she personally kept in touch with her nurses. She rarely went out, but they came to see her in her home at South Street where she lived for many years, and aided by her acute judgment of human character she quickly sized them up and her notes made at the time bear witness to her shrewd and crafty powers of observation. During her lifetime she became an almost legendary figure in English nursing. The growth of her reputation was not hampered by the eventual decline of her frail body. Her name continues to be the beacon light for our profession.

In 1893 she prepared a paper on "Sick Nursing and Health Nursing," which was read at the Chicago Exhibition of Women's Work at the World's Fair.

Many memorials have been erected to Miss Nightingale. National Hospital Day is

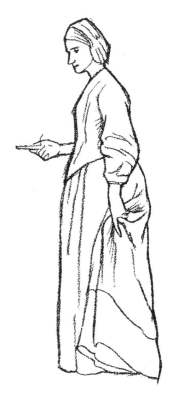

FLORENCE NIGHTINGALE FROM STATUE

The "Lady with the Lamp," immortalized by Longfellow in commemoration of her nightly rounds at Scutari, left an impact on nursing and hospitals that is felt today.

celebrated on her birthday; on the Sunday nearest that date nurses all over America hold memorial services. In 1912 it was proposed at the International Council of Nurses in Cologne that an international memorial be developed; a Florence Nightingale Foundation was set up for this purpose. Before World War II a group of nurses from many countries lived at Florence Nightingale International House in London for one year and acquired a better conception of international understanding while studying together in three courses: (1) public health, (2) nurse administration and teaching, and (3) social work. The courses were given at Bedford College in cooperation with the College of Nursing.

QUESTIONS AND STUDY PROJECTS FOR UNIT TWO

1. In what ways did the Crimean War affect nursing and the development of professional nursing?
2. To what other fields besides nursing did Miss Nightingale contribute? What were some of these contributions?
3. What were the basic principles upon which the Nightingale School was established?
4. Be prepared to discuss the life of Florence Nightingale under the following heads:
   a. Her early life and education
   b. Her preparation for nursing
   c. Her activities during the Crimean War
   d. Her contributions to the development of professional nursing
   e. Her contributions to public health
   f. Her writings
   g. Her influence on the first schools of nursing established in this country
5. Make an annotated bibliography of recent articles appearing in *The American Journal of Nursing, Nursing Outlook, Nursing Research,* and any other journals available in your library relating to the discussion in this unit.

REFERENCES FOR UNIT TWO

Andrews, Mary R.: A lost commander: Florence Nightingale, New York, 1938, Doubleday & Co., Inc.

Banworth, Calista: A living memorial to Florence Nightingale, American Journal of Nursing **40:**491-497, May, 1940.

Cook, Sir Edward: The life of Florence Nightingale (2 vols. in 1), New York, 1942, The Macmillan Co.

Editorial—Dedication of the American Nurses' Memorial, Florence Nightingale School, Bordeaux, France, American Journal of Nursing **22:**799-804, July, 1922.

Editorial—The dedication of the Bordeaux School Building, American Journal of Nursing **22:**635-636, May, 1922.

Editorial—The imperishable glory of Miss Nightingale, American Journal of Nursing **36:**491-492, May, 1936.

Extracts from letters from the Crimea, American Journal of Nursing **32:**537-538, 1932.

Florence Nightingale is placed among mankind's benefactors, American Journal of Nursing **50:**265, 1950.

Lee, Eleanor: A Florence Nightingale collection, American Journal of Nursing **38:**555-561, May, 1938.

McGinley, Phyllis: Saint-watching, New York, 1969, The Viking Press, Inc.

Noyes, Clara D.: American nurses complete fund for Memorial School in France, American Journal of Nursing **29:**1189-1191, October, 1929.

Nightingaliana: American Journal of Nursing **49:**288-299, May, 1949.

Pavey, Agnes E.: The story of the growth of nursing, London, 1938, Faber & Faber, Ltd., pp. 267-298.

Roberts, Mary M.: Florence Nightingale as a nurse educator, American Journal of Nursing **37:**773-778, July, 1937.

Scovil, Elisabeth R.: Florence Nightingale notes on nursing, American Journal of Nursing **27:**355-357, May, 1927.

Seymer, Lucy: St. Thomas' Hospital and the Nightingale Training School, International Nursing Review **11:**340-344, 1937.

Stephen, Barbara: Florence Nightingale's Home, International Nursing Review **11:**331-334, 1937.

Strachey, Lytton: Eminent Victorians, New York, 1963, G. P. Putnam's Sons.

Trevelyan, George Macaulay: History of England, London, 1928, Longmans, Green & Co., Ltd.

Whittaker, Elvi W., and Olesen, Virginia L.: Why Florence Nightingale? American Journal of Nursing **67:**2338-2341, November, 1967.

Woodham-Smith, Cecil: Florence Nightingale, New York, 1951, McGraw-Hill Book Co., Inc.

UNIT THREE
Early American Nursing

The humanitarian impulse that developed at the dawn of the
Christian Era resulted in many hospitals' being established. The
industrialization of the community emphasized the need for
hospitals and the training of personnel as a community as well
as a religious obligation. The concept of group responsibility
for the individual was beginning to develop.

CHAPTER 10 MEDICAL AND SOCIAL SETTING

■ Medical science was confronted by a host of problems. More than 100 years ago Louis emphasized the importance of the numerical method in medicine, but few doctors properly appreciated the necessity of the suitable application of statistical methods in determining effective treatment and in evaluating data. Tuberculosis, although its incidence was receding, was still a formidable enemy and required much preventive work and improvement of treatment during its early stages. Venereal disease, especially syphilis, was yet to be conquered; in this field, however, notable beginnings had been made by the discovery of the spirochete, the Wassermann reaction (1906), by further development of the specific drugs, salvarsan and its derivatives, by the use of the heavy metals, and by the general recognition of venereal disease as a public health problem. Maternal mortality was still too high for the country as a whole. Further advances in surgical technic were expected. (In this connection, however, we may remember that at a congress in England in 1872, just before Lister's work was generally appreciated, the opinion was expressed that surgery had then almost reached the limits of its achievement.) The greatest advances in the near future were expected in increased knowledge of the endocrine glands and of the vitamins, in the control of cancer, in mental illness, and in preventive medicine.

During the late eighteenth and nineteenth centuries scientific progress in all phases of diagnosis and treatment of disease had been very great. This increased knowledge had resulted in the beginning of specialization in all health activities. Increased knowledge meant the need for more and better equipment in doctors' offices, in clinics, and in hospitals. All these changes were beginning to increase the cost of medical care. As the community became educated in health matters and as confidence was created in hospitals, doctors, and nurses, increasing demands were being made on the health program of the entire United States. As health and disease became matters of public concern, we find that communities began to make plans for assuming certain responsibilities in these areas. This was observed particularly in countries in which socialism was advancing. Chancellor Bismarck was instrumental in working out a plan of compulsory insurance against illness in Germany in 1883. The German example of providing social insurance made quite an impression on other European countries. Compulsory health insurance for those of low incomes was adopted in Austria in 1888. Other countries in Europe adopting some type of compulsory health insurance or subsidizing voluntary societies were Sweden in 1891, Denmark in 1892, Belgium in 1894, Italy in 1898, and Switzerland in 1912. In Russia in 1918 a "People's Commissariat of Public Health" was established, and in line with other developments in the communist state almost complete state medicine developed. All these developments and their underlying social philosophies, naturally, were studied by and had some influence on other countries. England, although probably more individualistic politically than some of the continental countries, had become highly industrialized during the nineteenth century, and even the poorer classes were becoming better educated. In 1911 a National Insurance Act was adopted by the English Parliament. In England the state as well as employers and employees contributed to the cost. Patients had a free choice of doctors, and what has become known as the "panel system" developed.

EARLY AMERICAN MEDICINE

American medicine was still in its infancy in the eighteenth century. Many doctors came from Europe to settle in America, and many students went from this country to study in the European centers. Benjamin Franklin influenced American medicine not only by inventing bifocal glasses but also by preaching the use of fresh air and by helping in the foundation of the Pennsylvania Hospital.

Too, in America, medical teaching was for the most part at a low ebb. Only Philadelphia had attained any reputation; New York and Boston were still struggling into existence as medical centers. It was therefore simple and logical that American doctors should be divided into two groups: those with the ambition and resources that enabled them to visit Edinburgh, London, and Paris, from which they returned to become leading surgeons and physicians, mostly in the larger cities of the East, and those content with the preceptorship of an older practitioner—by far the majority.

The first medical schools in the United States were organized in the second half of the eighteenth century, the first one being the College of Philadelphia, now the University of Pennsylvania, founded by John Morgan, modeled after the Edinburgh School. The first American doctor of medicine degree was conferred in 1771 at the King's College School in New York, now the College of Physicians and Surgeons of Columbia University, founded in 1767. Harvard did not start a medical school until 1773. Other medical schools founded in this century were Dartmouth College and School and the Transylvania University School in Kentucky.

It is no wonder that with a few exceptions medical practice in the United States 100 years ago was very bad; it could not be otherwise. It is remarkable that in America, largely through the efforts of the American Medical Association, the profession has been raised to the level at which it stands today and that in spite of all handicaps, Americans have been able to make important and fundamental contributions to the science.

One such contribution was McDowell's operations on ovarian tumor. Having had his attention drawn to the problem when he was a student in Edinburgh under John Bell, Ephraim McDowell (1771-1830), when he became a backwoods practitioner in Kentucky, had the courage to perform the operation. He was successful and gained fame by several repetitions of his feat. So incredible was his achievement that when reports first reached Europe, they were simply not believed.

During the early nineteenth century a physiologist became noted because of his studies of gastric digestion and gastric motility, which formed the basis for all later work on the physiology of gastric digestion —William Beaumont (1785-1853).

On the morning of June 6, 1822, an accident happened on the little Island of Mackinac, north of Michigan, which was destined to bring fame to one man and a great increase of knowledge to the world. A young voyageur, Alexis St. Martin, happened to be in the way of a shotgun that accidentally went off 2 feet from his body. The entire charge entered his left side, tearing his clothing with it. At first the wound was thought to be fatal, but under the care of a regimental surgeon stationed at the fort the lad recovered. However, a fistula, or opening from the stomach to the surface of the body, remained. The surgeon, whose name was Beaumont, seized this opportunity for study of gastric function and attached the boy to his household for the next few years. He performed a series of experiments which have become fundamental in our knowledge of that organ, and Beaumont's name is now known to every young medical student. His studies were performed under primitive conditions, and the brilliant results are due to Beaumont's ability for research and not to his equipment. Alexis was an unworthy fellow who repeatedly left him, and at last Beaumont failed to recover him. In 1839 Beaumont was stationed in St. Louis. Later because of a difference with his superiors he retired from the army and entered private practice there, where his fame and ability soon made him the leading doctor of St. Louis.

Best known of all American doctors of the period was Benjamin Rush (1755-1813). He has been referred to as the "American Sydenham." His influence in furthering the clinical method in America continued long after his death; and his descendants are still practicing medicine in Philadelphia.

Perhaps the greatest medical advance made in America during this period was the use of ether for surgical anesthesia. For this great boon to medicine we are indebted to a Boston dentist named William T. G. Morton (1819-1868). Through careful research, Morton chose ether as the drug for his purpose. He demonstrated his discovery to the Boston surgeons, and it was soon broadcast all over the world. Along with the work of Pasteur and of Lister it made possible the great advance of modern surgery. It is a curious and sordid fact that Morton, instead of granting his gift magnanimously to the world as most medical benefactors did, tried to exploit it by patent rights. This soon in-

volved him in litigation, which broke him bodily and financially; so instead of reaping the laurels of fame his last years were spent in ignominious misery.

A historical figure in American medicine during the late nineteenth and early twentieth centuries, one whose influence is still felt today, was Sir William Osler (1849-1919). His activities were shared by three countries—Canada, the United States, and Great Britain. He combined with a thorough training in pathology outstanding clinical abilities, both as a teacher and as a diagnostician. Thus he came to be one of the founders of Johns Hopkins Medical School in Baltimore, and it was here he achieved his greatest fame.

The last years of his life were tragic. All through his life he had given of himself freely for the advancement of knowledge and love of mankind. For himself he had but one thing, a son, and that son was sacrificed in World War I. When Osler received the telegram from the war office, his spirit died within him, and his body survived but a few years. No more direct impression of the futility and bestiality of war could be given than that conveyed by the description of that father's grief for his son.

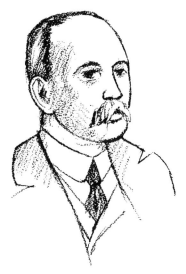

WILLIAM OSLER

In 1898 Pierre Curie and his wife, Marie, isolated radium, now used in the treatment of certain types of cancer. In 1910 Paul Ehrlich discovered a cure for syphilis in the form of arsphenamine. Large sums were being appropriated, particularly in America, for scientific investigation. In 1901 John D. Rockefeller endowed the Rockefeller Institute for Medical Research. Simon Flexner, an outstanding scientist, was director. He gathered about him outstanding scientists in medical and allied fields; many discoveries have come from that Institute.

In 1908 the Carnegie Foundation financed a study of medical schools in the United States and Canada, and on the basis of this report medical schools began to be graded in 1910 and have been graded ever since.

EARLY REFORMS IN NURSING

The first attempt at a regularly organized school of nursing was made in 1839 by the Nurse Society of Philadelphia under Dr. Joseph Warrington. It was inspired by the work of Elizabeth Fry in England. The instruction was elementary; there were regular courses, with lectures and demonstrations using a mannequin. After a stated period and evidence of proficiency the nurses received a "Certificate of Approbation." Dr. Warrington taught nursing students at the Philadelphia Dispensary together with medical students.

The nurses were called "pupils," and in 1849 they were housed in a home of their own. Another Philadelphia attempt was the school of nursing established in connection with the Women's Hospital of Philadelphia in 1861. The course was supposed to last for six months and was designed to appeal to the better type of young women in order to "train a superior class of nurses." Lectures were given in medical and surgical nursing, materia medica, and dietetics. These nurses were given a diploma at the successful termination of the course.

Another aspiration to form a nursing school was frustrated by the Civil War. Dr.

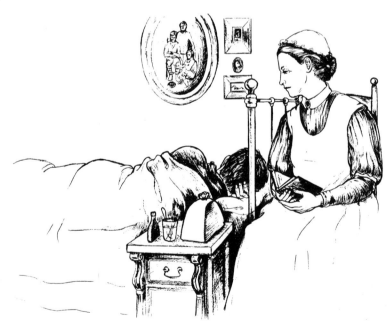

Formerly most sick persons were cared for at home where the nurse ministered to their needs.

Elizabeth Blackwell had closely studied Florence Nightingale's ideas and wanted to establish a school for nurses in connection tion with the New York Infirmary for Women. This school did not materialize.

The realization of the need for nursing reforms remained, but ideas were slow in maturing. The agitation that had been going on in England and the schools that were opened following the leadership of Miss Nightingale had become known in America. American reformers, inspired by visits to England and the continent, began investigating conditions at home. Attention was also paid to the struggling efforts to establish schools of nursing. The cause was not without the support of the medical profession, for in 1869 the American Medical Association accepted a report from its committee on the training of nurses. The chairman was an outstanding Philadelphia surgeon, Dr. Samuel Gross. The committee appreciated the importance of adequate training for nurses and recommended that schools of nursing be established in connection with hospitals all over the United States.

CONCLUSION

In the early nineteenth century a new era began in hospital construction and in medicine, which laid the foundation and emphasized the need for a trained group of nurses to meet the growing complexities of medicine and to staff the growing number of hospitals. One of the important hospitals of this period was the Massachusetts General Hospital. It was established in 1810 as the result of a letter circulated by 56 men of Boston who believed that Boston, too, should have a hospital for the poor. The movement was backed by leading Boston doctors and resulted in 1821 in the opening of the Massachusetts General Hospital. Ever since its opening, it has maintained standards often far ahead of its time. The deplorable conditions of nursing that developed in many of the hospitals at this time never existed here. Another hospital that led in nursing reforms was the Johns Hopkins in Baltimore, built in 1889. Many other communities built large hospitals because, with the growing industrialization, cities needed some place in which to house the sick. In America as in Europe, the process was largely a result of urban development occasioned by the growth of the Industrial Age. The main purpose of the hospital in the nineteenth century was to serve as a dormitory or a place of sojourn for the sick. It served incidentally as a convenient place for the practical training of the doctors and later of nurses. The events of the Civil War particularly emphasized the urgent need in the United States for adequate hospital facilities and for trained personnel.

CHAPTER 11 NURSING DURING EARLY AMERICAN WARS

■ The need for nurses has always been accelerated in wartime. During the Crusades and the wars of the Middle Ages, nursing orders such as the Knights of St. John, the Teutonic Knights, and the Maltese Knights were organized to meet the crises. In America the crisis of the Revolutionary War occurred before Miss Nightingale's day, but it is interesting to note that George Washington asked Congress for a matron and for nurses to care for the sick and wounded. However, we know that the number of women with any nursing experience was pitifully small and that many lay women volunteered their services more on a community level than anything else. The Catholic orders were the only organized groups with any actual knowledge of nursing, and they placed their hospitals and personnel at the disposal of the army. As was the custom of the time, wives, sisters, and mothers followed the men in the army and took care of them when they were sick and wounded.

REVOLUTIONARY WAR

During the Revolutionary War the Continental Army Medical Corps was not very successful at the beginning, and conditions were not improved until 1781 when Dr. John Cochran was appointed general director. Anesthesia and modern aseptic technic were unknown, the hospitals were unsanitary, and there was a shortage of food, medicine, and trained personnel. Epidemics were common in the army, and preventive medicine was unknown. It is interesting to note that during the Revolutionary War, chaplains from both the Catholic and Protestant faiths were appointed not only to improve morale but also to "recommend cleanliness as a virtue conducive to health." These conditions were common during all the wars of the nineteenth century and were not brought to the attention of the public in any organized and penetrating way until Miss Nightingale's efforts during the Crimean War.

CIVIL WAR

As was the case in England, the stimulus of a war was necessary to produce an effective demand for modern nursing. Some Americans had begun to hear about the Red Cross and Florence Nightingale's work during the Crimean War, but when the Civil War started, little organized information was available. We find that independently of M. Dunant's efforts at that time, the United States Sanitary Commission was established in April, 1861.

A branch of this commission opened a bureau in New York for the examination and registration of nurses for war service; about 100 applicants were offered as nurses to the federal army.

When the war finally broke out, this arrangement was totally inadequate, and the surgeon general agreed to the organization of its own sanitary commission as part of the army. The nurses for this arrangement were supplied largely by the Catholic orders: Sisters of Charity, Sisters of Mercy, and Sisters of St. Vincent. The Holy Cross Sisters, an Anglican Order, also supplied some.

Protestant nursing orders, including the deaconesses, did good work in the war, but all that organized nursing units could do proved insufficient after the big battles when experiences similar to those depicted in *Gone With the Wind* were reenacted all over the war-ridden area. Classic are the descriptions by Louisa May Alcott in her *Hospital Sketches*. She was one of the thousands of women who, anxious to aid the cause, signed up as nurses without other prerequisites than a warm heart and an eager hand. She vividly described her feelings when she was first faced with the invasions of bloody, filthy, smelly human wrecks, whose wounds were covered by remnants of uniforms matted with filth and clotted blood. Victims came in numbers far exceeding the capacity of the accommodations prepared for them. Somehow everybody had to go to work with soap and brushes and try to clean them up and get them ready for surgical attention. Food had to be provided, and when the confusions of the first rush had subsided there were hundreds of little jobs, apparently trivial, yet important to the patients or those they had left behind—letters to be written and valuables to be received and kept or transmitted to relatives.

Thus, in the American as in other armies, two types of nursing developed: a regular army nursing service, which was placed under the direction of Miss Dorothea Dix, and an organization sponsored by private citizens, at first tolerated, later supported, by the government.

Dorothea Lynde Dix (1803-1887) was known for her interest and activity in the field of reform for the mentally ill. She had studied in England and on the Continent and was a friend of both Elizabeth Fry and Mr. Rathbone. Returning to America, she had worked unceasingly to improve conditions for the care of the mentally ill.

In 1861 a meeting of interested women resulted in the formation of the Women's Central Association of Relief. Out of this activity grew the Sanitary Commission. Influential lay women and physicians became interested because it was necessary that they have some central organization through which supplies could be distributed. The Sanitary Commission attempted to bring together the relief work of many scattered organizations and groups. It was interested in recruiting and in everything associated with the health and welfare of the troops. It studied ways and means of supplementing government appropriations from private funds.

In some ways it might be said that this organization was a forerunner of the Red Cross. The Confederacy had no such type of organization, but as we know from official and unofficial stories, valiant work was done by lay women and religious groups. In 1861, although Dorothea Lynde Dix was not a nurse, she was appointed superintendent of female nurses, and then she proceeded to organize the first nurse corps of the United States Army. At this time Miss Dix was about 60 years of age, and by some her standards were considered very rigid and inflexible. She would not have any nurses less than 30 years of age, and they were preferably to be homely. Although no uniform was designated, somber colors were insisted upon, black or brown. An allowance of $12 a month was paid these nurses, Miss Dix herself serving without remuneration. Miss Dix found, as Miss Nightingale did in the Crimean War, that most of her nurses came from religious orders, both Protestant and Catholic.

Although eventually some 2,000 nurses participated in the Civil War, their number was entirely inadequate. Their equipment was worse than primitive, and hospital facilities were whatever could be found, although in this respect the Civil War contributed one thing: hospital ships were first placed in service at this time. Not only were hospital and nursing facilities insufficient but the hygiene was atrocious; there were in that war about 6 million medical hospital admissions, mostly from epidemic or contagious diseases, against about 425,000 surgical cases, that is, actual war casualties. It is no exaggeration to state that in those days war claimed more victims from disease than from bullets.

This experience made clear, especially in the light of what Miss Nightingale had done, the desperate need for organized schools of nursing; such schools were accordingly started in New York City, Boston, and New Haven.

SPANISH-AMERICAN WAR

At the turn of the century when trouble between America and Cuba was imminent,

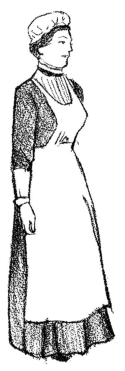

SPANISH-AMERICAN WAR NURSE

Congress authorized employment of nurses under contract. This was necessary because military nursing had not developed at all since the Civil War and because no mechanism existed by which the surgeon general could find nurses if needed. However, by 1898 when the Spanish-American War began, schools of nursing had been training young women for this profession for about 20 years. More than 500 schools of nursing had graduated about 10,000 nurses by the year 1900.

Dr. Anita McGee, at that time vice-president of the Daughters of the American Revolution, had interested the surgeon general, George M. Sternberg, with a plan for a nurse corps, which was to be organized with the D.A.R. acting as an examining board or a clearinghouse for all applications. Congress gave him authority to employ as many nurses by contract as would be needed. Nurses in the Spanish-American War received $30 a month plus ration allowances. In spite of the great need, not all medical officers were willing to accept army nurses in the beginning, but since they were carefully selected by Dr. McGee, assistant to the surgeon general, they gave satisfactory service, and the army doctors depended on them more and more. More than 1,500 nurses were accepted as army nurses during the Spanish-American War.

The Nurses' Associated Alumnae of the United States and Canada were disturbed with the nursing conditions at the outbreak of the Spanish-American War, and at a meeting its president, Mrs. Isabel Hampton Robb, suggested that the association offer its services to the government in an attempt to obtain more and better nurses. When this suggestion was taken to Washington, it was found that Dr. McGee had already been appointed and had set up her own standards. Several prominent superintendents of nursing schools volunteered to help in the organization of army nursing, among them Anna C. Maxwell, superintendent of nurses, Presbyterian Hospital in New York City. Miss

Maxwell was appointed chief nurse at the hospital at Chickamauga Park, Georgia.

In 1900, there were 202 nurses remaining in the nurse corps, and the Army Reorganization Bill presented to Congress in that year provided for a permanent nurse corps as part of the medical department of the army. The Army Nurse Corps was created by law on February 2, 1901.

CHAPTER 12 THE RED CROSS—ORGANIZATION AND EARLY DEVELOPMENT

■ All over the world the symbol of the Red Cross stands for help in wars or in civilian disasters. What is the history behind such a unique organization?

UN SOUVENIR DE SOLFERINO

In reviewing the life of Florence Nightingale, it was noted that her first great task was to care for the sick and the wounded of the battlefield. That accomplished, her attention turned to the general welfare of the men in the army. They had more coming to them than a cot, three meals a day, and small pay, and she began to organize all those recreational facilities that, as we know today, add greatly to the comforts of army life. Finally, after the war she turned her attention to many activities concerned with the health of the civilian population. In many respects the life of Miss Nightingale after 1854 epitomizes the later development of the Red Cross, which she inspired.

The story of this institution begins on June 24, 1859, near the town of Solferino in Northern Italy. About 300,000 men, Italians and French, were locked in mortal combat, and the carnage was terrific. Yet the work of Florence Nightingale but a few years previously had gone unheeded, and the provisions for taking care of the wounded were woefully insufficient. Hundreds died from inadequate attention. The appalling situation struck a tourist who accidentally happened to be there, to the point that he assembled such volunteers as he could gather, mostly women of Solferino, for the work of bringing succor to the wounded. The name of this gentleman was Jean Henri Dunant; he was Swiss, and he later described his experience in the classic *Un Souvenir de Solferino*.

Inspired by the work of Miss Nightingale in the Crimea, he then decided to devote his life to the prevention of a repetition of the needless horrors of Solferino. He traveled from country to country explaining his scheme to all responsible persons who could help him further it. In France, Napoleon III lent a willing ear, not knowing how badly he himself would need the services of the Red Cross but a few years later. Dunant's idea was to establish bands of volunteer helpers who would seek out and treat the wounded of the battlefield without regard to nationality and in complete neutrality under the protection of all the armed forces. Further, this establishment should be sanctioned by convention and respected by all belligerents. Dunant addressed international congresses, and finally M. Gustave Moynier, president of the Society of Public Utility of Geneva, Switzerland, convened a congress in October, 1863, of 36 representatives from 14 different countries, for the purpose of studying M. Dunant's proposal. At this meeting the fundamental principles of the Red Cross were established, and plans were laid for organizing Red Cross societies in various countries with organization and powers to render aid to wounded soldiers and other victims of war. The congress adjourned, and work progressed to secure for the movement the necessary international legal status and to devise an acceptable emblem that would be recognized everywhere.

THE GENEVA CONVENTION OF 1864

Even before it could be further organized, the young organization was put to a test. A short but bloody war broke out in the winter of 1863-1864 between little Denmark and Bismarck's newly organized Prussia. The Danish armaments were hopelessly outmoded, and the war was one long debacle for the Danes. However, it did offer the first opportunity for trying out the Red Cross, and when the Federal Council of Switzerland in August, 1864, convoked an international diplomatic conference, practical experience was available for the organization of what came to be known as the Geneva Convention of 1864. Dunant's original principles were established: the wounded must be respected, military hospitals must be considered neutral, and all persons, equipment, and buildings under the jurisdiction of the institution were to be marked with a red cross on a white background (the reverse of the Swiss flag).

In spite of some infractions, with many more accusations of infractions and few abuses, these original principles have been accepted and respected by almost all nations. At a conference held in The Hague in 1899, the principles were extended to sea warfare also, and at conventions held in 1906 and 1907, the Geneva and Hague conventions were revised. Curiously, Turkey, by special arrangement, has substituted for the red cross the crescent; and Iran, the lion and the rising sun. Thus, out of the Geneva Convention came the International Red Cross Committee, which is the coordinating agency of all the national Red Cross committees. Its purpose is to establish Red Cross committees in countries in which they do not exist, to act as a liaison between the various committees, and to endeavor to have the Geneva Convention accepted by all civilized countries and to ensure that it is observed. In time of war it establishes international agencies for the assistance of war prisoners and other victims of war, and in recent years it has added to this plans for relief during national disasters, such as floods and earthquakes. Thus the international committee acts in any matter that is beyond the scope of the national committees. In 1912 the international committee instituted the Florence Nightingale medal to be given to nurses who had especially distinguished themselves.

The national Red Cross societies are the component parts of the International Red Cross. They were originally formed purely for war service, but, as we shall see, their scope has been greatly widened. To be accepted by the International Red Cross, a national society must be recognized as an auxiliary to the army of its country by its government, which, in turn, must have subscribed to the Geneva Convention. It must accept the emblem of the red cross (with the exceptions noted above) and the organization must be open to all citizens of the country irrespective of sex, politics, or religion. It must also cooperate in all required respects with the international organization, which, in return, will recognize only one national Red Cross Society in each sovereign state. Within the country a national Red Cross society is autonomous and free to develop its own ideas.

It may thus be seen that the Red Cross has an important official standing. In war it becomes indispensable, and it has assumed so many peacetime activities that it is rapidly becoming one of the most important social agencies of the state, and yet it is entirely independent and supported by voluntary contributions.

FUNCTIONS OF THE RED CROSS

During war, then, the National Red Cross Society assists but does not replace the regular army medical service (which, however, also uses the emblem of the Red Cross in accordance with the Geneva Convention). It mobilizes nurses, nurses' aides, and voluntary helpers and sets up ambulance services, hospitals, hospital ships, canteens, libraries for the soldiers, entertainments, occupational therapy, and many other activities. It renders aid to war refugees and prisoners of war and may assist groups of citizens in devastated countries (for instance, by feeding children). When the war is over, the Red Cross becomes active in the identification and return of prisoners of war, resettlement of refugees, fighting postwar epidemics, reorganization for the next war, and relieving suffering arising from the war. It will see that disabled men get the best treatment and will train them by establishing orthopedic and other special clinics and by establishing trade schools. It may extend direct aid to widows and orphans of soldiers, or it may undertake to house permanently disabled men, as the British Red Cross does in The Star and Garter at Richmond, England.

These, then, are some of the principal activities of the Red Cross in connection with war. It is easily seen how many of these tasks concern nurses or are entirely dependent upon professional nurses. Nurses, therefore, form an important part of the organization, and any properly qualified nurse in good professional standing is encouraged to join the Red Cross reserve, which thus becomes the reserve upon which the military forces largely depend in time of war.

THE AMERICAN RED CROSS

So far we have considered the Red Cross as an international institution. The American Red Cross, however, has its own interesting history.

The Red Cross was organized in many European countries. Clara Barton went abroad and spent years studying the organization in various countries; she established close contact with Miss Nightingale, who later followed American developments with warm interest. Miss Barton's studies were very practical—during the Franco-Prussian War from 1870 to 1871, she actually accompanied one of the Red Cross ambulances into the field. She came back firmly convinced that America must have a Red Cross society that would adhere to the Geneva Convention. The result of her efforts was the incorporation in 1881 in the District of Columbia of an American Association of the Red Cross with Miss Barton as president. Ratification by the United States was accomplished in 1882.

The young organization was first put to the test in the yellow fever epidemic in Florida in 1888 and in the Johnstown flood in 1889. For the epidemic Miss Barton supplied around 30 volunteer nurses, mostly from New Orleans; they were supposed to be immunized to yellow fever, having had the disease. There was friction with the local board of health, and not without justification, for some of the volunteers were without previous experience in nursing. In the relief of the Johnstown disaster, Red Cross units

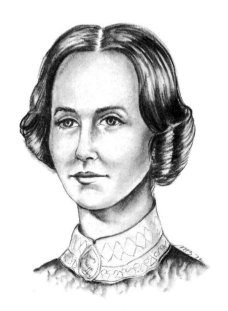

CLARA BARTON

came out from Philadelphia and worked under the direction of physicians.

During these years Miss Barton and others interested in the cause worked hard to develop the American Red Cross. An organization evolved with local committees and sections for the purpose of selecting and training volunteer nurses, so that in time of war they could be promptly mobilized and placed in active service. The American National Red Cross was established on a firmer basis in 1893, again with Miss Barton as president. The New York branch opened a hospital for the training of Red Cross nurses. The course was planned to take two years and three months, after which the nurse graduated as a Red Cross sister. This organization adhered to the Geneva Convention, and while on service the nurses devoted their full time to their work; they received no salary but were given the best maintenance obtainable. Gradually the Red Cross School of Nursing failed, because in the meantime the general education of nurses was advancing so fast that the purpose of the school was better fulfilled by some of the new modern training schools, which developed in connection with the larger hospitals.

Toward the end of the century, trouble was brewing in the Caribbean, and the war with Spain was approaching. The Red Cross was enlisting nurses for war service, and in March, 1898, the Cuban Relief Committee chartered the S.S. *State of Texas* as a Red Cross relief ship to sail under the Red Cross flag. Miss Barton was to meet the ship in Florida, but in the meantime war was declared, and the *Texas* sailed with an American convoy to be of aid to American soldiers.

Up until that time the American Red Cross had had no official standing, but its work became increasingly important. A special committee was set up to supply nurses, and in New York Mr. William Wardwell organized the American National Red Cross Relief Committee. Now the Red Cross obtained government sanction as the proper

and sole representative of the international committee in the United States. Its position was thus official.

The Red Cross nurses went to the war in Cuba under the direction of Miss Barton and nursed under her in American hospitals. However, the amount of nursing work increased beyond all expectations, and it became necessary to send for reinforcements. Before these could arrive, the entire staff, including Dr. Lesser, the staff surgeon, came down with yellow fever and, to make matters worse, the hoped-for reinforcements failed to arrive. At the same time the army organized its own regular nursing service; Dr. Anita Newcomb McGee was placed in charge directly under the surgeon general.

After World War I the Red Cross nurses were called upon in much reorganization work and in the fight against the epidemics and the pandemic of influenza that swept the war-torn world. The enlarged scope of the Red Cross was then generally appreciated; it participated in disaster relief and also in public health projects in areas in which local resources proved to be insufficient. This was accomplished particularly through the Delano Red Cross Nursing Service, established by the will of Miss Jane A. Delano, and has provided nursing service for several undeveloped and inaccessible regions.

However, disaster relief remains one of the chief peacetime tasks of the Red Cross Nursing Service, and since World War I there has not been a disaster of any magnitude in which that organization has not taken an important part in the rescue work.

Other activities of the Red Cross were developed about this time. Although instruction in home hygiene and care of the sick had been conducted by the Red Cross branch in the District of Columbia as early as 1908, these programs were not promoted nationally until 1913. The first edition of the Red Cross textbook on home hygiene and care of the sick was also published in 1913.

Public health nursing was first proposed

as a Red Cross program by Lillian D. Wald as early as 1908. It was financed mainly by Jacob H. Schiff, an officer of the New York branch. It was first confined to rural nursing but by 1913 extended to towns having populations as large as 25,000. This activity of the Red Cross was known as Town and Country Nursing Service. In 1915 the first plan for training nurses' aides was proposed. Although it was put into operation that year, it did not really develop fully until World War I. Miss Delano was, in 1917, appointed head of the new department of nursing. All phases of nursing service were included in this department—home hygiene and care of the sick, dietetics, public health nursing in rural areas and small towns, disaster nursing, and instruction of nurses' aides.

Miss Delano was succeeded by Clara D. Noyes, who had been her assistant since 1916. Miss Noyes was known internationally as well as nationally. She was twice elected first vice-president of the International Council of Nurses.

The basic international policies under which the Red Cross was first organized have permeated the national programs in all countries recognizing the Red Cross. The American Red Cross Nursing Services assist in various nursing activities all over the world. It cooperates with the director of the Nursing Bureau of the League of Red Cross Societies. It shares knowledge and resources with Red Cross societies of other countries, including provision for visitors to study in this country.

The American Red Cross method of teaching instructors has been adapted to the needs of many countries and is being used in more than 20 Red Cross societies. The opportunities for nursing service and nursing education under the banner of the Red Cross are a challenge to all nurses interested in working toward *One World for Nursing*.

The Red Cross Nursing Service no longer assumes responsibility for recruiting nurses for the army or navy. Legislation in 1947 establishing a permanent nurse corps for the armed forces, including the maintenance of nurse reserves, did away with the need for the Red Cross to maintain a roster of reserve nurses. Since then, local Red Cross chapters have enrolled nurses for community services, including local and national disasters.

Since 1945 Red Cross home nursing instruction has become part of the curriculum in many secondary schools. At first instructors for these courses were nurses, but since 1948 the Red Cross has authorized for this task not only nurses but also teachers and others with teacher-training experience, who complete the instructor's course given by the Red Cross. In 1947 the new blood program was established by the Red Cross, and in 1948 an intensive training program was begun for volunteer registered nurses. By 1956 more than 60,000 registered nurses has been trained in some phase of blood collection activity.

The various services that have developed within the Red Cross since World War II are provided to communities through approximately 3,700 Red Cross chapters throughout the nation. Each of these local chapters is an administrative unit of the Red Cross, operating within the limits of a charter granted by the national organization. A volunteer board of directors and volunteer committees direct the work of the chapter. One of the important committees in every community is the nursing services committee. This committee is responsible for planning and carrying through the nursing programs within the Red Cross, in accordance with community needs and demands. The nursing programs within the Red Cross are planned in close cooperation with recognized health groups, such as the National League for Nursing, the American Nurses' Association, the Children's Bureau, and the United States Public Health Service.

Contemporary programs of the Red Cross Nursing Service are planned to meet the present-day needs of American communities and include disaster nursing, home nursing, including mother and baby care, the instruction of volunteer nurses' aides, enrollment of graduate nurses in local chapters in community service, the blood program nursing, and educational and technical assistance to nurses in Red Cross societies in other countries. Some fine educational materials in the form of bulletins describing the work of the Red Cross nurse, to be used in the recruiting of graduate nurses for these activities, have been prepared.

CHAPTER 13 EARLY SCHOOLS AND NURSING LEADERS—PAST AND PRESENT

■ During the nineteenth century a greater sense of social responsibility for community health and welfare developed. Medical science was advancing more rapidly than ever before in the history of medicine. Traditional concepts of the woman's place in society and of her educational needs were changing. It was time for the development of a formal education for nursing. Close association between Florence Nightingale and early leaders in America resulted in many similarities between the early schools in the United States and those in England.

PRINCIPLES OF THE EARLY SCHOOLS OF NURSING

Finally, in 1873, three important schools appeared, almost simultaneously. All of them were destined to influence the development of modern nursing. These schools were organized more or less in accordance with Miss Nightingale's ideas. Some of these ideas later tended to be forgotten. The main principle was that the school must be considered primarily an educational institution, not a source of cheap labor. The earliest schools of nursing in America were created independently of hospitals by boards or committees with power and freedom to develop the school. However, mainly because of lack of endowment the schools were early absorbed into the hospitals with which they were connected. Therefore the history of

nursing in America is inextricably bound up with the growth and development of hospitals, and most of the schools were created and conducted by hospitals to serve their needs, and the education of the nurse became a by-product of her service to the hospital.

As schools of nursing developed rapidly during the years that followed, many hospitals, especially the smaller ones, discovered that a school of nursing under the guise of "practical experience" could be made a valuable source of free, or almost free, labor. Consequently formal instruction was often neglected, and it was not until the modern reform movements became effective that this principle again became firmly established. Now it is increasingly realized that Miss Nightingale was right when she said that the education of nurses, like that of doctors, is a public duty and emphasized that a school of nursing must be endowed or supported by public funds—it cannot be self-supporting and remain a good school.

The second principle was that the school of nursing must be administratively independent although closely connected with the hospital. The head of the school, whether she is called "matron" as in England or "director" as in America, should be a nurse, responsible only to the hospital or school of nursing board. This point has been highly disputed. Another school of thought would have the director of nursing responsible to the hospital superintendent for the nursing care and—under a separate budget—the instruction of nurses. Only through an independent connection with the hospital can the education of nurses be ensured, free of interference by interests that may disrupt orderly planning of the course.

It was generally thought advisable that student nurses live in a nurses' home. Hours of work were often irregular, and discipline of necessity was strict. This arrangement was, however, not always considered necessary during preclinical courses or postgraduate work.

The importance of the head nurse, or the "sister" as she is called in England, was also an integral part of Miss Nightingale's scheme. She is a professional nurse responsible for the administration of a ward or a division and for the teaching of the student nurses that come under her care. Much of the clinical instruction is thus her responsibility.

The young schools that came into existence could not fill all these requirements—in fact many modern schools are still striving to solve these problems—but they were ideals at which they could aim, and during the next few years notable progress was made.

BELLEVUE HOSPITAL SCHOOL OF NURSING

When American women interested in the Sanitary Commission no longer had to worry about the war, they turned their interests to domestic eleemosynary institutions. They formed the New York State Charities Aid Association under which the Bellevue Hospital Visiting Committee operated, directed by Louisa Lee Schuyler. Reference has been made to the shocking revelations of that committee, and it was realized that improvement of the nursing was one of the essential requirements for hospital reform. In all this the committee met the resistance of most of those in authority, but that did not stop it. It publicly appealed for funds; Dr. Gill Wylie, who had been an intern in the hospital and who was sympathetic to the reform movement, was sent abroad to learn

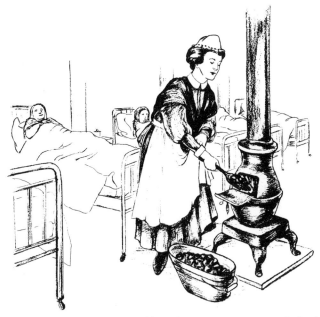

In earlier times custodial jobs such as stoking the stove were part of the hospital nurse's regular duties.

what he could directly from Miss Nightingale and from the schools that she had helped to organize. Consequently the plan for organization of the school of nursing at Bellevue followed closely Miss Nightingale's principles; in America the system became known as the "Bellevue system."

There was some difficulty in finding someone to take charge of the new school. Public announcements were made, in response to which Sister Helen of the Order of the Holy Cross offered her services. She was accepted, and the school was established May 1, 1873.

Sister Helen (Miss Bowden), a member of the Sisterhood of All Saints, had been trained at the University College Hospital in London, when nursing there was in the hands of the Order of the Holy Cross. Later she had extensive experience in workhouse infirmaries, in epidemics, and during the war between France and Germany in 1870-1871. At the time of her application she was in residence at the Community House in Baltimore. Therefore she brought to Bellevue Hospital a thorough training, and although she was not a Nightingale nurse, she was fully conversant with the principles of that school. She carried out these principles successfully until the school was well estab-

lished in 1876, when she went to South Africa to take part in pioneer nursing there. She was a strict, austere woman with profound knowledge of human nature and of politicians, for whom she was always fully a match.

Under her direction the pupil nurses were housed in a building rented for the purpose. Although many of the old nurses applied for acceptance, they were refused; an attempt was made to recruit young girls from above the servant class in order to make nursing attractive as a career. Their training was planned but included no regular classwork or lectures. In the beginning only a few wards were placed at the disposal of the new school for instructional purposes. This proved to be so successful that more were soon added. Although the school did publish a *Manual of Nursing* in 1876, the formal instruction left much to be desired.

In 1874 Miss Linda Richards, America's first "trained nurse," came from Boston to become night superintendent. She instituted the system of keeping written records and orders, which has since become a requirement in all nursing schools. After a while, uniforms were introduced; the nurses were reluctant to wear them until someone had the idea of encouraging one of the pupil nurses from a very good family to wear one. Then a general clamor for uniforms arose. It was readily gratified.

Thus the school, founded through the efforts of Louisa Lee Schuyler, flourished and became a leading school of nursing. It has had many brilliant alumnae, notably Jane A. Delano, Isabel Hampton, and Lavinia L. Dock. In 1967 the diploma program was closed, and the school became an integral part of the Department of Nursing of Hunter College of the City University of New York.

EARLY BOSTON SCHOOLS OF NURSING

The New England Hospital for Women and Children attempted to form a school in

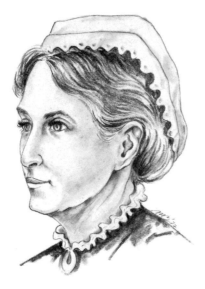

LINDA RICHARDS

1861 but was not successful until it was re-formed in 1872. Dr. Marie Zakrzewska, who studied in Berlin but took her medical degree in Cleveland, Ohio, urged that the New England Hospital be given a school of nursing. A charter for a training school for nurses was included in the hospital charter of 1863. She personally took active part in the training of nurses, but it remained on a rather informal basis until the hospital was rebuilt in 1872 and placed under the charge of Dr. Susan Dimock who, like most good American doctors of the time, had been trained in Europe. She had been to Kaiserswerth, and when the reorganized school opened in 1872, it largely followed that pattern. The course lasted one year and included both practical instruction and lectures. The school achieved its greatest fame because one of its alumnae became one of the leaders of nursing throughout the following generation.

Miss Linda Richards began her nursing career in the Boston City Hospital. Eager for training and advancement she entered in the first class of the New England Hospital and graduated one year later. After graduation she worked for a while as night superintendent at the Bellevue Hospital; she later returned to Boston and took over the school at the Massachusetts General Hospital. When this school was well organized, she resigned to study English methods. During this period she became personally acquainted with Miss Nightingale. On her return she began a remarkable career reorganizing the nursing services of hospitals throughout the country; in 1885 she was called to Japan where she organized and for five years led the first Japanese school of nursing at Kyoto. Back in the United States she took up the organization of mental hospitals and spent the remainder of her long and remarkable career moving from one mental hospital to another, improving their nursing services. She has left a record of her experiences in her *Reminiscences,* published by Whitcomb and Barrows.

The nursing instruction at the New England Hospital as described by Miss Richards was largely practical, hours were long, and time off was limited to an afternoon every two weeks. There were no night nurses. Very sick patients could interfere seriously with the nurses' sleep, for their rooms were between wards. In this early school there was little formal teaching, and there were no textbooks. Some bedside instruction was provided by women interns.

As we note from the general tenor of such descriptions, which practically applied to other Boston hospitals as well, they were a far cry from the medieval conditions at Bellevue and many other places. Nursing was to a certain extent systematized, and a measure of cleanliness and acceptable care was extended to the patients. There was still plenty of room for reform.

Perhaps even better conditions obtained at the Massachusetts General Hospital. In fact, according to those times a nursing reform was not urgently needed; both governors and medical staff prided themselves on the care that their patients received. Nevertheless the spirit of nursing reform, which the Civil War had engendered, extended to Boston where the Women's Educational Union appointed a committee to look into the opportunities that nursing could offer women as a career. We note here the appearance of professional aspiration, for on the committee were ladies of the best families of Boston. They were looking not for hospital reforms but for opportunities for career women. Purely on the strength of the social and intellectual standing of the women on this committee the hospital trustees and doctors accepted the experimental establishment of a school of nursing in the Massachusetts General Hospital. It was opened on November 1, 1873; six pupil nurses enrolled.

The equipment was elementary, but there was an organized attempt at formal instruction closely supervised by the members of the committee, and certain innovations were actually tried. It is to this school that we may trace the first "preliminary course" in America. In spite of all this the young school had difficulties getting started. The early superintendents seemed to lack vision and were unable to break with the old ways. Long hours and menial duties interfered with the efficiency of the students. It was necessary to establish the proper leadership. Miss Richards, then in New York, was selected. She accepted, and within a year conditions were much improved; classes were organized, and the proper emphasis was placed upon the training that was the purpose of the whole undertaking. The more menial tasks were gradually relegated to attendants, and the doctors began to recognize the advantage of having properly trained nurses. After a year's trial under Miss Richards' guidance the school was accepted by the hospital, and it has ever since maintained the highest standards and traditions. This feat was all the more remarkable when we compare Miss Richards' professional training with minimum requirements today. After some preliminary work at Boston City Hospital she had received such formal training as was possible in the first class of the New England Hospital; her "postgraduate" experience was limited to what she had been able to learn as night superintendent at the newly reorganized Bellevue. She herself realized that she still had much to learn, and after two and one-half years she resigned to visit England and Miss Nightingale and to study the work that was being done overseas.

CONNECTICUT SCHOOL

Among the three early schools of nursing, the Connecticut School was the first to receive its charter, but for some time it admitted no pupils. In 1872 the New Haven Hospital appointed a committee to investigate the feasibility of organizing a training school for nurses. In their study they heavily relied upon the report of Dr. Wylie, which had just become available. They were remarkably farseeing in adopting one of Miss Nightingale's principal ideas: they did not want the hospital to start a school, but

they wanted a school organized independently of the hospital, which then would serve as a field for the practical training. By such an arrangement they made it difficult for the hospital to use the nurses as cheap labor. After extensive advertising for potential students they finally were able to open on October 1, 1873.

It was an immediate success; the number of pupils rapidly increased, and soon the school was a source of superintendents for other hospitals. In 1879 it published the *New Haven Manual of Nursing,* a textbook created by the committee, which consisted of both nurses and doctors; it was a comprehensive text and soon found wide acceptance among the nursing schools, which by then were being organized all through the country. The New Haven school has retained its leading position. Later, when it became endowed and obtained university affiliation, it made another important contribution to nursing.

All the more important schools have their history, but because of limited space a detailed description cannot be included here.

EDUCATION IN THE EARLY SCHOOLS TO ABOUT 1900

The period that followed was one of quiet progress in nursing education. To it we trace the early development of many movements that later were to become important, including the Red Cross, army nursing, and some of the functions of public health nursing, but these will be considered in later chapters.

There was also a steady growth of nursing schools. The growth was closely associated with development of modern surgery and medicine, which, as we have seen, occurred very rapidly as the result of Pasteur's and Lister's work and the advances in bacteriological knowledge. As it was realized that so much new work could be done if hospital facilities were available, hospitals grew rapidly in number and size all over the country. Now they changed their function from

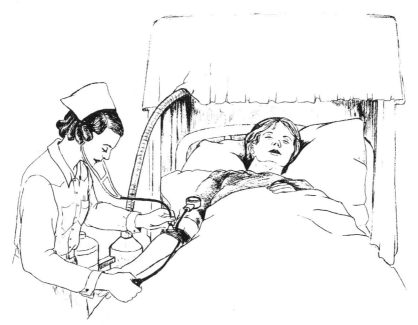

Prior to the discovery of antibiotics and other modern miracle drugs, many patients had to be cared for in croup tents.

being refuges of the destitute to becoming the natural work grounds for surgeons and physicians whenever patients demanded more than the most general care. Facilities had to be created and organized to provide for all classes of the population, and part of the original function of the hospital was taken on by the infirmary. With such increase in both the quality and quantity of hospital work the demands for trained nursing care grew accordingly. Nursing developed largely as an inevitable consequence of these circumstances. It was fortunate that within its membership the necessary leaders existed to carry it through this formative period.

The improvement in educational standards occurred in several areas. Originally one year had been considered sufficient for the training of a nurse; that was Miss Nightingale's idea, and it was the accepted period of training in the early schools. It was probably sufficient for the needs of the times. We must realize that most of the items of a modern nurse's education are necessitated by contributions to medical knowledge and to public health, which have received practical application since the first schools were opened. So, as more knowledge and more skill became necessary, the course had to be extended. At first it was done by adding a few months for special work. Soon, however, it became necessary to reorganize the courses completely, and courses were planned for two and eventually for three years. The full three-year course was, however, not generally accepted until well into the present century.

The problem was not merely one of lengthening the course; it was also one of the student nurse's understanding. It is not enough that the nurse be told that she must not touch the instruments on the operating table, she must understand why she must not touch them; she must understand why it is dangerous, and not just unpleasant, to have a diphtheria patient or a tuberculous patient cough into her face. She can administer a dietary or drug treatment far better if she knows something about the physiology and pathology of the diseased organs and about the action of the drugs. The nurse's place in the whole structure of the care of the sick is occupied much better if she understands rather than if she slavishly follows directions. To the modern reader this sounds like a statement of the obvious, and yet it was not at all accepted outside of nursing circles. Actually, 70 years ago medications in some hospitals were dispensed by number in order that their contents remain secret to all but the initiated—which did not include the nurses.

As nursing has evolved, there has been a constant struggle against the attitude that modern nurses are being "overtrained." It was argued that by knowing too much the nurses became unfit for the essential nursing task or that we were wasting our time educating a group of "semi-professionals." This attitude among members of the medical profession and among others upon whom the nurses must rely for advancing their standing has been the chief obstacle against which they have had to fight. However, it rather strengthened than weakened their fight because it made it necessary for every advance to possess the vitality of inherent value to survive. Since 1872 the education of nurses has advanced in spite of this opposition. It still has to show that a nurse is efficient as a result of education and an understanding of what she is doing. Inadequate nurses are generally so because they are not suited to nursing, not because they are overeducated. Some are inadequate because they have not had a good basic course in nursing.

Thus we see an increasing demand that promised lectures actually be delivered, that lecture courses be split up and lengthened, and that new subjects be added to the curriculum. In the beginning, pupil nurses attended lectures for medical students; later, lectures were prepared especially for them. Better and better choice was made of instructors. Not all nursing lectures were best given by doctors. Specially prepared instructors, themselves nurses, were preferable for many subjects. It was found essential to add courses that were not strictly technical but which dealt with ethical and professional problems and attitudes. In some respects the preparation of nurses has a broader base in the social and behavioral sciences than is required of medical students. The period with which we are dealing was very much concerned with the germination and growth of these trains of thought.

Because of these advances it became necessary to provide the proper equipment. The early pupil nurses often slept in rooms between the wards, where they were readily available for nocturnal emergencies; some were housed in special buildings. The facilities for instruction were meager, and the requirements for equipment were simple: a few mannequins and models of limbs, upon which to learn how to apply bandages, a skeleton, a blackboard, and a few books. As standards rose, demands rose with them, and gradually beds, ward equipment, laboratories, and up-to-date libraries became essential if schools were to meet even minimum standards.

EARLY LEADERS

The early leaders were consistent in their wish to improve the educational program in these schools because of their feeling that the professional nurse could not fulfill her responsibilities to the patient and the community until she was really prepared to do so. Two names stand out in connection with almost every development of professional nursing. One woman was the product of the nineteenth century but was farsighted enough to envision the possibilities and tireless enough to try to improve educational facilities. The name of Isabel Hampton Robb is linked with almost every type of nursing organization, every plan, and every activity at the turn of the century. One of her outstanding students at the Johns Hopkins Hospital was Mary Adelaide Nutting. Miss Nutting complemented Mrs. Robb in many ways and lived long enough to carry out many of the plans and programs that had been the dreams of her teacher. Also important were Lillian Wald, Mary Eliza Mahoney, Mary Sewell Gardner, Annie W. Goodrich, and Isabel Maitland Stewart.

There were other leaders in nursing too numerous to mention. In fact, every school had its leaders during the period of organization, growth, and change which every good school experiences in meeting the changing needs of the nursing profession.

Isabel Adams Hampton (1860-1910)

Miss Isabel Adams Hampton was born in Canada in 1860 and began her career as a schoolteacher. This, however, did not satisfy her, and she applied for nurse's training at Bellevue, from which she was graduated in 1883. In 1886, following two years in Italy, she became superintendent of nurses at the five-year-old Illinois Training School for Nurses. During her three years of office in Chicago she introduced two important reforms. She began a graduated course of clinical experience and classwork, so that nurses

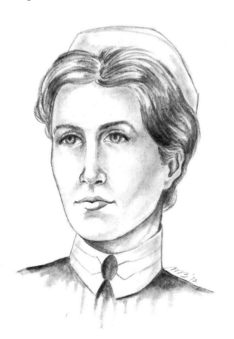

ISABEL HAMPTON ROBB

advanced step by step, and she arranged for affiliation of her students with other hospitals that possessed advantages, especially in private nursing, not obtainable at Cook County Hospital. When the school of nursing at Johns Hopkins opened in 1889, she was made its "principal" (a term then used for the first time in this connection). Her chief contributions here were in better organization of the work so that the pupil nurse's day could be limited to 12 hours, including two hours off for recreation. Both the hospital and Miss Hampton earned the highest reputation. She was made chairman of the nursing section of the Congress of Hospitals and Dispensaries that was held at Chicago in 1893. She read a paper on nursing at the meeting. When, at the subsequent meeting, the Society of Superintendents was formed, she was one of the leading organizers and became the first president. The next year she married Dr. Hunter Robb and resigned from active administrative work. Her interest in nursing continued as is evidenced by the two texts that she wrote at this time (*Nursing, Its Principles and Practice for Hospital and Private Use and Nursing Ethics*) and by her further organizational activities.

In 1896 she became the first president of the newly formed Nurses Associated Alumnae of the United States and Canada; as such she was active in the scheme of offering the services of that association in the Spanish-American War. Her next important activity was the part she played in the work for establishing university affiliation for nursing education and postgraduate courses. At first courses were offered in hospital economics in the Department of Science. Officially the Department of Nursing and Health began some 11 years later in 1910 at Teachers College, Columbia University. After the turn of the century she again came into prominence as one of the founders and original stockholders of *The American Journal of Nursing*. Her authority and prestige did much to bring the young journal through its first difficult years. When she died in 1910 in a street accident, at the relatively early age of 50, she had in a short career of less than 30 years in nursing done more for American nursing than any other person. It will be noted from studying the subsequent pages that there was no important nursing enterprise during the years when she was active in which she did not take a leading part.

Mary Adelaide Nutting (1858-1947)

When Mrs. Hampton Robb resigned from her post at the Johns Hopkins Hospital, her place was taken by Miss Adelaide Nutting, a graduate of the first class of the school. A warm friendship developed between Miss Nutting, a Canadian by birth, and her teacher Isabel Hampton (later Mrs. Robb). As superintendent of nurses and principal of the School of Nursing at the Johns Hopkins Hospital she carried out many of the reforms initiated by her predecessor. Early in the year of 1896 she established the three-year course and the eight-hour day for stu-

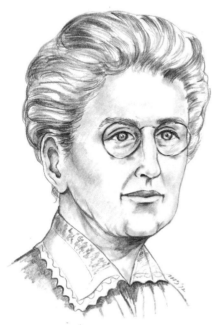

M. ADELAIDE NUTTING

dent nurses and abolished the monthly allowance to students. In 1901 she initiated a six months' preparatory course, which served as a model for many other schools. A lasting memorial to Miss Nutting is her unique collection of works on the history of nursing. From this interest emerged the four-volume *History of Nursing* written in collaboration with Miss Lavinia Dock.

Miss Nutting was convinced early that progress in nursing education would be slow until two reforms could be brought about: the provision for endowments or other financial support for schools of nursing and the separation of schools of nursing from hospital ownership and control.

Perhaps she is best known for her work in the creation and development of the Department of Nursing and Health at Teachers College, Columbia University. When she resigned her position at Johns Hopkins in 1907 to take the new Chair at Columbia University, she became the first professor of nursing in the world. She held that professorship until her resignation in 1925, when she was succeeded by a former student and colleague, Miss Isabel Stewart.

Miss Nutting's interest in all aspects of nursing education and her vital personality have made a deep impression on nursing throughout the world. She took a prominent part in nursing organizations and through her interest in international developments was influential in the formation of the International Council of Nurses.

Lillian Wald (1867-1940)

Lillian D. Wald was graduated from the New York Hospital School of Nursing in 1891. She became interested in the need for nursing among the poor, and in 1893 Miss Wald and a friend, Mary Brewster, rented a tenement in Henry Street, New York. This tenement developed into the famed Henry Street Settlement. These two women soon recognized what many leaders had seen: the need for nursing was just one of the many needs of these people. And so the social aspects of nursing began to develop, and modern nursing in the community began. Miss Wald was one of the lecturers at the new Department of Nursing Education at Columbia University and was a leader in most of the activities of public health nursing during her lifetime.

Her activities at Henry Street Settlement are those for which she is most famous, and the story is dramatically told in her two books, *The House on Henry Street* and *Windows on Henry Street*. When the National Organization for Public Health Nursing was organized in 1912, Miss Wald was elected its first president. She was interested in legislative reforms. The result of her interest and suggestions were the organization of the Children's Bureau, the development of the Nursing Service Division of the Metropolitan Life Insurance Company, and the organization of the Town and Country Nursing Service of the American Red Cross.

On September 12, 1971, Lillian Wald—founder of the Henry Street Settlement House and of what is now the Visiting Nurse

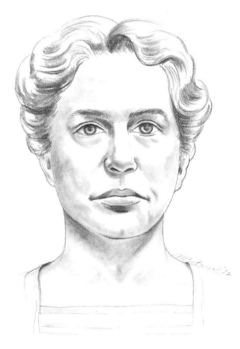

LILLIAN D. WALD

Service of New York—became the first nurse, the tenth woman, and the ninety-fifth person elected to the Hall of Fame for Great Americans. She enjoys the further distinction of having been elected the first time she was proposed. However, no mention of Lillian Wald as a nurse is involved in the citation, and she is listed in the Hall of Fame directory as a "reformer."

Mary Eliza Mahoney (1845-1926)

The first professional Negro nurse in the United States entered the New England Hospital for Women and Children in 1878 and completed the 16-month course in 1879. Miss Mahoney had a good record at the school, and after graduation did private nursing mainly in Boston and its suburbs. Miss Mahoney gave the address of welcome at the first conference of the National Association of Colored Graduate Nurses in 1909. She died in the New England Hospital in January, 1926, at 81 years of age. After her death the Mary Mahoney medal was established by the National Association of Colored Graduate Nurses and was first presented in 1936 to a member of the organization making an outstanding contribution to nursing. Throughout her more than 40 years of professional activity, Miss Mahoney gave devoted service to her patients and the nursing profession and did much to further intergroup relationships so that the Negro nurse could become a vital part of the community.

Mary Sewell Gardner (1871-1961)

Probably one of the most outstanding nurses in the history of public health nursing is Mary Sewell Gardner. She was born in 1871 in Massachusetts and was graduated cum laude in 1905 from the Newport Hospital Training School for Nurses. Soon after her graduation, she became the director of the Providence District Nursing Association, Rhode Island, a post she held until her retirement in 1931.

She is probably best known for her influence on the development of the National Organization for Public Health Nursing. She was one of the nursing leaders who helped to initiate the National Organization for Public Health Nursing in Chicago in 1912. Miss Lillian Wald was the first president, and Miss Gardner was the first secretary. In 1931 she was made honorary president of the organization, which she had done so much to develop.

Miss Gardner was instrumental in the transactions that resulted in the taking over of the *Cleveland Visiting Nurses' Quarterly* when it was offered to the National Organization for Public Health Nursing as an official journal, and as the *Public Health Nurse* it became the monthly magazine of this new public health organization.

Miss Gardner was also responsible for helping to develop public health nursing services in the American Red Cross. In 1912 she was given leave of absence from the Providence District Nursing Association for a year and became temporary director of the Town and Country Nursing Service, the Public Health Nursing Service in the Red Cross. After World War I she visited many European countries as special adviser to the nursing service work being done by the American Red Cross.

Miss Gardner is well known for many articles published in the *Public Health Nurse, The American Journal of Nursing,* and many other magazines. However, in nursing literature she is best known for her book, *Public Health Nursing,* first published in 1916, which has become a classic. A second revision of this book was published in 1924 and was translated into French, Chinese, Spanish, and Japanese. A third and last edition of this book was published in 1936. For the lay readers she wrote *So Live We* in 1942, and in 1946 *Catherine Kent* was published, which contained many autobiographical experiences.

Annie W. Goodrich (1876-1955)

Annie Warburton Goodrich was graduated from the New York Hospital Training School for Nurses in 1892. She was one of the pioneer leaders who actively helped nursing develop from an apprenticeship to a profession. She was an outstanding and inspired nurse educator. Her first important position was as superintendent of nurses at the New York Post-Graduate Hospital, a position she held for seven years. Then she was superintendent of nurses at St. Luke's Hospital in New York and then superintendent of nurses at the New York Hospital. She left the New York Hospital in 1907 to become superintendent of Bellevue and Allied Training Schools for Nurses. In 1910 she resigned to become state inspector of nurse training schools in New York. In 1914 she went to Teachers College as assistant professor.

All during these years she had worked with other leaders in nursing organizations, both national and international, to develop the nursing profession. She was president of the International Council of Nurses from 1912 to 1915. She had always been interested in public health and in 1916 became director of the Visiting Nurse Service of the Henry Street Settlement. During these years of great developments in nursing, Miss Nutting, Miss Wald, and Miss Goodrich were often referred to as "the great trio." All three were associated with every great idea and movement of the young profession.

In 1918 she was given leave of absence from Henry Street to make a survey of the military hospitals with the Nursing Department of the United States Army. When the Army School of Nursing was organized in 1918, she was appointed dean. At the same time she was instrumental in developing the Vassar Training Camp Program.

After the war she returned to Henry Street and continued her activities in nursing education. She was particularly interested in the Goldmark study, "Nursing and Nursing Education in the United States." In 1923 she was appointed dean of the new school of nursing at Yale University, endowed by the Rockefeller Foundation, a position that she held until 1934. Miss Goodrich received many honors and was one of the outstanding nurse educators of this century.

Isabel Maitland Stewart (1878-1963)

The influence of Miss Stewart as an educator, writer, organization worker, and important figure in international nursing affairs for over 40 years is just now being recognized. She took her basic training at the Winnipeg General Hospital Training School and, being attracted by an article written by Miss Nutting in *The American Journal of Nursing*, entered the course in hospital economics at Teachers College, Columbia University, in 1908. She was the first nurse to receive a master's degree from Columbia University. She remained at Teachers College for the rest of her professional career, holding the position of assistant instructor, assistant professor, and finally in 1925 succeeding Miss Nutting as the Henry Hartley Foundation Professor of Nursing. She was keenly aware of new concepts in the field of general education and always tried to evaluate new developments in relation to the specialized field of nursing. She was very active on the Education Committee of the National League of Nursing Education. While she was chairman, the curriculum committee first published the original guide to curriculum upgrading in 1917, with revisions published in 1927 and 1937 under her guidance.

She served as chairman of the Vassar Training Camp Program during World War I and wrote a pamphlet for general circulation on this and on other wartime activities. In July, 1940, when the National Nursing Council for National Defense was organized, mainly as the result of Miss Stewart's suggestions, one of the important committees appointed was that on educational policies and resources with Miss Stewart as chairman. She was interested in international affairs and was very active on the Committee on Education of the International Council of Nurses. She prepared a pamphlet called *The Educational Program of the School of Nurs-*

ing, which was translated into English, Spanish, German, and French by the Nursing Bureau of the League of Red Cross Societies. In 1950 she finished a study of postgraduate education in nursing for the international council. As author and editor she is well known to nurses all over the world for her books *Education of Nurses* and *A Short History of Nursing,* which she coauthored with Lavinia Dock.

In 1916 she became the first editor of the Department of Nursing Education of *The American Journal of Nursing.* She participated in the founding of the Association of Collegiate Schools of Nursing and in the early developments of the National League of Nursing Education, the International Council of Nurses, and the Florence Nightingale International Foundation.

CONTEMPORARY LEADERS

Other nurse leaders who have made significant contributions to nursing in recent years include the following.

Faye G. Abdellah

Faye Abdellah is presently chief nurse officer of the United States Public Health Service. She was one of the first two women to receive the commission of admiral in the USPHS.

Dr. Abdellah graduated as an R.N. in 1942 from Fitkin Memorial Hospital School of Nursing, New Jersey. She received her B.S., M.A., and Ed.D. degrees from Columbia University, New York. In 1967 she received an L.L.D. degree from Case Western Reserve University, Cleveland, Ohio.

Dr. Abadellah began her career as a nurse researcher for the federal government in New York City. She served on the faculty of Yale University School of Nursing and was a research fellow and member of the faculty at Teachers College, Columbia University, from 1948 to 1949. From 1949 to 1959, she was chief of the Nursing Education Bureau, Division of Nursing Resources, United States

Public Health Service, Department of Health, Education and Welfare, Washington, D. C., and was a senior consultant in nursing research from 1959 to 1962. Dr. Abdellah was a consultant for the Western Interstate Commission for Higher Education and a recipient of the Federal Nursing Service award, 1964.

She is a fellow of the American Psychological Association and a member of the American Nurses' Association and the National League for Nursing.

Dr. Abdellah is the author of many articles in the field of nursing and is recognized as one of the ablest researchers in the nation. She wrote *Patient-Centered Approaches to Nursing,* published in 1960, and *Better Patient Care Through Nursing Research,* published in 1965. She also was director of health education of the Child Education Foundation, New York City.

Pearl Parvin Coulter

Pearl Coulter was formerly dean of the University of Arizona College of Nursing, Tucson. She received her A.B. degree in 1926 and her M.S. degree in 1927 from the University of Denver. She attended the University of Colorado School of Nursing in 1935 and received a certificate in public health nursing from George Peabody College, Nashville, Tennessee, in 1936.

Ms. Coulter was educational director of public health nursing at the Nashville Health Department from 1939 to 1941. Her teaching experience includes the positions of instructor, assistant professor, and associate professor at Peabody College, associate professor of nursing at the University of Wisconsin School of Nursing, associate professor at the University of Colorado School of Nursing, and later professor at the same school.

Ms. Coulter was a board member and was elected president of the Arizona State Board of Nursing in 1964. She was also president of the Colorado League for Nursing and the Colorado State Nurses' Associtaion and was a board member of the American Journal of Nursing Company and the National League for Nursing.

Ms. Coulter received the Public Health Nurse of the Year award from the American Nurses' Association in 1962 and was chairman of the Mary Roberts Scholarship Committee.

She has written many magazine articles and is the author of *The Winds of Change, A Progress Report on Regional Cooperation in Collegiate Nursing Education in the West,* published in 1962, and *The Nurse in the Public Health Program,* published in 1954.

Ruth B. Freeman

Ruth Freeman was president of the National League for Nursing from 1955 to 1959. She graduated from the Mount Sinai Hospital School of Nursing, New York, and received her M.A. and Ed.D. degrees from New York University, New York. Dr. Freeman was professor of public health administration, School of Hygiene and Public Health, Johns Hopkins University, Baltimore, from 1950 to 1962. She was a member of the World Health Organization's expert advisory panel on nursing and a member of the White House Conference on Children and Youth from 1959 to 1960. She has served as a consultant on nursing for the medical and natural sciences program of the Rockefeller Foundation. Dr. Freeman was national administrator of the American National Red Cross Nursing Services and consultant to the National Security Resources Board.

She has received many awards, including the National League for Nursing Mary Adelaide Nutting award, Pearl McIver Public Health Nurse award, and annual nursing award of the Department of Nurse Education, New York University.

Lulu Wolf Hassenplug

Lulu Hassenplug is professor and dean emeritus of the School of Nursing, the University of California at Los Angeles.

She is a graduate of the Army School of

Nursing, Washington, D. C., and received her bachelor's degree from Teachers College, Columbia University, New York, and her master's degree in public health from Johns Hopkins University, Baltimore.

The Los Angeles Times in 1958 named her Los Angeles Woman of the Year in Education. She has received many awards, among which are the National League for Nursing Mary Adelaide Nutting award in 1965 for her constructive devotion and contribution to the development of nursing as a professional discipline within the system of higher education in America. The University of New Mexico and Bucknell University have awarded her honorary doctor of science degrees.

Governor Reagan of California has appointed her for a four-year term (1971-1975) to the Advisory Committee on Physician's Assistant Programs of the California Medical Board. As part of the Nursing Advisory Committee of the National Institute of Mental Health, she served as a civilian nursing consultant. Ms. Hassenplug served as a member of the Surgeon General's Consultant Group on Nursing whose report was the basis for the Nurse Training Act of 1964 granting federal aid to nursing education.

Ms. Hassenplug has held the teaching positions of professor of nursing, Vanderbilt University, Nashville, Tennessee; associate professor, the Medical College of Virginia; educational director, the Jewish Hospital School of Nursing, Philadelphia; and instructor in nursing, the Piedmont Hospital, Atlanta.

Inez Haynes

Inez Haynes was general director of the National League for Nursing for ten years. She holds the United States Legion of Merit and the Distinguished Service award of the University of Minnesota.

Ms. Haynes began her army career in 1932 as second lieutenant, serving as operating room nurse in Texas and the Philippine Islands. She advanced to administrative and supervisory positions with the army in the United States, Europe, and the Far East. In 1959 she was chief of the Army Nurse Corps, holding the rank of colonel, which was the highest rank for a nurse to achieve at that time.

Ms. Haynes received her nursing degree at Scott and White Memorial Hospital School of Nursing in Texas and her bachelor's degree from the University of Minnesota.

Ms. Haynes was a member of the board of directors of the National Council of Homemaker Services and a member of the Nursing Advisory Committee of the United States Department of Defense and of the executive committees of the National Health Council and the National Assembly for Social Policy and Development. She was active in the American National Council for Health Education of the Public, Pilots International, the Council of Federal Nursing Services, and Sigma Theta Tau. Ms. Haynes was vice-president of the Citizens Committee for the World Health Organization.

Lucile Petry Leone

Lucile Petry Leone held the position of chief nurse officer and assistant to the surgeon general of the United States Public Health Service in 1949. She was the first woman in the United States to hold the rank of brigadier general.

In 1927 Ms. Leone graduated from the Johns Hopkins School of Nursing. She has held teaching positions at many universities, including the University of Minnesota, Texas Woman's University, the New York Hospital School of Nursing, where she was dean, and Yale University School of Nursing.

Ms. Leone was director of nursing education of the United States Public Health Service, administering the Cadet Nurse Corps program and was a consultant for the USPHS on nursing problems of enrollments at schools of nursing. She was a technical expert on nursing in Geneva in 1948 at the second assembly of the World Health Organization. She was also the chairman of the Joint Committee on Unification of Accreditation Activities.

In 1966 the USPHS established a Lucile Petry Leone award for the contribution she has made to nursing and nursing education through her leadership.

R. Louise McManus

Louise McManus has been active in nursing for 45 years and is recognized as the designer of the first national testing service for the nursing profession, which is considered the second largest educational testing program in the country.

Dr. McManus received her nursing degree at Massachusetts General Hospital, Boston, and her B.S., M.A., and Ph.D. degrees at Columbia University, New York.

Dr. McManus advocated experimentation with a two-year academic nursing program in junior and community colleges and arranged for establishment of a national cooperative research project at Teachers College, Columbia University, to assist in developing programs in nursing in community and junior colleges to test the quality of the programs. She also helped establish the Institute of Research and Service in Nursing Education at Teachers College, which serves as a training center for research workers in nursing, as well as being an agency for research.

Dr. McManus was honorary consultant to the Bureau of Medicine and Surgery of the United States Navy from 1949 to 1953 and an adviser to the surgeon general in the National Advisory Health Council. She also served on the Defense Advisory Committee on Women in the Services and was consultant in nursing at the Walter Reed Army Institute of Research in Washington, D. C., in 1956.

Dr. McManus was chairman of the Nursing Council of the Florence Nightingale International Foundation and served as director of the Department of Nursing Education at Teachers College, Columbia University. Before going to Teachers College, she was director of nurses at Waterbury Hospital School of Nursing, Waterbury, Conn.

Dr. McManus is the author of *The Effect of Experience on Nursing Achievement* and co-author of *The Hospital Head Nurse*. She also has written many articles for nursing journals.

Mildred L. Montag

Mildred Montag was professor of nursing education at Teachers College, Columbia University, for 20 years from 1952 to 1972. She received her A.B. degree from Hamline University, St. Paul, Minnesota, her B.S. and M.A. degrees from the University of Minnesota, Minneapolis, and her Ed.D. degree from Teachers College, Columbia University, New York.

Dr. Montag held the position of instructor of nursing arts at Lincoln General Hospital School of Nursing, Lincoln, Nebraska, at the University of Minnesota School of Nursing, and at St. Luke's Hospital School of Nursing, New York. She was director of the School of Nursing, Adelphi College, Garden City, New York, staff nurse at the Henry Street Visiting Nurse Service, New York, and assistant director of the Nurse Testing Division, Psychological Corporation, New York. She became a member of the faculty of the Division of Nursing Education, Teachers College, Columbia University, in 1950. From 1952-1957 she was director of the Cooperative Research Project in Junior and Community College Education for Nursing.

Dr. Montag has been the recipient of many awards, among which are the Outstanding Achievement award of the University of Minnesota; Distinguished Alumni award, Hamline University; Linda Richards award, National League for Nursing; Achievement award, School of General Studies, Brooklyn College, New York; and Ella Goldthwaite award, University of Texas, School of Nursing.

Two honorary degrees have been conferred on Dr. Montag—the degree of doctor of laws from the University of Bridgeport, Connecticut, and the degree of doctor of humanities from Adephi University.

Dr. Montag has written many books and articles; they include *Fundamentals in Nursing Care, Education of Nursing Technicians, Community College Education for Nursing,* and *Pharmacology and Therapeutics.*

Helen Nahm

Helen Nahm has recently retired as dean of the School of Nursing, the University of California at San Francisco.

Dr. Nahm received her masters and doctoral degrees from the University of Minnesota and is a graduate of the University of Missouri School of Nursing.

Dr. Nahm was awarded the National League for Nursing Mary Adelaide Nutting award in 1967 for outstanding leadership and achievement in nursing. She was also cited specifically for her efforts in creating a national accrediting service for schools of nursing.

Dr. Nahm has served on the Commission on Nursing Education of the American Nurses' Association. She is also a member of the American Psychological Association. She has received many citations, among which are a Citation of Merit from the University of Missouri and a Distinguished Service award from the University of Minnesota.

Dr. Nahm served on the Board of Directors of the National League for Nursing from 1959 to 1967 and was second vice-president from 1959 to 1963. She was the first director of the National Nursing Accrediting Service, which became a program of NLN upon its founding in 1952. For four years Dr. Nahm was director of the Division of Nursing Education of the NLN. She has written many articles for important publications.

Martha E. Rogers

Martha Rogers is presently professor and head of the Division of Nurse Education New York University, New York.

Dr. Rogers received her doctoral degree in 1954 from Johns Hopkins University, Baltimore; she was graduated from the Knoxville General Hospital School of Nursing, Knoxville, Tennessee, in 1936, and received her B.S. degree from George Peabody College, Nashville, Tennessee in 1937, her M.A. degree from Teachers College, Columbia University, New York, in 1945, and her M.P.H. degree from Teachers College, Columbia University, in 1952.

Dr. Rogers is a member of the National League for Nursing's Commission on Historical Source Materials in Nursing and was president of the New York State League for Nursing.

Dr. Rogers has received many awards, among which are an award from New York University for her outstanding contribution to nursing in 1965 and an award for inspiring leadership in intergroup reaction.

Dr. Rogers has been executive director of the Visiting Nurse Service, Phoenix, Arizona, secretary of the Arizona State League for Nursing, assistant educational director and assistant supervisor of the Visiting Nurse Association, Hartford, Connecticut, and staff nurse and rural public health nurse at Children's Fund of Michigan. She was a research assistant at Johns Hopkins University from 1953 to 1954.

Dr. Rogers is the author of numerous articles and books, including *Educational Revolution in Nursing* and *Reveille in Nursing.*

Jessie M. Scott

Jessie Scott now holds the positions of assistant surgeon general and director of the Division of Nursing, National Institutes of Health, Bethesda, Maryland. She was one of the first two women to receive the commission of admiral in the United States Public Health Service.

Ms. Scott received her nursing diploma from Wilkes-Barre General Hospital School of Nursing, Pennsylvania, in 1936, her B.S. in education from the University of Pennsylvania, and her M.A. degree from Teachers College, Columbia University, New York, in 1949. She has been in nursing for over 30 years, and her experience is in many specialty areas.

Since coming to the Public Health Service in 1955, Ms. Scott has been with the Division of Nursing continuously, acting as consultant to many States and conducting surveys defining their nursing needs. She has conducted many workshops to teach hospital staffs how to curtail the loss of professional nurse time.

Ms. Scott was assigned to India to counsel on problems of nursing shortages and education and to promote improved utilization of nursing personnel. She helped plan for a national survey of nursing needs and resources. Ms. Scott also was the only nurse on a five-member team from the Public Health Service and the American Hospital Association that made an on site study of the organization of services for the chronically ill in England and Scotland in 1961. She also was a member of a team that studied health needs and services in Liberia.

Ms. Scott was assistant executive secretary of the Pennsylvania Nurses' Association for six years. She taught at Jefferson Medical College Hospital, Philadelphia, St. Luke's Hospital, New York, and the University of Pennsylvania. She was educational director at Mt. Sinai Hospital, Philadelphia, and has been a visiting lecturer at graduate seminars.

Ms. Scott is a member of the American Nurses' Association, the National League for Nursing, and the American Public Health Association and is active on many Public Health Service committees, including the committee on career development for nursing.

Judith G. Whitaker

Judith Whitaker was executive director of the American Nurses' Association for ten years, from 1959 to 1969. She increased the membership of the ANA during her tenure as executive director and more than doubled its staff and operating budget. She extended its activities and functions on behalf of nursing in the public interest.

Ms. Whitaker has visited and worked with constituent associations and has served on national and international commissions dealing with all aspects of nursing.

Ms. Whitaker received her nursing degree from Nebraska Methodist Hospital School of Nursing, Omaha, Nebraska, and received her M.A. and B.S. degrees from Columbia University, New York.

QUESTIONS AND STUDY PROJECTS FOR UNIT THREE

1. How did the investigations of the New York State Charities Aid Association during the nineteenth century affect the development of nursing?
2. What were the principles upon which the early American schools of nursing were founded?
3. What was the origin of the Red Cross?
4. What are the functions of the Red Cross?
   (a) In times of war?
   (b) In times of peace?
5. Discuss the activities of the Sanitary Commission during the Civil War and compare them with the activities of the American Red Cross during World War I.
6. Discuss the first schools of nursing established in this country following the Nightingale system. What was the effect of the Nightingale system on nursing education and nursing service?
7. Discuss revolutionary changes in medicine of this period and show how these changes and their combination with the development of social conscience in matters of health set the stage, so to speak, for the emergence of nursing at this time.
8. Be prepared to describe the life history of six nursing leaders of this period. Tell why you selected these individuals as the six outstanding nursing leaders and show how their backgrounds and training helped them to take their place in the nursing service and education.
9. Make an annotated bibliography of recent articles appearing in *The American Journal of Nursing, Nursing Outlook, Nursing Research,* and any other journals available in your library relating to the discussion in this unit.

REFERENCES FOR UNIT THREE

A century of nursing. Reprints of four historic documents, including Miss Nightingale's letter of Sept. 18, 1872, to the Bellevue School; Foreword by Isabel M. Stewart and Agnes Gelinas, for the National League of Nursing Education, New York, 1950, G. P. Putnam's Sons.

American National Red Cross: The American Red Cross: a brief story, Washington, D. C., 1951, American National Red Cross.

Baker, Nina Brown: Cyclone in calico, the story of Mary Ann Bickerdyke, Boston, 1952, Little, Brown & Co.

Baker, Rachael: The first woman doctor (Elizabeth Blackwell), New York, 1944, Julian Messner, Inc.

Barton, William E.: The life of Clara Barton—founder of the American Red Cross (two vols.), Boston, 1922, Houghton Mifflin Co.

Blackwell, Elizabeth: Pioneer work for women, New York, 1914, E. P. Dutton and Co., Inc.

Blanchfield, Florence A., and Standlee, Mary W.: Organized nursing and the army in three wars.

Unpublished manuscript on file, Historical Division, Office of the Surgeon General of the Army, Washington, D. C.

Brockett, L. P., and Vaughan, Mary C.: Women's work in the Civil War: a record of heroism, patriotism and patience, Rochester, New York, 1867, R. H. Curran.

Christy, Teresa E.: Portrait of a leader: Lavinia Lloyd Dock, Nursing Outlook **17:**72-75, June, 1969.

Christy, Teresa E.: Portrait of a leader: M. Adelaide Nutting, Nursing Outlook **17:**20-24, January, 1969.

Christy, Teresa E.: Portrait of a leader: Isabel Hampton Robb, Nursing Outlook **17:**26-29, March, 1969.

Christy, Teresa E.: Portrait of a leader: Isabel M. Stewart, Nursing Outlook **17:**44-48, October, 1969.

DeBarberey, Helen: Elizabeth Seton, New York, 1931, The Macmillan Co.

Dock, Lavinia L., and others: History of American Red Cross nursing, New York, 1922, The Macmillan Co.

Dubos, Rene J.: Louis Pasteur: free lance of science, Boston, 1950, Little, Brown & Co.

Dulles, Foster R.: The American Red Cross: a history, New York, 1950, Harper & Brothers.

Epler, Percy H.: The life of Clara Barton, New York, 1919, The Macmillan Co.

Gladwin, Mary E.: The Red Cross and Jane Arminda Delano, Philadelphia, 1931, W. B. Saunders Co.

Greenbie, Majorie Barstow: Lincoln's daughters of mercy, New York, 1944, G. P. Putnam's Sons.

Gumpert, Martin: The story of the Red Cross, New York, 1938, Oxford Press.

Kernodle, Portia B.: The Red Cross nurse in action, 1882-1948, New York, 1949, Harper & Brothers.

Livermore, Mary A.: My story of the war, a woman's narrative of four years' experience as a nurse in the Union Army, Hartford, Conn., 1888, A. D. Worthington Co.

Marshall, Helen E.: Dorothea Dix, Chapel Hill, 1937, University of North Carolina Press.

Pickett, Sarah Elizabeth: The American National Red Cross, New York, 1924, Century Co.

Roberts, Mary M.: American nursing history and interpretation, New York, 1961, The Macmillan Co.

Stimson, Julia C.: Earliest known connection of nurses with army hospitals in the United States, American Journal of Nursing 25:15, 1925.

Stimson, Julia C.: Medical Department of the United States Army in the World War, vol. 13, part II. The Army Nurse Corps, Washington, D. C., 1927, United States Government Printing Office.

Stimson, Julia C., and associates: History and manual of the Army Nurse Corps, Medical Field Service School, Carlisle Barracks, Pa., 1937.

Stimson, Julia C., and Thompson, Ethel C. S.: Woman nurses with the Union forces in the Civil War, Military Surgeon, January, February, 1928.

The American National Red Cross: Jane A. Delano: a biography, ARC 781, Washington, D. C., 1952.

Tiffany, Francis: Life of Dorothea Lynde Dix, Boston, 1890, Houghton Mifflin Co.

Williams, Blanche Colton: Clara Barton, daughter of destiny, Philadelphia, 1941, J. B. Lippincott Co.

UNIT FOUR
Expansion of nursing

With better hospitals, better medical practice, better education of doctors, nurses, and all health workers, and more effective health teaching throughout the community, the welfare of the group has emerged as a definite concept. Modern medicine is interested in protecting every individual from the hazards of life, particularly diseases, by scientific knowledge. In order to do this the health of the individual becomes the concern of many groups in the society. Thus we have the development of sanitary legislation, city and state public health societies, and the organization and support of many private health organizations, particularly in the fields of tuberculosis, cancer, heart disease, and mental illness. In some countries medicine is being socialized. In other countries, such as the United States, public and private enterprises are working together to control disease and to provide the best care possible for every individual.

Organizational developments and specialization were evident in the professionalization of nursing. Nursing education has become established in universities, and the profession has become vocal through its publications.

CHAPTER 14 ORGANIZATIONAL DEVELOPMENTS

■ The period up to 1900 is, in nursing, characterized by the rapid increase in the number of schools, by improvement and extension of the courses, by better equipment, by the early beginnings of libraries and textbooks, and finally, although perhaps it was not so obvious at the time, by the appearance in the nursing world of a group of women who were to bring about the next two great reforms. These reforms, the organization of nursing schools by the universities, and the organization of the nursing profession, culminated in the formation of the American Nurses' Association and the National League of Nursing Education, which definitely established the nursing profession.

Professional societies can be developed in two ways. Someone can decide that it would be well for the members of a certain group to be organized for the purpose of controlling conditions of training, of work, and of compensation and of controlling new knowledge concerning the group. On the other hand, persons who have lived closely together during a period of training and education may wish to meet or at least keep in touch with each other when they scatter after graduation. This sentiment is the primary cause for the organization of alumni associations. Both of these purposes can be found in the organizations of the young nursing profession.

It is not possible for professionals to form organizations until certain basic concepts have been accepted by the members. It is not strange to learn that the earliest American nurses' association of which we have knowledge is the Philomena Society formed in New York in 1886. Only its name is known, for it disbanded after a year, leaving no records. Professional nursing organizations did not develop until almost ten years later. Small local groups and alumnae associations began to be organized in the late eighties and early nineties. In a short time these joined together and formed the basis for a national association.

As one studies the purposes and activities of the two major professional nurses' associations, it is evident that from the beginning the members understood the real meaning of professional organization. The function of a professional organization in general is to protect the members and the public it serves. Specifically, this is done by formulating and imposing a code of ethics upon its members and assuring the public of the proficiency of its members by testing their ability before allowing them to practice. The evolvement of educational standards and the licensing of professional nurses developed early and are controlled by the profession. The professional organization is pledged to safeguard its members from unfair competition, to guarantee conditions of employment, and to ensure a fair remuneration. Study the program of the American Nurses' Association throughout the years.

ALUMNAE ASSOCIATIONS

As the nursing schools developed, the alumnae formed associations; the first were those of Bellevue (1889), Illinois Training School (1891), and Johns Hopkins (1892). It may be more than a coincidence that these were the very schools with which Miss Hampton had been connected, for, as we noted, she became their first president when they were consolidated into a national association. These associations must not be looked upon as being primarily social in purpose. In a few years these groups had joined together to become the Nurses' Associated Alumnae of the United States and Canada. The purpose was enlarged and became national in scope to embrace the general betterment of the profession. This occurred especially because the advancement of educational standards was being sponsored by the Superintendents' Society, which also was active in organizing the Associated Alumnae. As soon as the greater scope was considered, incorporation became necessary. For legal reasons Canadian nurses then had to organize a separate society, which, however, continued to cooperate cordially with the sister society south of the border. The aims and purposes of the two societies remained similar.

As the society developed as a national organization, it naturally became organized into city, county, and state societies, and it affiliated with similar groups in other countries into an international association.

AMERICAN NURSES' ASSOCIATION

It became clear that as the Alumnae Association developed it no longer fitted its old name. It was no longer primarily an alumnae association, and besides the old name was rather clumsy. So in 1911 the association made a new departure under the name the "American Nurses' Association." As such it has continued to grow and is largely responsible for the reforms that developed during the following periods. In December, 1962, its membership was 168,912. When it was organized in 1897 the purposes of this association were (1) to establish and to maintain a code of ethics, (2) to elevate the standards of nursing education, and (3) to promote the usefulness and honor, the financial and other interests of the nursing profession.* Throughout the years the association has continued its work. Its program has been altered and shaped by the continuous changes that have taken place in nursing as the profession has developed.

The American Nurses' Association has continued to help the individual nurse. Uniform licensing laws in the states have been developed in order to protect both the nurse and the public. Today professional nurses of every state have to be registered; the registration of practical nurses is also being developed.

The membership in the American Nurses' Association is open to all graduate nurses registered in the state, who join through their local district or who join directly with the State Nurses' Association if the state is not districted.

The platform of the American Nurses' Association, adopted at the biennial in Chicago in 1948, emphasized the expanding role of the American nurse in world affairs, increased participation of the nurse in national affairs, and provided for the rapid expansion in nursing service to meet the health needs of the American people.

NATIONAL LEAGUE OF NURSING EDUCATION

Another nurses' society was organized in order that nurses could work more efficiently. When, in 1893, Chicago decided to celebrate the March of Civilization toward the West with a World's Fair, a Women's Building was in the plans. One exhibit in this building was to be sponsored by British nurses under the direction of Mrs. Bedford-

---

*The A.N.A. and you, New York, 1941, American Nurses' Association, p. 2.

Fenwick. Knowing the difficulties that the British nurses had surmounted when organizing their society, Mrs. Fenwick suggested that a place be provided where American nurses could meet and get acquainted. She visited Miss Hampton, and as a result the superintendents of 18 training schools for nurses met and formed a section under the chairmanship of Miss Hampton. As could be expected, the heterogeneous nature of nursing education was then revealed. Although most schools had been patterned from the Kaiserswerth or Miss Nightingale's ideas, the whole program was still so young that the various courses could not be compared, so much had they been shaped by local circumstances. If a profession were to be created, certain standards had to be universally accepted, and new departures had to be watched and controlled.

For this purpose plans were made toward forming a permanent organization, and in January, 1894, the American Society of Superintendents of Training Schools came into being. In the beginning, membership was limited to the heads of the larger schools, but it gradually became apparent that it would be for the good of the profession to include the smaller schools also. Later it was also decided to extend the membership to others interested in nursing education even though they were not heads of schools. It is this society that has sponsored the reforms in nursing education that have gradually evolved and that are still going on. The work has particularly been along the lines of (1) higher minimum entrance requirements in order to attract an even better class of student into nursing, (2) improvement of living and working conditions, and (3) increased opportunities for postgraduate and specialized training. In 1952 the National League of Nursing Education, in conjunction with the National Organization of Public Health Nurses and American Association for Collegiate Schools of Nursing joined to become the National League for Nursing.

ORGANIZATION OF PUBLIC HEALTH NURSES

The appearance of a new group of nurses with different interests—the public health nurses—demanded some form of organization. This did not happen, however, until 1911 when a joint committee was appointed by the two national nurses' organizations, the American Nurses' Association and the American Society of Superintendents of Training Schools, for the purpose of standardizing nurses' services outside the hospital. The chairman of the committee was Lillian D. Wald and the secretary was Mary S. Gardner. After thorough consideration of the problem, it was decided that what was needed was a brand-new organization that in its own right could answer the needs of the new profession. So the committee invited all the 800 agencies, which they knew to be engaged in public health nursing activities, to send delegates to the forthcoming meeting of the two established nursing organizations in Chicago in June, 1912. At the meeting the interest was great, and a most heated discussion continued for two days. One of the difficulties was to find a suitable name for the new organization. Finally at noon on June 7, the National Organization for Public Health Nursing was unanimously voted into existence, with Lillian D. Wald as its first president. That the discussion during the proceedings must have been heated in more than one respect is apparent from Miss Gardner's description, for she refers to the "hot morning of June seventh."

The purpose of the new society was to standardize public health nursing activities on a high level and coordinate all efforts in the field. Although primarily a nurses' organization, membership was not restricted to registered nurses but included all whose work properly concerned this field. The organization was ready to cooperate with all other groups having mutual interests. It soon grew quickly, and it has almost ideally served its purpose, for its growth has intimately reflected the growth of public health nursing in America.

CHAPTER 15 DEVELOPMENTS IN NURSING SERVICE

■ Until the time of Florence Nightingale, nursing as a profession had not been sufficiently developed to make worthwhile differentiation between nursing services within and those outside the hospital. She, however, developed the nursing school, with resultant better nursing in the hospital, the opening of hospital careers, and the consequent organization of nursing service and nursing education. As the schools of nursing attracted more and better prepared young women, the nursing service in the early hospitals sponsoring such schools improved.

Not all sick people go to the hospital; in fact, we saw that for many centuries none but the poor went to the hospitals, and even the improvements that followed Miss Nightingale's reforms still left a great field of nursing service outside the hospital among both the rich and the poor.

In "private nursing" the patient bears the entire cost of the nursing. If he cannot do so, the cost is borne partly or entirely by the community either in the form of some private organization or by some public body. This latter form of nursing was at first called visiting nursing. Later, as the emphasis changed, it was called public health nursing.

A hundred years ago people who were ill had nurses in their homes. They were women often with vast practical experience but without formal training because none existed at that time. Naturally, as young women received such training and acquired special skill in attending the sick and carrying out doctors' orders, which were becoming ever more technical in nature, people who could pay for their services would demand them, and nurses trained in hospitals would go into private homes. There was nothing striking or dramatic about such a development, and it leaves no historical landmark. In the early days of many schools, student nurses did private duty in both hospital and home. The hospital usually collected the fee.

About the turn of the century, emphasis on prevention of disease began to emerge as a principle underlying all health care, including nursing service. In many instances the reason disease is not prevented is not always poverty but often ignorance of the simplest rules of health. The difference in cost between simple, clean, and healthy living and squalor is not as great as one would think. So it became impressed upon these young professional nurses, as they worked in the slums or in the wilderness, that if people knew a little more, much suffering could be avoided.

This was a period of changing social outlook. The duty of the state to improve and to protect the health of the citizens who cannot do so themselves was just beginning to be emphasized. Furthermore it is good business to do so, for it is ultimately the state that stands to lose through sickness and premature death of its citizens. It is cheaper to prevent an obsterical complication than to have the mother of a family a chronic invalid for years; to have a child properly fitted with glasses than to spend money on his education, which he partly misses because he cannot see; to have a tuberculous patient isolated than to lose years of work from others who have become contaminated because the patient was allowed to go about his business when he should have been in a sanatorium; or to treat and to cure early syphilis rather than to have the loss and expense later of keeping the patient for years in a mental hospital or to have him die prematurely from syphilitic heart disease. The age of "rugged individualism" was giving way to a sense of social responsibility.

Thus the obligation of the community was readily recognized once it was pointed out, but who was to bear the expense? Charity (for "free" preventive medicine is a form of charity) to a large extent, has been borne by private organizations. The visiting nurses' societies were private enterprises; the Rockefeller Foundation was promoting public health, and so was the Red Cross. On the other hand the local communities were establishing health departments. Problems vary so much from locality to locality that prevention of disease is often best handled locally by municipalities or state governments. The United States Public Health Service was developing quickly, and there were many health problems that definitely were nationwide, such as harbor quarantine and maintenance of food and drug standards in interstate commerce. Later, the prevention of spread of certain infectious diseases, such as leprosy and syphilis, was deemed to be a federal problem. All these arguments had something in their favor, and all classes of agents sponsored health services, so we now have work done by private organizations, by municipal and state governments, and by the federal government, all of them needing the aid of nurses. Often they cooperate; sometimes they act independently of each other.

PRIVATE DUTY NURSING

Hospitals a half century ago would retain the private duty nurse on their payroll and collect the fee for services rendered. It was satisfactory to the nurse because it provided her with security and occupation between private cases. As private nursing grew, this arrangement was found to be unsatisfactory. A system of nursing through "registers" or employment offices developed. A certain percentage of the wage was retained as a commission. Sometimes such registers provided not only private cases but permanent appointments, and some of them are still doing well in this respect. Registers for private nursing, however, sometimes fell into unscrupulous hands, and the nurses were exploited. Therefore they often placed the register in the hands of someone whom they cooperatively employed or with their professional organization. These methods reduce the cost to a minimum and are extensively used now.

Another aspect of private nursing that had become a serious problem was the cost to the individual patient. As the nurse's education and skill became more complicated, her expected financial return naturally had to be greater. With the introduction of the eight-hour day, 24 hours of private nursing became quite expensive. Three attempts were made to overcome this difficulty: "hourly nursing," admission to private hospitals in which nursing service could be obtained from general duty nurses, and insurance. This leaves only the more serious cases still requiring full-time private nursing.

In "hourly nursing," the nurse, like the doctor, goes from patient to patient in the home, carrying out the procedures that require extensive nursing skill, leaving the simpler tasks to an attendant or member of the family. The most common practice today is admission to private hospitals. As well as the nursing service, it offers many other advantages, such as the services of laboratories, diet kitchen, and resident physicians. Insurance schemes to pay for the rising cost of nursing are also gaining ground, especially in the form of group insurance, which lowers the overhead cost. In historical perspective, private nursing was at its height during the halcyon days of the twenties. In the subsequent depression many private duty nurses fell into dire need.

Today the concept is all but extinct and has litttle or no appeal for the young graduate, even though the group has a fairly solid organization.

NURSING DEVELOPMENTS IN THE COMMUNITY

It is important that the American nurse understand the development of nursing in the community, for although the first organized attempts at visiting nursing began quite early in this country, the movement was slow to gain momentum, and many influences can be traced back to English beginnings.

In 1842 an early Philadelphia institution established a Nurse Society for the purpose of supplying nurses alternately to indigent sick and to those who could pay for them. This service was similar to what we now call visiting nursing. Then in 1877 the Women's Branch of the New York City Mission established a nursing service for the sick poor by graduate nurses. However, their usefulness may have been somewhat impaired by the fact that while nursing they were supposed to actively proselytize for the church. Although the religious motive in nursing always has been and always must be highly respected, it has been the general experience that the cause of God has always been better served by the gentle, loving example than by aggressive agitation. This very factor may have induced the Ethical Society of New York to place four nurses in New York Dispensaries for the purpose of spreading the gospel of healthful living, thus establishing early in New York a service that was not to become general for several years.

During this period visiting nursing in England had passed through its initial stages,

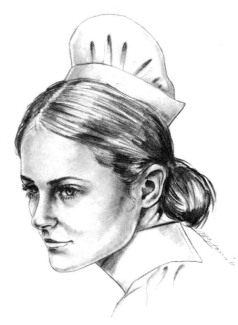

LENOX HILL GRADUATE NURSE—NEW YORK

had been under scrutiny, and now was developing into a valuable social service. With such an example before them it is not surprising that various American communities established similar societies. During the middle eighties visiting nurses' associations developed in Buffalo, Boston, and Philadelphia. Although the first of these were started under the auspices of the Presbyterian church, all of them soon became independent societies organized solely for the purpose of maintaining visiting nurses. These societies, inspired partly by those in England and partly by those in New York, have survived to become some of the leading organizations of this kind in our day. The example was soon followed by New Bedford, Chicago, and Kansas City.

THE SETTLEMENT

A new development occurred in the year 1893 that was to have an enormous influence on work among the poor, for much of public health and social service actually stems from the first American settlement. The "settlement" was not a new idea. For years English philanthropists had gone to live among the poor, but this was the first time that an American nurse brought her special training to the task. Miss Lillian D. Wald and her friend, Miss Mary Brewster, settled in Henry Street, one of the poorest neighborhoods in the metropolis, in order to give their lives to the betterment of the conditions of the poor. In other words, their scope extended far beyond nursing the sick; it even extended beyond preventing disease; they aimed at rectifying, so far as it was in their power, those causes that were responsible for poverty and misery. That, in its essence, is social service. The experiment was so successful that Miss Wald became an accepted authority on all subjects within this sphere, and the place itself, Henry Street Settlement, has become the field-ground for training and experience in social work for students from Columbia University and other educational institutions.

The social aims, however, were not pursued to the neglect of nursing or preventive medicine. All of them are considered important, and the institution itself has become the prototype of others of its kind elsewhere in the country. Among the first to follow were the nurses' settlements in Richmond, Virginia (1900), San Francisco, California (1900), and Orange, New Jersey (1903).

SCHOOL NURSING

School nursing has become one of the most important public health functions. In the nineteenth century, when compulsory schooling became general, it was necessary to pass certain health measures that eventually became centered in the periodic medical inspection of premises and pupils. In 1872 in the school of Wild Street, Drury Lane, London, a desire arose to have a nurse look into the method of feeding the schoolchildren. A request was made to the Queen's Nurses, and Miss Amy Hughes, then their superintendent, decided to look into the matter herself. Her investigation revealed much unnecessary suffering among schoolchildren, and she began at once to place Queen's Nurses in London schools. However, the London schoolboard was slow to see the value of this service, and eventually it became necessary for the London County Council itself to appoint a staff of municipal school nurses. This did not happen until 1904. By then, Liverpool had already an 11-year-old school nursing service financed by voluntary subscription. However, by 1902 when Miss Wald visited in England, school nursing there had reached such a high level of development that she returned, inspired to fight for the institution of a similar service in the New York schools.

In those days children were barred from school if the teacher found reason to do so, but no effort was made to see that such exclusion was on sound medical grounds or that the children excluded received proper care. Miss Wald was able to convince the authorities of the inefficiency of this method. In 1903 she was permitted to place a nurse experimentally in each of the four schools showing the highest incidence of exclusions. The nurses' work was so successful that in the experimental schools the exclusion fell some 90%. Such a result naturally led to the employment of school nurses throughout New York and other large cities, Los Angeles following suit as early as 1904. School nursing is now universal. The nurse supplements the work of the doctor, and she can handle most routine matters. She can follow cases during treatment until recovery, and she can make the necessary contacts and readjustments within the home. This leaves the doctor time to do physical examinations and diagnostic work and to direct treatment. Such activity has since been adopted in many schools other than those of the municipal school system, and it is practically the pattern of the health service of private and special schools as well as colleges and universities. Nowadays an American college would be unthinkable without its health service.

Miss Gardner pointed out that school health service has passed through three stages. At first, it was thought sufficient for the health officer to conduct periodic "inspections" of school children, thereby to discover those who obviously needed medical care. When it was realized how inefficient such a method was, it was supplemented by periodic examinations of the individual children to discover defects not immediately apparent, such as defective vision, poor teeth, or heart murmurs. This was a great step forward but did not realize the full scope of health service, which is essentially the preservation of health, that is, prevention of disease. So now a great emphasis is placed on this phase, by instruction in hygiene and inoculation against preventable communicable disease. This instruction should not stop in the classroom but should be carried to the very homes of the children when necessary.

QUESTIONS AND STUDY PROJECTS FOR UNIT FOUR

1. Why was the National Organization for Public Health established?
2. Who was its first president?
3. What are the functions of your school nurse?
4. Discuss the early professional nursing organizations. How do these organizations differ from labor unions? To what leaders do we owe most in the early days of these organizations?
5. Make an annotated bibliography of recent articles appearing in The *American Journal of Nursing, Nursing Outlook, Nursing Research,* and any other journals available in your library relating to the discussion of this unit.

REFERENCES FOR UNIT FOUR

A new magazine for nursing (editorial), American Journal of Nursing **52:**1077, September, 1952.

American Journal of Nursing, 1900-1940, American Journal of Nursing **40:**1085-1091, October, 1940.

Bird's-eye view of nursing history (twentieth annual convention of The American Nurses' Association), American Journal of Nursing **17:**958-966, 1917.

Blair, Mary Stewart: Social trends and nursing organizations, American Journal of Nursing **34:**141-148, February, 1934.

Chayer, Mary Ella: School nursing, New York, 1937, G. P. Putnam's Sons.

New magazine for nurses: American Journal of Nursing **51:**664, November, 1951.

Presenting Nursing Outlook (editorial), Nursing Outlook **1:**21, January, 1953.

Story of our magazine, Public Health Nursing **25:**162, March, 1953.

Vreeland, Ellwynne M.: Fifty years of nursing in the federal government nursing services, American Journal of Nursing **50:**626, October, 1950.

Wald, Lillian D.: Windows on Henry Street, Boston, 1934, Little, Brown & Co.

UNIT FIVE
Nursing education

The continuous changing and upgrading of nursing education is the cornerstone for the delivery of health services to all Americans.

The care demanded by all, not as a privilege but as a right, can only be accomplished by advances in nursing education. These changes and advances began before the turn of the century and continue constantly but now at an accelerated rate.

Nursing, as it has in the past, will meet the challenges of the next two decades.

CHAPTER 16 MISS NIGHTINGALE'S INFLUENCE ON NURSING EDUCATION

■ It is hard for us to realize that recognized preparation for modern nursing and the real beginning of nursing education began with the establishment of the Nightingale School at St. Thomas's Hospital.

The cardinal principles upon which she established that first school were the following:

1. Nurses should be technically trained in hospitals organized for that purpose.
2. Nurses should live in "homes" fit to form their moral lives and discipline.

The direction of her school was largely accomplished through the efforts of others, but she was consulted often about what was being done in the school. She rebuked head nurses who were not giving enough time and thought to teaching students. She also recognized the need for appointing a nurse instructor for classroom teaching. Some of the following points that she made are quite modern.

1. In addition to her salary received from the hospital, the Ward Sister should be paid by the Fund (The Nightingale Endowment Fund) for training these probationers.
2. It was recorded that remuneration was to be paid also to medical instructors.
3. Weekly records of the work of the probationers were to be kept by the head nurses and monthly records by the matron.
4. Diaries (as previously noted) were to be kept by probationers.
5. Miss Nightingale emphasized the need for cor-relation of theory and practice (although she did not use that phrase).
6. Probationers, she said, must be taught to know symptoms—and the reasons why and they must be given time to learn "the reason why."*

Miss Nightingale established the custom of sending an annual letter to her students. In some respects similar messages are now given at commencement time. Quotations from these letters demonstrate that they contain not only helpful ideas but also encouragement and inspiration. Many of them are applicable to students in nursing schools today.

A woman who takes a sentimental view of nursing (which she calls "ministering" as if she were an angel) is, of course, worse than useless. A woman possessed with the idea that she is making a sacrifice will never do; and a woman who thinks that any kind of nursing work is "beneath a nurse" will simply be in the way.

For us who nurse, our nursing is a thing, which, unless in it we are making progress every year, every month, every week, take my word for it we are going back. The more experience we gain the more progress we can make. The progress you make in your year's training with us is as nothing to what you must make each year after your training is over. A woman who thinks of herself "Now I am a full nurse, a skillful nurse. I have learnt all there is to be learnt," take my

---

*Roberts, Mary: Florence Nightingale as a nurse educator, American Journal of Nursing **37**:775, July, 1937.

word for it, she does not know what a nurse is, and she will never know: she has gone back already. Conceit and nursing cannot exist in the same person.*

The principles upon which this first school of nursing was established exerted great influence as the need for trained nurses increased. These graduates went out to establish schools and to become matrons in hospitals throughout England and her colonies and in the United States of America. Because of inadequate financial arrangements few schools remained separate from the hospitals even if they had been organized as distinct units. They were all soon part of the hospital and controlled by its administration. This important principle of Miss Nightingale's, namely, that the school be considered as an educational and not as a service institution, is being revived today in the recent reorganization of nursing schools.

It was natural that there should have been opposition to Miss Nightingale. There was a growing need for nurses, and many believed that the type of training demanded,

*Pavey, Agnes E.: The story of the growth of nursing, London, 1938, Faber & Faber, Ltd., p. 296.

the close supervision, and the strict regulations insisted upon would never produce enough nurses to meet the need. In 1866 a committee of the Hospital Association proposed that an independent body of examiners should be created to set an examination and that when a nurse had passed it, her name would be placed on a register of nurses. Thus the public would be protected from incompetent or unscrupulous nurses. Miss Nightingale opposed this step because she thought nursing was still too young and too unorganized for such a standard examination and because she did not believe that any examination could test the character of the nurse, which she held to be so very important. She believed that only a certificate from the matron in the nursing school would be a guarantee that the nurse had the necessary qualities of character as well as the technical skill. An examination conducted by strangers, she thought, could never test this important aspect of the nurse's qualifications. This controversy continued between Miss Nightingale and a few of her royal matrons for some years. Later the British Nursing Association was granted a royal charter but not in the terms they had sought, so that actually neither side won.

CHAPTER 17 AMERICAN BEGINNINGS

■ In 1896 the maximum hours of theory in the few good schools of nursing were 105. The standard course included 38 hours practical nursing, 36 hours anatomy and physiology, 4 to 6 hours gynecological nursing, 4 hours obstetrical nursing, 1 hour each in eye, ear, nose, and throat, and 2 hours in hygiene. When one compares this with the course suggested in *A Curriculum Guide for Schools of Nursing* and with the course being taught in good schools today, some measure of the progress made in nursing education in over 74 years may be appreciated.

The curriculum committee of the National League of Nursing Education made an outstanding and tangible achievement in the compilation of *A Curriculum Guide for Schools of Nursing.* It was originally titled *A Standard Curriculum for Schools of Nursing,* published in 1917. This publication offered concrete suggestions on how standards in schools could be improved, included outlines for courses, mainly in the theoretical subjects, and outlined the classwork for the three-year course.

In 1927 a revision was published under the title *A Curriculum for Schools of Nursing,* embodying the advances in nursing education since the first edition and emphasizing courses in public health, prevention of disease, and sociology, which began to be included in the basic course in the 1920's. The third edition was published in 1937 under the name *A Curriculum Guide for Schools of Nursing.* The revision contained two important changes:

1. It no longer laid down hard and fast rules. Recognizing the varying conditions of different schools, it called itself a "curriculum guide" rather than a "curriculum."
2. To counteract the charge that the many classes would render the nurses' course too theoretical, it was proposed to move the instruction back into the wards as "ward teaching."

The latter suggestion has proved practical, and much effort is now being expended to develop this practical form of teaching, which compares with some of the most important parts of the training of medical students.

When the schools of nursing developed, as they did toward the end of the century, under the leadership of ambitious and far-seeing women, it was natural that these leaders should strive for the highest standards for their young profession. They were favored by an ever-increasing demand for well-qualified nurses and an ever-increasing number of tasks that nurses could do if they were properly prepared. All this called for increased basic experience in nursing. On the other hand there remained the noneducational duties of making beds, giving bed baths to convalescent patients, and many tasks of hospital housekeeping, which required some training for their expert per-

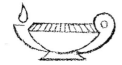

NURSING EDUCATION LAMP

formance. The problem then developed about whether all nurses should receive the highest possible professional education and to an increasing extent relegate simpler tasks to less trained attendants or whether there should be established various degrees of nursing education.

It was soon realized that nurses wishing to prepare for administrative and teaching positions must have certain experiences not offered in the organized courses to train themselves for such tasks. These principles evolved fairly promptly and have in the course of time obtained general acceptance, but the major problem still remains: how far should the nurse's basic preparation go? The question is to some extent answered by its economic aspects: there must be a certain proportion between the expense involved in obtaining an education and the financial reward that can be anticipated.

The American Society of Superintendents of Training Schools soon realized that there were three ways of establishing university standards for nurses: (1) they had to establish leadership, (2) they had to improve the student body by raising entrance requirements, and (3) they had to improve the quality of the schools by endowments and through recognition by the universities. It was not enough to establish the schools in university hospitals. This had already been done repeatedly without any appreciable effect on the course offered in nursing.

The first step was taken about 1894 when the University of Texas established its school of nursing as a regular division of its medical department. However, its leadership proved insufficient, and the requirements of this school did not meet the general requirements for university students. The plan was frustrated, and the effort has only historical interest now.

TEACHERS COLLEGE, COLUMBIA UNIVERSITY

The first effort of enduring value was the establishment of a course in hospital economics at Teachers College, Columbia University, in 1899. In 1898 Mrs. Robb had read a paper before the American Society of Superintendents of Training Schools recommending that a committee be appointed to study how special instruction could be provided for nurses who wished to prepare themselves for advanced positions. The committee was appointed with Mrs. Robb as its chairman. After having surveyed the field, it approached Dr. James S. Russell, dean of Teachers College, Columbia University, in New York, with its plans. As a result the college was opened to qualified nurses, who could attend all courses that they required. Courses specifically for nurses had to be organized and maintained by the Society.

In retrospect it is hardly possible to realize what a tremendous advance this was. Here was a group, which 30 years before had had little if any professional education or standing, now actually transformed into a group qualified by general and special education to aspire to university degrees. With the opening in 1899 of the course in hospital economics the revolution was practically complete. The work of the following generations consisted merely of extending the advantages thus gained and in building on a firmly established foundation.

Although only two students registered for the new course, the superintendents went to work with great enthusiasm; they gave freely and often gratuitously of their time and efforts to make the course successful. Gradually more nurses registered.

In 1907 Mrs. Nutting became the first professor of nursing in a university. She established "a new department of household administration which included the division of hospital economics."* Under her guid-

*Roberts, Mary May: American nursing: history and interpretation, New York, 1954, The Macmillan Co.

ance the department rapidly developed and achieved international fame, attracting students from abroad who later were to lead nursing developments in their own countries. The first actual head of a training school for nurses in Denmark was a graduate of the New York Presbyterian Hospital and had studied at Teachers College, Columbia University. One of the most important activities of the new department was to establish the Henry Street Settlement in order to develop public health nursing. To accomplish its task, money was necessary. The department was fortunate in receiving an endowment of $200,000 from Mrs. Helen Hartley Jenkins. In 1925 Miss Isabel M. Stewart, who had been Miss Nutting's assistant since 1909, became head of the department.

The purpose of this department was to offer thorough and advanced courses for nurses destined to become heads of nursing schools and who were to seek other advanced positions in teaching and hospital administration. Until the fall of 1964 it offered short refresher courses for persons who had had some experience in the field. It has succeeded eminently in these tasks and remains the leading institution of its kind in the country and perhaps in the world In the course of time other colleges and universities have established postgraduate courses of varying scope, many of them excellent, but none of them as completely organized as those of Teachers College, Columbia University.

CURRICULUM ORGANIZATION

Another step in advancing nursing education was the gradual improvement of entrance requirements.

While it became known that higher entrance requirements would make for better nurses, it also became clear that a graduate course could best be undertaken if it were preceded by a preliminary course given in the classroom. This was originally a Scotch plan that had been tried in Boston and was reintroduced into this country by Miss

Nutting at Johns Hopkins Hospital in 1901. It was found so eminently satisfactory that by 1912 there were 114 schools in the United States giving preliminary courses. These varied in time from a few lecture courses to a regular six-month course. Some included physical and social sciences and practical work, either on mannequins or in the wards themselves, so that when the students entered the wards, they felt more confident and could more quickly adjust to hospital routine. Sometimes the preliminary course is given at a college that is not an integral part of the school of nursing. In some countries, notably in Finland, this has led to a central school for these preliminary courses, after which the students are distributed to their separate schools. The system of preliminary courses greatly increased the efficiency of the whole course. The principal objection to it has been its cost. It does appear expensive at first sight, although this point may be questionable when the gain in efficiency is considered.

EDUCATION OF THE PUBLIC HEALTH NURSE

Special training was required for the nurse who was to do visiting nursing, but much more special knowledge was required of the nurse who was to take up preventive medicine. It is one thing to make a bed or to care for the physical needs of a patient, but quite another to examine a class of children and spot the ones who are developing the measles or to visit in a home and evaluate tuberculosis contacts. This was soon realized, but there is, even now, a great deal of argument about what type of preparation public health nurses should have. Various methods are being tried in various countries. Rather than enumerate in detail how different countries have approached the problem, we shall trace the various lines of thought that have been advanced to solve it.

Many views were advanced, and each has prevailed to some extent. Some have strongly favored complete specialization for all tasks that require but a simple technic. They do not consider basic education in nursing necessary. It has been argued that, to do district midwifery only, it is not necessary to have had a full nurse's course; and many countries have midwives who are not nurses and who are trained not only to see that nature takes her normal course but also to know and recognize complications and to prevent those that can be prevented. Other similar arrangements have been made when a task was big enough to occupy a person's full time and yet special and simple enough to be done without extensive knowledge other than that immediately pertaining to the job. This principle has not gained wide acceptance in the United States.

Most tasks in preventive medicine were not simple. It was generally admitted that the majority of them required some knowledge of anatomy, physiology, hygiene, or pathology, such as was included in the modern nursing course. On the other hand it was admitted that with the growing importance of public health, almost every nurse would sooner or later come up against some problems of public health. To answer both of these demands it was deemed advisable to include some public health instruction in the undergraduate course. This was done either by affiliation with a visiting nurses' association or through a district nursing service maintained by the hospital. Because the emphasis was mainly on hospital training, most of these arrangements were not very satisfactory until the importance of public health was properly appreciated by the teaching staff of the hospital and until the curriculum of the schools had developed to a point at which such a course could be integrated without the curriculum's being unduly crowded. The first undergraduate courses in this field were given in Boston.

Then as the scope of public health nursing expanded, it was realized that the more or less casual undergraduate contact with the field was not enough. There was enough to learn to justify organized postgraduate courses, and in 1914 Miss Nutting offered a postgraduate course in public health nursing at Teachers College in affiliation with the Henry Street Settlement. This was successful, and soon the city of Boston began the special training of public health nursing which, by 1914, had developed into an eight-month course at Simmons College. Later other centers, mostly university schools, developed public health courses. Now public health nursing is an integral part of all higher education curriculums for nurses. Thus, as public health nursing has increased in importance, the educational facilities in the field have developed also.

For many years leaders in the nursing profession believed that schools of nursing should be more closely affiliated with educational institutions. In 1908, mainly through the efforts of Dr. Richard Olding Beard, the school of nursing at the University of Minnesota became part of that university. Particularly since World War I, studies and surveys have been made to determine the position schools of nursing should have in the educational structure of this country as far as both administration and financial support are concerned. The first major study, published in 1923, is called "Report of the Committee for the Study of Nursing Education" made under the direction of Josephine Goldmark. As a result of this study, the Rockefeller Foundation endowed the school of nursing at Yale University.

Continuing interest in the study of nursing education was shown by the Committee on the Grading of Nursing Schools, which worked under the direction of May Ayers Burgess beginning in 1925. One report of this committee, "Nursing Schools Today and Tomorrow," published in 1934, set the blueprint for the organization of the diploma school of nursing.

CHAPTER 18 STUDIES BETWEEN WORLD WAR I AND WORLD WAR II

■ In 1920, standards in the best schools of nursing were high, but the greatly increased demands for nursing students during and after World War I had forced many schools to relax their entrance requirements in order to attract more students. Thus many less desirable applicants were admitted to the schools, resulting in such heterogeneous educational standards that before anything serious could be undertaken, the current state of affairs had to be recorded and analyzed. Then recommendations could be made for standardization and improvements.

The trend was to place even greater emphasis on public health and preventive medicine. This happened to be the exact field in which the Rockefeller Foundation was much interested. It became possible for the foundation to finance the Committee for the Study of Nursing Education, which was organized in 1918 as a result of a meeting called by the foundation and attended by about 50 persons, including doctors, nurses, and others interested in public health. The committee was headed by Professor C. E. A. Winslow of Yale University, but most of the work was done by its secretary, Josephine Goldmark, who by her previous training in social research was especially well fitted for the task. Sometimes the committee has been called after her—the "Goldmark committee." Originally the task of the committee was to study educational require-

ments for health nursing, but by 1920 it had become clear that this problem was so inextricably tangled with other aspects of nurses' preparation that at a second meeting the inquiry was extended to encompass the entire field of nursing education. Accordingly the investigation proceeded along wider lines; especially 23 hospital schools of nursing, representative of all types and localities, were carefully analyzed, as well as all nursing activities, with emphasis on public health nursing.

FINDINGS OF THE COMMITTEE

The entire investigation resulted in the publication in 1923 of *Nursing and Nursing Education in the United States*. The following three important points were brought out by the investigation:
1. There was widespread neglect of the field of public health.
2. Many schools were deficient in technical facilities for the teaching of nurses and had instructors inadequately prepared for their tasks. The course was unstandardized, especially in the relationship of theory to practice.
3. It was general practice for the chief nurse of the hospital also to be the head of the school of nursing. The cause of nursing would be better served by having these two duties vested in separate persons.

The committee then made several recommendations, some pertaining to public health nursing. It was recommended that public health nurses needed a sound basic hospital training of about two and one-third years plus an eight months' course in public health nursing. Although the number of nurses had increased from about 83,000 in 1910 to over 149,000 in 1920, shortages were still apparent in certain areas. This committee pointed out that the old apprenticeship type of training was outmoded in the preparation of the nurse. The committee also recommended that the training of attendants should be developed further. The requirement of a grammar school education and a training program of about eight months' in a good hospital was suggested.

Other recommendations concerned the general education of nurses. The current tendency to lower requirements should be discontinued and efforts made to raise the general standards of nursing education to the level of the best schools. Instructors and other officers of schools of nursing should receive special training to fit them for their tasks. The development of university associations with schools of nursing should be strengthened, and schools should be given adequate financial backing. It was further suggested that "subsidiary nurses" be trained for eight or nine months to carry out non-nursing tasks in institutions and to take charge of patients who do not need skilled nursing care. This meant the introduction of a group of subsidiary workers with a certain elementary training. Within the past few years this group has increased in number and, together with attendants and orderlies, pages, clerks, and secretaries, it has been added to ward personnel to do work formerly done by nurses, while nurses now perform those duties requiring special skill and technic.

The recommendations of this committee have profoundly affected the education of nurses in America. They immediately led to the endowment of the Yale School of Nursing by the Rockefeller Foundation. Their indirect effects extended much farther, and there are few schools of nursing throughout the country that are not better for its efforts.

CHAPTER 19 THE COMMITTEE ON THE GRADING OF NURSING SCHOOLS

■ At the beginning of the century the training of medical students in America was very poor. Although some of our doctors were among the best in the world, thousands were so poorly trained that they should not have been entrusted with the simplest medical responsibilities. Yet they were graduates of "accredited" schools. Because there was no law to force these schools out of business, the American Medical Association, about 1910, investigated all medical schools and graded them A, B, and C. Without legislative efforts the results of this grading were miraculous. A prospective medical student realized that if he graduated from a grade B or grade C school, it would lower his professional standing. As a result, poor medical schools either improved to meet acceptable standards or discontinued the course.

The plan was so successful that in 1925 nurses decided to sponsor a committee on the grading of nursing schools. Its scope was somewhat wider than was suggested by its name, for besides grading schools the committee was also to study in detail the work of nurses and to define the duties belonging within the scope of nursing. It was also to study the supply of nurses and the demands for nursing services, including the problems of public health nursing. In other words, the committee was to carry further the task that had been started by the Rockefeller commit-

tee. The grading committee, however, was only in part financed by outside sources; the nurses raised among themselves $115,000 over a five-year period. The chairman was Dr. William Darrach, but Dr. May Ayres Burgess, a trained educator and statistician, was actually in charge of the work.

The committee was naturally comprised of representatives of the three national nursing associations, the National League of Nursing Education, the American Nurses' Association, and the National Organization for Public Health Nursing, and also representatives from the American Medical Association, the American Hospital Association, and the American Public Health Association. Besides these there were representatives of the general public and educators. Miss Mary M. Roberts, editor of *The American Journal of Nursing,* placed the columns of this nursing publication at the disposal of the committee.

The committee worked for about seven years finding facts that were published in three reports. The first, a preliminary report, was *Nurses, Patients, and Pocketbooks,* which appeared in 1928. In 1934 *An Activity Analysis of Nursing,* a partial report comprising the studies of Ethel Johns and Blanche Pfefferkorn was published. The final report was *Nursing Schools Today and Tomorrow,* which goes into great detail concerning all the problems involved.

FINDINGS OF THE COMMITTEE

The grading of nursing schools, which was the original purpose of the committee, was not carried out by this committee. In the beginning it was thought that without personal visits to each school by the grading committee a just grading would not be feasible, and such a scheme would be too expensive. Later questionnaires were sent out to the schools and, after a study of these, each school was shown how it stood in relation to other schools. In 1932 a second survey of the schools proceeded along similar lines. The first questionnaire brought to light a great many facts—some of them new even to the trustees of the nursing schools—concerning requirements, equipment, and costs. The result was that many smaller schools decided their effort was not worth the cost and the schools were discontinued. Others realized their defects and had them remedied, with the gratifying results revealed in the second survey.

Although the immediate results may not have been as striking as they would have been by grading schools as the medical schools had been graded, this analysis had a profound effect upon the schools during the next ten years, and reforms of various kinds were greatly supported by it. The actual grading of schools was later started by the accrediting committee. It was recommended that courses in nursing schools should be on a college level, that entrance requirements for schools of nursing and for colleges should be similar, that close cooperation between the schools should be encouraged, and that they should advance along similar but not identical lines, lest nurses' preparation be frozen; there were still many probems to be solved by experiments. It was also pointed out that improved standards of instruction would lead to improved and greater opportunities for the nurse.

In a practical way the survey inquired minutely into what actual nursing was in the eyes of those who could form an opinion on the question, such as hospital adminis-

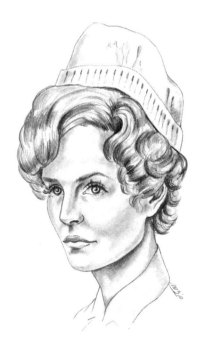

JOHNS HOPKINS GRADUATE NURSE

trators, nurses, doctors, and patients. It also studied the conditions of work, including working hours, remuneration, and opportunities for advancement.

The practical results were the elimination of inferior schools and a temporary decrease in the number of students admitted, with nine tenths of the schools admitting only high school graduates. The decrease in the number of students led to more graduate nurses being employed in the hospitals. The instruction passed into better qualified hands. Also the entire course is gradually being fitted to the students' needs rather than to the hospitals' requirements.

In this whole reform movement the American Nurses' Association and the National League of Nursing Education have worked closely together. To further improve this coordination the NLNE has since 1932 acted as the educational department of the ANA.

ACCREDITING OF SCHOOLS OF NURSING

The Committee on the Grading of Nursing Schools did not, as pointed out, actually grade schools as medical schools had been graded into A, B, and C schools. Too much material had to be studied and evaluated because of the great variety of standards and working conditions found in schools in the United States. However, all this study did lead eventually to the accrediting of nursing schools being undertaken as a project of the National League of Nursing Education.

The aims that were formulated by the accrediting committee were stated as follows:

1. To stimulate through accrediting practices the general improvement of nursing education and nursing practice in the United States.
2. To help those responsible for the administration of schools of nursing to improve their schools.
3. To give public recognition to schools that voluntarily seek and are deemed worthy of professional accreditation.
4. To publish a list of accredited schools for the purpose of guidance of prospective students in their choice of schools of nursing and to aid

secondary schools and colleges in their guidance programs.
5. To serve as a guide to state accrediting agencies in further defining their standards for recognition of schools and to promote interstate relationships in professional registering of nurses.
6. To make available to institution administrators, students or graduate nurses advanced standing information that will help in evaluating credentials.
7. To provide information which may be made available to lay and professional groups for purpose of developing an understanding of the ideals, objectives, and needs of nursing education.*

The accrediting committee worked hard on standards for the evaluation of nursing schools. The school, as a whole, was to be judged, and the list of accredited schools would be those that had satisfactorily met the criteria set up by the committee. The

*Editorial: Field work of the accrediting committee begins, American Journal of Nursing **38:** 461-462, April, 1958.

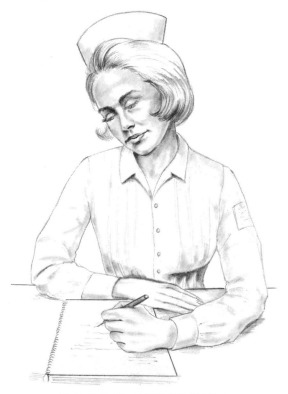

COLLEGIATE STUDENT NURSE

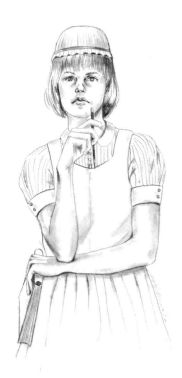

FORMER BELLEVUE STUDENT NURSE

accrediting committee would visit schools at their request and examine them. The individual school would pay the cost of such evaluation, and the individual school must apply to the committee for accreditation. In 1941 the first list of schools accredited by the National League of Nursing Education was published. Although the war slowed down the work of the committee, it did not entirely stop it; however, because of lack of finances and lack of personnel, the program moved rather slowly during the war years.

CONCLUSION

The period between World Wars I and II is considered by many people as an armistice. However, in the United States the wish of the people to do away with warlike activities as soon after any war as possible was observed in, among other things, the reduction of nurses in the army and navy corps during the 1920's and 1930's.

All surveys that were made during this period pointed to the fact that the nursing profession was aware that it needed to change in order to meet, on the one hand, demands being made by the community for good nursing service and, on the other hand, demands being made by prospective students for a better professional course. A monograph, *Nursing as a Profession,* prepared by Dr. Esther Lucile Brown under the auspices of the Russell Sage Foundation, published in 1936 and revised in 1940, focused attention on some of the problems such as the control of nursing education. In 1936 the National League of Nursing Education published a manual, *Essentials of a Good School of*

Nursing. In the same year in cooperation with the Division on Nursing of the Council of the American Hospital Association and a committee of the league, a manual called *Essentials of Good Hospital Nursing Service* was published. These publications pointed out that the major aims of nursing schools and nursing services are different and that these differences must be planned for in the organizations and programs of each.

One of the great handicaps in carrying out some of these programs in nursing education was lack of trained personnel. Again the league tried to help schools and nurses all over the country by publishing, in 1933 a manual, *The Nursing School Faculty: Duties, Qualifications and Preparation of Its Members.* This was revised in 1946. The curriculum in schools of nursing was being readjusted to meet the modern situation. More emphasis was placed on the social sciences. The preventive and social aspects were being integrated in the clinical programs, as well as were mental hygiene and health teaching. More community experiences were recommended for all students. All these changes brought up the question of cost. A study made jointly by a committee of the league and the American Nurses' Association resulted in a pamphlet, *Administrative Cost Analysis for Nursing Service and Nursing Education,* published in 1940. The accrediting program of the league was progressing, and collegiate programs were increasing in number. More money, although not nearly enough, was being made available for nursing education, from private endowments and from public sources. This then was the situation at the beginning of World War II.

QUESTIONS AND STUDY PROJECTS FOR UNIT FIVE

1. Describe the Nightingale influence on American education? How were her original concepts altered?
2. What were some of the outstanding developments in nursing in the period between World Wars I and II?
3. How has the Committee on the Grading of Nursing Schools affected the entire progress of nursing?
4. Show how developments in medicine, public health, and other related social activities in the community affected nursing between World Wars I and II.
5. Make an annotated bibliography of recent articles appearing in *The American Journal of Nursing, Nursing Outlook, Nursing Research,* and any other journals available in your library relating to the discussion in this unit.

REFERENCES FOR UNIT FIVE

Accrediting moves forward, American Journal of Nursing 39:647-648, June, 1939.

Brown, Esther Lucile: Nursing as a profession, ed. 2, New York, 1940, Russell Sage Foundation.

Darrach, William: Implications for nursing in the findings of the grading committee, National League of Nursing Education, New York, 1932, pp. 53-60.

Deming, Dorothy: The practical nurse, New York, 1947, The Commonwealth Fund.

Gelinas, Agnes: Nursing and nursing education, New York, 1946, The Commonwealth Fund.

Green, Margaret, Vendegrift, Willie, and Bouwhuis, Clara: Progress and development of the Veterans Administration Nursing Service (mimeographed outline), August, 1948, Washington, D. C., Veterans Administration.

Heinzelman, Ruth, and Deming, Dorothy: How federal civil service works, American Journal of Nursing 46:319, May, 1946; 46:379, June, 1946.

Hodgson, Violet H.: Public health nursing in industry, New York, 1933, The Macmillan Co.

Investigation of problems in nursing education, Nursing Education Bulletin, new series no. 4, New York, 1941, Bureau of Publications, Teachers College, Columbia University.

Koch, Harriett Berger: Militant angel, New York, 1951, The Macmillan Co.

National League of Nursing Education: Annual reports and proceedings, from 1933 on, and other publications including:

A curriculum for schools of nursing, 1927.

Administrative cost analysis for nursing service and nursing education (in cooperation with the American Hospital Association), 1940.

Curriculum guide for schools of nursing, 1937.

Essentials of a good school of nursing, 1942.

Fundamentals of administration in schools of nursing, 1940.

Manual of essentials of a good hospital nursing service (pamphlet, in cooperation with the American Hospital Association), 1942.

Nursing school faculty: duties, qualifications, and preparation of its members, 1933.

Nursing and nursing education in the United States. Report of the Committee for the Study of Nursing Education and Report of a survey by Josephine Goldmark, New York, 1923, The Macmillan Co.

Nursing schools today and tomorrow. Final report of the Committee on the Grading of Nursing Schools, New York, 1934, Committee on the Grading of Nursing Schools.

Petry, Lucile: One hundred fifty years of service, American Journal of Nursing 48:434-435, July, 1948.

Stewart, Isabel M.: The Association of Collegiate Schools of Nursing, American Journal of Nursing 36:45-47, January, 1936.

Stewart, Isabel M.: The philosophy of the collegiate school of nursing, American Journal of Nursing 40:1033-1036, September, 1940.

Stewart, Isabel M.: The Indian Service in Alaska, American Journal of Nursing 42:1114, October, 1942.

Stewart, Isabel M.: The education of nurses, New York, 1943, The Macmillan Co.

Twenty-five years of nursing education in Teachers College, 1899-1925, Teachers College Bulletin, seventeenth series no. 3, New York, 1926, Bureau of Publications, Columbia University.

Vreeland, Ellwynne M.: Fifty years of nursing in the Federal Government nursing services, American Journal of Nursing 50:626, 1950.

Wiedenbach, Ernestine: Toward educating 130 million people, American Journal of Nursing 40:13-18, January, 1940.

Witte, Frances W.: Opportunities in graduate education for men nurses, American Journal of Nursing 34:133, 1934.

UNIT SIX
Changing patterns in education for nurses

Modern nursing has evolved from the religious, militaristic, and social backgrounds described earlier. Because of the Nightingale type of preparation in the United States, nursing education developed within the hospital. Much of this education, until the last quarter of the century, was based on the apprenticeship system; the student worked in the hospital and by doing more work than was necessary for her nursing education, paid for her room and board and part of her instruction. A similar system exists in some schools of nursing today. Other nursing schools have worked out a type of affiliation with an educational institution in which the student's program is based on her educational needs. Hospital schools, to meet the requirements set by the state and the accreditation standards established by the National League for Nursing, have carefully worked out educational programs.

The first schools of nursing in the United States were organized on "the Nightingale system." When the schools first tried to become independent under the support of committees of women, the economic problem of supporting them became too great. Therefore the pattern in America was for hospitals to support and control schools of nursing. When a hospital sponsors a good school of nursing, however, it finds that funds must be set aside for this purpose. Although nursing schools originally developed as educational institutions, they were not supported or administered by educational institutions, but by hospitals, whose main focus of interest and concern must always be the care of the patients. It was within this setting that the diploma programs, the oldest form of nursing education in the United States, developed. In 1973 there were 553 such programs in the United States. Baccalaureate programs, in which a student enrolls as a regular college student and earns a college degree as well as being eligible to sit for licensure examinations, were the second form of educational program in nursing to develop. Originally most of these were five years in length, and consisted of two years of college and three in a hospital. There has been extensive change in the curricula of these schools, particularly since the end of World War II. Most students study nursing as well as other subjects in a program that may vary from four academic to five calendar years.

CHAPTER 20 STUDIES AND PROGRAMS

■ At the end of World War II there was no indication that professional nursing was going to settle back into any kind of complacency for a long, long time. As soon as hostilities ceased, all the national nursing organizations set up planning committees. The National Nursing Council for War Service, Inc., initiated a domestic postwar planning group, which in 1944 developed into the National Nursing Planning Committee. This committee was composed of presidents, executive secretaries, and other representatives of national nursing organizations. It outlined objectives and defined areas in which programs for study should be developed. The results of its deliberations are to be found in "A Comprehensive Program for a Nationwide Action in the Field of Nursing."* In general the areas for study and action were (1) the improvement of nursing services, (2) the total program of nursing education, practical as well as professional, (3) the distribution of nursing services, (4) the study of standards and the improvement of public relations, and (5) general information about nursing.

THE BROWN REPORT—NURSING FOR THE FUTURE

The National Nursing Council for War Service, Inc., might have abruptly ceased

*American Journal of Nursing, September, 1945.

its activities at the end of World War II. However, members of this committee believed that a comprehensive study of nursing education was indicated. They requested and received financial support for the study from the Carnegie Corporation of New York. Dr. Esther Lucile Brown, director of the Department of Studies in Professions of the Russell Sage Foundation, served as the director of the study. This study was published in 1948 and is known either as the Brown Report or *Nursing for the Future*. In this study Dr. Brown approached the problem of what provisions should be made for the nursing and health needs of society. Programs for the future of nursing education could be worked out only in the light of meeting these needs. Few reports have had such a tumultuous reception as the Brown Report. Nurses, hospital administrators, and doctors have been loud in their approval or disapproval of it. The report was made, and, from the findings, programs and plans for the future were studied and implemented.

Important findings of the Brown Report

The Brown Report recommended that the term "professional" when applied to nurses should be used only for those who have studied in a school designated as "an accredited professional school." The education, financial support, and legislation for the training of practical nurses were discussed and recommended. This report also pointed out that schools of nursing should be nationally classified and accredited; that faculty standards, such as those formulated by the Association of Collegiate Schools of Nursing, be accepted in all schools; and that the nursing courses as given in the hospital school should be both shortened and improved, particularly as central schools of nursing in connection with teaching resources of colleges and universities were better utilized. It pointed out that the rapidly expanding demands of the nursing function could be satisfactorily met only when the nurse had made a place for herself on the health team, or with allied professional groups, such as physicians, health officers, social workers, and teachers. It pointed out that nursing education needs financial support from both private and public sources. It recommended that state and regional planning for nursing service and nursing education should be started immediately so that plans for the future could be worked out on the basis of need.

Two major changes suggested by Dr. Brown's recommendations were that schools of nursing should have affiliation with universities and have separate school budgets. Since about 553 schools of nursing in this country are still hospital schools, and many of these have very little if any affiliation with any educational institution, far-reaching changes were indicated. Dr. Brown pointed out that the inadequacy of nursing service in most hospitals exists because nurses have been poorly trained in schools of nursing that are inadequate for participation in any educational program. There has been a great deal of criticism about this report by nurses, particularly about the recommendation made that professional nurses be college-trained and that in order to relieve the nursing shortage two-year courses in collegiate nursing be established. Many registered nurses believed that if this program were carried out, many of them would be demoted to the status of a practical nurse.

Tangible results of the Brown Report

One important and constructive result of this report has been that nurses, doctors, hospital administrators, and the lay public have studied the whole question of nursing service and nursing education with a thoroughness seldom seen before. To stimulate thinking about the situation, the National Nursing Council for War Service, Inc., sponsored three regional conferences in 1948 in connection with the study. The results have been published in a book, *1000 Think Together*. The bringing together of nurses, doctors, hospital administrators, and interested lay people was most constructive. Incidentally the technic of group dynamics was used, and to many in the nursing field this was a first experience with a new technic in conducting conferences.

The National Nursing Council for War Service, Inc., which had stimulated this study, *Nursing for the Future,* later changed its name to National Committee for the Improvement of Nursing Service.

THE ROCKEFELLER FOUNDATION— THE COMMONWEALTH FUND

The influence of the Rockefeller Foundation has been somewhat different in that it supported largely educational efforts and was even more international in scope than the Red Cross. The foundation has liberally supported schools of nursing that emphasized the health aspects of nurses' education. We have mentioned what it has done for Yale and Toronto Universities in this field. As this activity was part of an international scheme, it is in line with the work the foundation has done all over the world. It has been active in furthering education in public health in Brazil, China, Czechoslovakia, and France, to mention but a few countries. Its scope following World War II was broadened in many areas. It also supplied traveling fellowships for the exchange of public health nurses, and it has supported the work of the Nightingale Foundation. Of all the great institutions interested in public health, the Rockefeller Institution takes the widest view of the problem.

The Commonwealth Fund has done similar work. Its activities are, to some extent, international in scope. Most outstanding is the work done in Austria following World War I, especially to further the health of children. In the United States, also, the furtherance of child welfare has been foremost among its activities.

The Commonwealth Fund has been in-terested in rural health conditions. In 1934 it helped to finance a survey of rural health by the National Association for Public Health.

Many other fields were opening for nurses, but they have developed so naturally and without fanfare and they are still so young that they have no "history." Many nurses now find careers as assistants in doctors' private offices, in department stores, in transportation, in industry—in brief, almost anywhere that people congregate.

CHAPTER 21 THE JUNIOR/COMMUNITY COLLEGE

THE JUNIOR COLLEGE

■ The junior or community college has evolved over the last half century into the most dynamic force in higher education today. Some of the early colleges limited their role to providing the first two years of a baccalaureate program. The original plan has been altered by the social forces of population and the postwar demand for college opportunity for all youth. Thus, although the original concept of liberal arts and general education courses for transfer purposes is still a part of the junior college, most of the institutions now emphasize studies that prepare men and women to take jobs immediately in industry, government service, and service occupations—such as hotel management. This basic change in philosophy is dramatized by the growth of junior colleges within the last decade. Over 300 junior colleges have been established since 1952, when there were 597, bringing the number to over 1000 in 1972. This basic change in philosophy made it possible for nursing education to establish itself within this arm of higher education.

COMMUNITY COLLEGE EDUCATION FOR NURSING RESEARCH

The first programs in nursing within the framework of community colleges followed the publication of Dr. Mildred Montag's doctoral thesis, *Education of Nursing Technicians,* 1951. In 1952 a national research project was started to determine the feasibility of developing this new type of nursing education. The project, the Cooperative Research Project in Junior and Community College Education for Nursing, was under the direction of Dr. Montag. One purpose of the project was to develop and test this new type of program preparing young men and women for those functions commonly associated with the registered nurse. Before the five-year project with the geographically selected schools was completed, the concept had more or less mushroomed; programs in community colleges were developed from coast to coast and there are now over 520 programs. The curriculum is generally offered in a two-year academic period, in accordance with college policy and regulations of the various state licensing agencies. The surgeon general's report, "Towards Quality in Nursing—Needs and Goals," anticipated a 445% increase in the number of graduates from associate degree programs by 1970—which was reached.

The characteristics of associate degree nursing programs are described in a set of *Guiding Principles for the Establishment of Programs in Nursing in Junior and Community Colleges* as follows:

1. It is desirable that only junior colleges that are accredited by the appropriate regional educational associations establish associate degree programs in nursing.
2. The junior college assumes the same responsibility for the nursing program as it does for other programs; that is, it has complete control

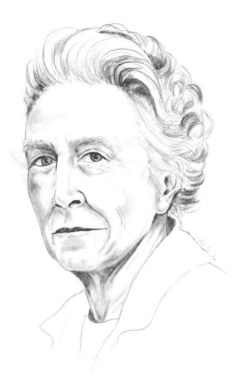

PROFESSOR MILDRED L. MONTAG

of the program and is wholly responsible for its quality.

3. The structure and organization of the junior college are such as to make possible the effective performance of its total function and to permit inclusion of nursing education as part of that function.

4. The administrative leadership in the junior college fosters a democratic environment throughout the entire institution, providing opportunities for the faculty and students of the nursing department to participate in the affairs and life of the college in the same way as do members of other departments.

5. The junior college provides competent leadership for the nursing program, selecting a qualified nurse educator as head of the nursing department and a qualified faculty in nursing.

6. The administration of the junior college takes the initiative in the organization of such lay advisory committees as may be deemed essential to assist the nursing department to achieve a quality program.

7. The junior college provides appropriate resources and facilities for the nursing program.

8. When a junior college makes arrangements with a hospital or other cooperating agencies for the use of facilities in which the college provides instruction for its students, there is an established formal relationship.

   a. This relationship is entered into only after the groups involved have thoroughly studied and reached agreement on the ways in which the facilities are to be used and the conditions governing their use.

   b. This relationship is clearly defined in a written statement approved by the appropriate boards of control.

   c. The junior college sees to it that the policies established and the mutual obligations specified in the formal agreement are implemented.

9. The junior college assumes full financial responsibility for providing a quality educational program in nursing and has the financial resources to meet such commitments.

   a. The student in nursing is not expected to bear any greater portion of the direct and indirect cost of the program than is required of any other student in the junior college.

   b. The junior college has a sound budgetary procedure for its nursing program as well as for all other programs.

   c. There is opportunity for the nursing faculty and administrative staff to participate with others in the preparation of the budget and in other financial matters.*

---

*Committee of the National League for Nursing and the American Association of Junior Colleges: Guiding principles for junior colleges participating in nursing education, New York, 1961, National League for Nursing.

CHAPTER 22 SCHOOLS OF NURSING IN UNIVERSITY OR COLLEGE SETTINGS

■ Nursing entry into the framework of higher education is historically relatively recent. The first collegiate school of nursing was established at the University of Minnesota in 1909 with a three-year curriculum pattern whose graduates were awarded a diploma but no degree. In 1916 the University of Cincinnati and Teachers College, Columbia University (in conjunction with the Presbyterian Hospital School of Nursing), established five-year programs leading to a baccalaureate degree in nursing. This pattern was followed by colleges in establishing nursing programs until the end of World War II.

In 1953 Bridgman observed that the growing interest of colleges and universities in providing nursing education has not always been accompanied by a thorough study of the nature and responsibilities assumed.

The problem of developing a professional curriculum that did not consist of three years of hospital school training girded or overloaded with two years of liberal arts has been a persistent one. In 1961 Rogers pointed out that preparation for professional practice required "substantial knowledge in the liberal arts, the biological, physical, and social sciences, and nursing theory." The curriculum needed to be planned and taught by a knowledgeable nursing faculty whose qualifications were comparable to those of any other faculty in the institution.

Hoexter demonstrated in her study using

the faculty members from 29 generic baccalaureate programs that even today (1967) faculty members in nursing are not acculturated to the academic community.

Montag's study, "The Education of Nursing Technicians," proposed a new type of worker, a nursing technician, and a new type of education consisting of two years in junior or community college.

In the 22 years since the first technical nursing program was opened at Orange County Community College, Middletown, New York, to October, 1971, there have been 552 associate degree nursing programs opened.

In her report of the four-state, five-year Kellogg project to develop associate degree nursing education, Anderson predicts that the shortage of qualified faculty for these programs will increase rapidly. White, in her study, found that the teacher in an associate degree nursing program needed graduate preparation in nursing as well as general education beyond that being offered in most master's programs in nursing. It seems relevant to extrapolate from Hoexter's statement that "no matter what may be its material resources and programs, a college or university cannot rise above the level of the quality of its faculty," nor can a community college.

Qualifications for associate degree nursing educators require additional exploration so that obstacles to the educators' securing sufficient preparation for their task may be better understood. It may be that existing graduate programs are not adequately developed for this population, and consequently nurses with master's preparation tend to gravitate to other educational or service settings.

In small communities the faculty is often drawn from a group of married women whose personal and family obligations take precedence over their professional education responsibilities. An examination of the faculty vitae sheets of numerous colleges frequently reveals that all members of the faculty are married women who hold only a baccalaureate degree and who give no indication of intention to matriculate for a higher degree. Despite the social revolution of today and the effort of many to create a basic change in the role and status of women, nursing education may well continue to be a "second job" for a woman who is a wife and mother. The magnitude and scope of the problem, however, obviously demands rigorous scientific investigation and less speculation.

CHAPTER 23 THE FEDERAL GOVERNMENT AND THE FINANCING OF NURSING EDUCATION

■ The participation of the federal government and the financing of nursing education culminated in the Cadet Nurse Corps. This participation was made possible by the Bolton Act (sponsored by Mrs. Frances Payne Bolton, congresswoman from Ohio who had been interested for years in nursing education), which was passed in July, 1942. However, a great deal of planning and work had been done before July, 1943. The need for more nurses had been apparent long before Pearl Harbor. In early 1940 nursing organizations, government agencies, hospital administrators, and interested people in the community were beginning to think and to plan toward alleviating the nurse shortage. The needs of the country had been defined as follows:

1. To step up recruitment of student nurses.
2. To educate further and better prepare graduate nurses.
3. To induce professional, inactive nurses to return to service and if necessary to take refresher courses.
4. To train and use voluntary nurses' aides under professional supervision.*

The first national inventory of nurses was taken in 1941, directed by Pearl McIver of the United States Public Health Service and

*Federal Security Agency, United States Public Health Service: United States Cadet Nurse Corps, 1943-1948, Washington, D. C., 1950, Government Printing Office, p. 4.

largely financed by that agency. The cost of the survey was $100,000, of which the American Red Cross contributed $5,000 and the Health and Medical Committee $10,000. This inventory showed that in 1941 there were 289,286 registered nurses in the United States. Of these, 171,055 were actively practicing nursing.

FEDERAL AID BEGINS

During World War I the army had its own school of nursing, and the Vassar Training Camp helped to increase the number of nurses. It was felt, however, that similar efforts would not be adequate during World War II. As a result the federal government appropriated more than $175,000,-000 for nursing education during World War II. Most of this was used for student nurses in the cadet corps. The first proposal for federal aid resulted in $1,200,000 being appropriated in the Labor-Federal Security Agency Appropriation Act of 1942, seventy-seventh Congress. This act provided for three types of education: (1) refresher courses for inactive registered nurses, (2) postgraduate education in special fields for graduate nurses, and (3) increased student enrollment in basic nursing schools. The surgeon general of the United States Public Health Service had authority to establish regulations for the administration and allotment of funds. This was two years before the creation of the Cadet Nurse Corps. Institutions offering postgraduate training had to meet standards equal to those recommended by the National League of Nursing Education and the Association of Collegiate Schools of Nursing. Criteria for standards were those published by the National League of Nursing Education in *Essentials of a Good School of Nursing* and *Essentials of a Good Hospital Nursing Service*. Schools of nursing associated with hospitals having a daily average of 100 or more patients in the four basic services were eligible to apply for aid. These funds were used for tuition scholarships for the maintenance of students added to the normal enrollment for the school, for necessary additional instructors and instructional facilities, and also for affiliation in special services. Funds could not be used for the construction of buildings but could be used for securing additional living quarters. Cash allowances to students were not provided at this time, although they were later under the Cadet Nurse Corps.

CADET NURSE CORPS

The Bolton Act became law on July 1, 1943. It provided for a uniformed Cadet Nurse Corps and for grants for postgraduate education. Any state-accredited school was eligible to apply for funds, provided a three-year course was accelerated to 30 months. Under the act the school arranged for senior cadets to serve in either a federal hospital or other health agency. The federal government paid for tuition, fees, and maintenance of students for the first nine months of training. An initial appropriation of $65,-000,000 was begun July, 1943.

This program was administered in the United States Public Health Service under the surgeon general. To handle the administration, a Division of Nursing Education was established in July, 1943, with Lucile Petry director of this new division. Some of the outstanding nurses who worked with her in

this program were Eugenia K. Spalding, Mary J. Dunn, and Pearl McIver. With this accelerated program the following regulations were established to maintain standards. The school must fulfill the following requirements:

1. Be state accredited.
2. Be connected with a hospital approved by the American College of Surgeons or with a hospital of equivalent standards.
3. Maintain adequate institutional facilities and personnel.
4. Provide adequate clinical experiences in the four basic services—medicine, surgery, pediatrics, obstetrics.
5. Provide maintenance and a stipend of $30 for all senior Cadet nurses or arrange for their requested transfer to federal or other hospitals.
6. Provide satisfactory living facilities and an adequate health service for students.
7. Provide for an accelerated program.
8. Restrict its hours of practice.*

Standards devised by the National League of Nursing Education were used. The goal of 65,000 new students for the year was set, and a total of almost 170,000 cadets joined the corps during its short existence. Of these, 65,986 withdrew before finishing the course. This was a loss of about 33%, which was slightly lower than that reported for all students enrolled in nursing schools during the same period and only 4% higher than the prewar rate. The reasons for withdrawal were the usual ones—some slightly accentuated by the war—homesickness, marriage, failure in studies, health reasons, and, of course, when hostilities ceased many left the program.

One of the main objectives of the Cadet Nurse Corps was to accelerate the length of the course. Acceleration of such programs had become common during the war—for example, medicine and engineering. Because many states required 36 months for gradua-

*Federal Security Agency, United States Public Health Service: United States Cadet Nurse Corps, 1943-1948, Washington, D. C., 1950, Government Printing Office, p. 23.

tion, planners for the accelerated program were faced with a dilemma. The compromise made was that a senior cadet period of six months be spent in a military or essential hospital or health agency. The acceleration of the program resulted in a great deal of discussion both during and after the war. Many leaders believed that two years was adequate time for the nurse course, if so-called noneducational duties were kept to a minimum. Others believed that the shortened period was justified only during the emergency.

The Bolton Act provided that the program should be open to all regardless of race, color, or creed. It is interesting to note that 21 Negro schools of nursing participated in the program and that 38 other schools admitted Negro girls as regular students. This precedent has continued and the process accelerated by the community college movement in recent years.

With the great increase in the number of nursing students, dormitory facilities were vitally needed. Under the Lanham Act (National Defense Office), funds were made available for living quarters, libraries, and class and demonstration rooms in nursing schools. It is interesting to note that $29,-657,785 was appropriated for this purpose. At the end of the war, many schools of nursing had better physical facilities than they had ever had before.

The Nurse Training Act of 1943 created the Cadet Nurse Corps and also provided for the continuation of refresher and postgraduate training of graduate nurses, which had been begun as part of the war effort. These programs for graduate nurses had to meet the standards of or be approved by the National League of Nursing Education, the National Organization for Public Health Nursing, and the Association of Collegiate Schools of Nursing.

When Japan surrendered in August, 1945, recruitment to the cadet corps was terminated at once, and no more students were admitted after October 15, 1945. Provision was made for students already in training to complete their course, and the last cadets were graduated in June, 1948. In the Cadet Nurse Corps, 169,443 student nurses had been enrolled in 1,125 nursing schools; of these, 124,065 graduated.

After World War II the G.I. Bill of Rights made it possible for many nurses who had served during the war to attend college and to become better qualified as leaders in the field. The federal government, through Public Law 911, provided grants to graduate nurses and to schools so that an increasing number of graduate nurses could become better prepared for the demands made of them.

FINANCING OF NURSING EDUCATION

One great stumbling block in the development of collegiate programs in nursing has been finances. The traditional pattern was that the student through an apprenticeship or internship gave service to the hospital and thus paid for her education. In many diploma schools, tuition is very low or, in some cases, nonexistent.

As nursing education moves from the hospital-controlled schools into colleges or universities, students must assume financial responsibility for their education. In the United States, state and city colleges provide less expensive education than private institutions. Many scholarships, loan funds, and fellowships exist for students of nursing as well as for other students.

Most leaders in the health related occupations and professions believe that education should be the responsibility of the educational institutions of the country, both public and private, and that preparation for nursing should be considered as education rather than as work experience. They believe that these programs should be administered and controlled by educational institutions, that money from public and private sources should be available for all nursing education,

TABLE 1. Statistics for state-approved schools of nursing—R.N., 1973*

Type of program	Programs 10/16/71 to 10/15/72		Number of students							
			Admissions 8/1/71 to 7/31/72		Graduations 8/1/71 to 7/31/72		Fall admissions 8/1/71 to 12/31/72		Enrollment 10/15/72	
	Number	Percent	Number	Percent	Number	Percent	Number	Percent	Number	Percent
Baccalaureate	293	21.3	27,357	29.1	11,027	21.3	26,627	28.8	73,890	34.7
Associate degree	541	39.3	36,996	39.3	19,165	37.0	37,366	40.4	67,543	31.7
Diploma	543	39.4	29,801	31.6	21,592	41.7	28,422	30.8	71,694	33.6
Total	1377†	100.0	94,154	100.0	51,784	100.0	92,415	100.0	213,127	100.0

*Adapted from state-approved schools of nursing—R.N.—1973, ed. 14, New York, 1973, National League for Nursing.
†Represents 1363 schools, 14 double programs.

and that funds should be available for the development of instructional facilities and for research. The question may be asked, "Who should pay for nursing education? The student? The patient? Educational institutions? The public?" The public pays a large share of the bill for educating teachers and preparing workers for other professions; it must also be prepared to pay for the education of nurses. Nursing service is one of the greatest needs in all communities today. Communities should be prepared to bear the expense of preparing workers in this field. Many experiments are currently being conducted in this field. Reevaluation of old types of programs and experimentation with new forms are evident in many places. For example, tuition cost for students enrolled in nursing curricula located within most community colleges is borne one third by the student, one third by the local community, and one third by the state.

Many schools of nursing have reported in the last few years that they cannot enroll as many nursing students as they would like because of the lack of qualified faculty. In 1956, the *Professional Nurse Traineeship Program* under Title II of the Health Amendment Act (Public Law 911) provided funds for graduate nurses for advanced preparation in teaching, administration, and supervision. This program is administered by the Division of Nursing Resources of the United States Public Health Service. It was designed to help relieve the shortage of well-prepared nurses in these three important positions.

In a statement released in June, 1964, Surgeon General Luther Terry reported that over 24,000 registered nurses had studied under this program. Ten thousand nurses pursued full-time academic study at colleges and universities to prepare for teaching or administration or both, and 14,000 nurses took intensive short-term courses to improve and update their skills. Dr. Terry said, "The training of nurses is a national concern because nurses now require more knowledge than ever before, to be able to use the advanced techniques which modern medical science makes possible."

Each trainee receives tuition and fees, transportation to the institution and to and from field practice centers, and an allowance for living expenses and for legal dependents. In 1969 the stipend allowances were radically revised. Baccalaureate and higher degree programs have protested this action. By January, 1974, this program is to be phased out entirely under the present federal budget arrangements.

To be eligible for this program a graduate nurse must be a citizen of the United States or have declared the intention of becoming a citizen, must be a graduate of a state-approved school of nursing, and must be enrolled in a program preparing the nurse to become a clinical specialist, teacher, supervisor, or administrator. Another program, under Title I of Public Law 911, provides funds for graduate nurses to prepare for staff level positions in public health nursing.

In 1964 Public Law 88-591 was passed by Congress and signed into law. It became known as the Nurse Training Act of 1964. Its purpose was to increase the supply of well-prepared nurses in the United States through a program of federal assistance to schools of nursing and students of nursing. The major points of the law consisted of the traineeship program, project grants for improvement in nurse training, nursing student land program, payments to diploma schools of nursing, and construction grant programs for schools of nursing. It was a giant step in giving nursing education a broader financial basis from which to move in providing better and more knowledgeable patient care.

The act was originally intended to last for five years, but from the evaluation report submitted in the spring of 1968, there was every indication that it would be renewed and expanded.

The Nurse Training Act amendments signed into law on August 16, 1968, continued the programs, with changes, through fiscal year 1971. Major changes are a system of institutional grants and scholarship grants to schools of nursing.

ACCREDITATION

Of great interest to junior colleges is the change in accreditation requirements incorporated into the 1968 act.

Under the new amendments the present system of program accreditation will be augmented with accreditation of the institution as a whole by a regional accrediting body— a state agency or other accrediting body.

The commissioner of education is directed by the act to publish a list of recognized accrediting bodies and of state agencies that he determines to be reliable judges of the quality of training. This expanded definition of "accreditation" will make it possible for some 500 previously excluded schools of nursing to participate in the benefits of the Nurse Training Act's programs. The new law will make the act's provisions available to all accredited schools, whether they have program accreditation of nurse training or regional accreditation of the institution as a whole.

On November 18, 1971, President Nixon signed the Nurse Training Act of 1971 (Public Law 92-158). This act continues with modifications the authorities for nurse training provided in earlier acts. Major features of the new act include extension and amendments of student assistance; grant and contract authorities for special projects for improvement in nurse training; start-up grants for new nurse training programs, and capitation grants to encourage expansion of enrollment and preparation of nurse specialists.

The act authorizes assistance to schools in the form of construction grants, loan guarantees and interest subsidies for construction, financial distress grants, and capitation grants; it also authorizes assistance to schools and other institutions for special project grants and contracts to strengthen educational programs, and for start-up grants for new nurse training programs. Assistance to students is authorized for traineeships, loans, and scholarships. There is also provision for grants and contracts to recruit individuals with potential for nursing.

The general provisions affecting implementation of the legislation include the following:

1. Increase in the membership of the National Advisory Council on Nurse Training from 16 to 19. Three of the appointed members will be full-time students enrolled in schools of nursing; they will be appointed for one-year

terms and will be eligible for reappointment to the council.

2. Prohibition against discrimination by schools on the basis of sex. The secretary may not make a grant, loan guarantee, or interest subsidy, or enter into a contract unless the school of nursing furnishes assurances that it will not discriminate on the basis of sex in the admission of individuals to its training programs.

3. No change in definition of schools of nursing. Diploma, associate degree, and collegiate (baccalaureate and higher degree) schools of nursing are defined as programs of nursing education, but only if they are accredited.

4. No change in definition of "accredited." A program of nurse education is accredited if the program is accredited, or if the institution in which the program is located is accredited, by recognized bodies or state agencies approved for such purpose by the commissioner of education; or if there is reasonable assurance of accreditation.

This period of rapid changes in nursing coincides with rapid changes in social and economic conditions in the United States. Nursing education today must prepare the nurse to meet the challenge that is made by society. It may be said that the future of nursing education in America is likely to be characterized by changes in line with the general system of education.

CHAPTER 24 PROFESSIONALIZATION OF NURSING AND THE NURSING TECHNICIAN

■ Many articles in nursing literature, particularly in *The American Journal of Nursing* and *Nursing Outlook,* discuss nursing as a profession. Many people have tried to answer the question, "What makes an occupation a profession?" Sociologists point out that professionalization of an occupation arises to protect both the worker and the public. When great responsibility and trust as well as technical knowledge are involved, practice must be limited. The professions well established for centuries were medicine, law, and the ministry. Only individuals properly qualified by training and by character were allowed to enter these professions. During the twentieth century many other occupations have become professionalized. Nursing is one of these. The selection of candidates to practice nursing is complicated. Professional nursing organizations are constantly alert to standards of education and standards for practice.

It is emphasized by scholars of history and other social sciences that professional organizations have a responsibility to their members and the public to set standards for admission, to control education, to impose a code of ethics, and to safeguard the conditions under which its members practice. The standards set by the profession benefit the public served.

Brown describes the professional nurse as follows:

In the latter half of the twentieth century the professional nurse will be one who recognizes and understands the fundamental health needs of a person, sick or well, and who knows how these needs can best be met. She will possess a body of scientific nursing knowledge which is based on and keeps pace with general scientific advancement and she will be able to apply this knowledge in meeting the nursing needs of a person and a community. . . .

She must be able to exert leadership in at least four different ways:
1. In making her unique contribution to the prevention and remedial aspects of illness
2. In improving those nursing skills already in existence and developing new nursing skills
3. In teaching and supervising other nurses and auxiliary workers
4. In cooperating with other professions and planning for positive health of community, state, national and international levels. . . .

The professional nurse must be able to evaluate behavior and situations readily and to function intelligently and quickly in response to their variations. She must recognize physical symptoms of illness that are commonly identified with organic changes. She must also recognize the heretofore less considered manifestations of illness such as anxieties, conflict, and frustrations which have a direct influence on organic changes and are now thought to be the result of an incompatible interaction between a person and his environment. . . .

The nurse must be able to direct her actions and her verbal expressions on the basis of a sound understanding of human behavior and human relationship.*

The struggle to differentiate the functions and practice of the technical and professional nurse is reflected in the number of meetings, seminars, and studies devoted to this subject.

Dr. Ruth Matheney, in a historic paper presented at a meeting of the Councils of Associated Degree Program and Baccalaureate and Higher Degree Programs at the National League for Nursing Convention in 1967, lists several functions of the technical nurse. These include the following:

1. Identifying nursing problems; for the technical nurse this includes the common, recurring problems (e.g., maintenance of oxygen, nutrition, elimination; prevention of cross infection).
2. Selecting appropriate nursing action; for the technical nurse this includes listening, observing, environmental manipulation, feeding, and other nursing measures.
3. Providing continuous care for the individual's total health needs; for the technical nurse this includes referral to other members of the health team and to other health agencies.
4. Providing care to relieve pain and discomfort and promote security; for the technical nurse this means measures of physical hygiene, maintenance of body alignment, keeping channels of communication open, and avoiding adding to patient stress.
5. Adjusting nursing plans to the patient as an individual; for the technical nurse this includes recognizing and utilizing the significance of the patient as a person and a social being.
6. Helping the patient toward independence; for the technical nurse this means helping the patient to help himself when he is ready.
7. Supporting nursing personnel and family in helping the patient to do for himself that which he can; for the technical nurse this means listening, suggesting, and informal teaching with nursing personnel and patient families and referral to other members of the health team (such as the professional nurse or physician) where indicated.

8. Helping the patient to adjust to his limitations and emotional problems; for the technical nurse this means creating an invironment where the patient is free to focus on feelings and reactions, and referrals to appropriate members of the health team where indicated.

Dr. Shirley Chater, director of a funded study entitled A Study of Content Differentiation Between Technical and Professional Nursing Education and Practice, concludes "that technical and professional nursing are different, and that each is dependent upon the complementary to the other. We believe that it is professional nursing particularly that requires further definition and elaboration if the status quo of nursing practice and patient care is to be bettered and not simply maintained. A most critical and immediate need is the clarification and demonstration of professional nursing practice."*

THE ANA POSITION PAPER

In December, 1965, the American Nurses' Association, through its committee on education, set forth the following position concerning education for the practice of nursing:

The education for all those who are licensed to practice nursing should take place in institutions of higher education.

The minimum preparation for beginning professional nursing practice at the present time should be baccalaureate degree education in nursing.

The minimum preparation for beginning technical nursing practice at the present time should be associate degree education in nursing.

The education for assistants in the health service occupations should be short, intensive, preservice programs in vocational education institutions rather than on-the-job training programs.†

*Brown, Esther Lucile: Nursing for the future, a report prepared for the National Nursing Council, New York, 1948, Russell Sage Foundation, pp. 73-74.

*Chater, Shirley, Wilson, Holly Skodol, and Waters, Verle H.: Differentiation between technical and professional nursing–an annotated bibliography, New York, 1972, The National League for Nursing, League Exchange No. 97.
†American Nurses Association first position for nursing education, American Journal of Nursing, December, 1965, pp. 107-108.

After months of discussion by units across the country the House of Delegates of the American Nurses' Association unanimously approved the work of the education committee at the San Francisco convention in May, 1966.

THE NLN POSITION

In May, 1965, at the biennial convention, the following resolution was adopted by the National League for Nursing membership:

The NLN in convention assembled recognizes and strongly supports the trend toward college-based programs in nursing. The NLN recommends community planning which will recognize the need for immediate expedition of recruitment efforts which will increase the numbers of applicants to these programs and implement the orderly movement of nursing education into institutions of higher education in such a way that the flow of nurses into the community will not be interrupted.

To forward the continuing professionalization of nursing reflected in this statement, the National League for Nursing shall sponsor a vigorous campaign of interpreting the different kinds of programs for personnel prepared to perform complementary but different functions.

The NLN strongly endorses educational planning for nursing at local, state, regional, and national levels to the end that through an orderly development a desirable balance of nursing personnel with various kinds of preparation become available to meet the nursing needs of the nation and to insure the uninterrupted flow of nurses into the community.

IS NURSING A PROFESSION?

In 1915 Dr. Abraham Flexner read a paper before the National Conference of Charities and Correction in which he set down certain criteria that have ever since formed a basis for judging whether an occupation has attained professional status. According to his interpretation of the professions:

. . . (1) they involve essentially intelectual operations accompanied by large individual responsibility; (2) they are learned in nature, and their members are constantly resorting to the laboratory and seminar for a fresh supply of facts; (3)

they are not merely academic and theoretical, however, but are definitely practical in their aims; (4) they possess a technique capable of communication through a highly specialized educational discipline; (5) they are self-organized, with activities, duties, and responsibilities which completely engage their participants and develop group consciousness; and finally (6) they are likely to be more responsive to public interest than are unorganized and isolated individuals, and they tend to become increasingly concerned with the achievement of social ends.*

STATE BOARDS

In most states today licensure is required to practice nursing. Licensing is necessary for the protection of the nurses as well as the patients, the community, and employment agencies. Until 1944 each state made up its own examinations; as a result they were quite varied. An important educational advance was made when the National League of Nursing Education (one of the organizations that became the National League for Nursing in 1952) developed, through its evaluation and guidance service, examinations that could be used by all the states. These examinations are composed by experts and distributed to the states, where they are administered in local centers. The papers are returned to headquarters for grading and evaluation. This is known as the State Board Test Pool and is controlled by the Council of State Boards, which is under the jurisdiction of the American Nurses' Association. At the present time some states are developing strong departments or divisions of education. The state boards automatically come within this central control with some of the lines of authority not clearly defined.

The rapidly expanding junior college programs have, in many instances, encouraged the state boards and nurse educators to re-examine minimum requirements and the

*Is social work a profession? In Proceedings of the National Conference of Charities and Correction, 1915, pp. 578-581.

methods in which to achieve the educational goals.

The basic purpose of all nursing education is to prepare qualified graduates to meet the current and future challenge of nursing. Basically a school of nursing must meet the requirements set up by the state board of nursing. Many nursing schools now meet the higher standards required for accreditation by the National League for Nursing. Many nursing programs in colleges are accredited along with the other college curricula by the appropriate regional accrediting board, such as the Middle-States Association of Colleges and Secondary Schools. At the present time students may learn nursing in three general types of schools: diploma, associate degree, and baccalaureate. The first two prepare for technical practice, the last for professional practice.

QUESTIONS AND STUDY PROJECTS FOR UNIT SIX

1. When was the first collegiate school of nursing established?
2. When was the first Nurse Training Act established by law? List ten results of this act.
3. What does program accreditation mean to you?
4. Compose your own definition of professional and technical nurse.
5. From the discussion in this unit and from your readings, list major trends affecting (a) nursing service and (b) nursing education. Show how these trends are linked to the general social and economic picture in our country.
6. If you are a student in a collegiate program, are there any major differences between your program and that of other undergraduate students in professional programs? Be prepared to discuss the differences and similarities in the programs.
7. If you are a student in a hospital school of nursing, are you aware of the differences between nursing service and nursing education? Discuss with your instructors, both in the hospital and in the school of nursing, the differences and similarities between the two programs.
8. Study an organizational chart of (a) your school of nursing and (b) the nursing service in the hospital or hospitals in which you receive clinical experience. Be prepared to discuss these organizational charts in class.
9. Describe the current concept of profession in the United States. Does nursing qualify.
10. Make an annotated bibliography of recent articles appearing in *The American Journal of Nursing, Nursing Outlook, Nursing Research,* and any other journals available in your library relating to the discussion in this unit.
11. Name some postwar trends affecting nursing service and nursing education.
12. Why was the study, Nursing for the Future, made?
13. Evaluate the comments for and against the Brown Report?
14. In what ways is there evidence of joint action in professional nursing today?
15. What is the direct result of Dr. Mildred Montag's doctoral thesis, "Education of Nursing Technicians"?
16. List six characteristics of associate degree nursing programs.
17. How do these characteristics differ from the program you are now enrolled in?

REFERENCES FOR UNIT SIX

Abdellah, Faye G., Beland, Irene L., Martin, Almeda, and Matheney, Ruth V.: Patient-centered approaches to nursing, New York, 1960, The Macmillan Co.

Allen, Virginia O.: Community college nursing education, New York, 1971, John Wiley & Sons, Inc.

American Nurses Association: First position paper on education for nursing, American Journal of Nursing 65:106-111, December, 1965.

Anderson, Bernice E.: Nursing education in community junior colleges, Philadelphia, 1966, J. B. Lippincott Co.

ANA facts about nursing, New York, published yearly by American Nurses' Association.

ANA standards for organized nursing services, American Journal of Nursing 65:76, March, 1965.

Andreoli, Kathleen G., and Stead, Eugene A., Jr.: Training physicians' assistants at Duke, American Journal of Nursing 67:1442-1443, July, 1967.

Ashkenas, Thais L.: Aids and deterrents to the performance of associate degree graduates in nursing, New York, 1972, The National League for Nursing, League Exchange No. 99.

Berry, Elizabeth J.: Hope docks in Guinea, American Journal of Nursing 66:2238-2242, October, 1966.

Bixler, G. K., and Bixler, R. W.: The professional status of nursing, American Journal of Nursing 45:730-735, September, 1945.

Blakeney, Hazle: The associate degree nurse in the health care delivery system—now and in the eighties. In Associate degree education—current issues, 1972. Papers presented at the Fifth Conference of the Council of Associate Degree Programs, Dallas, Texas, March 1-3, 1972, New York, 1972, The National League for Nursing.

Bloom, Samuel W.: The doctor and his patient—a sociological interpretation, New York, 1963, Russell Sage Foundation.

Boguslawski, Marie, and Judkins, Barbara: Contemporary guidelines in teaching, Journal of Nursing Education 10:3-11, April, 1971.

Bridgman, Margaret: Collegiate education for nursing, New York, 1953, Russell Sage Foundation.

Bridgman, Margaret: On types of programs, American Journal of Nursing 60:1465-1468, October, 1960.

Bridges, Daisy C.: A history of the International Council of Nurses: the first sixty-five years—1899-1964, Philadelphia, 1967, J. B. Lippincott Co.

Brown, Esther Lucile: Nursing as a profession, ed. 2, New York, 1940, Russell Sage Foundation.

Brown, Esther Lucile: Nursing for the future (Brown report), New York, 1948, Russell Sage Foundation.

Brown, Esther Lucile: Newer dimensions of patient care, Part I, New York, 1961, Russell Sage Foundation.

Brown, Esther Lucile: Newer dimensions of patient care, Part II, New York, 1962, Russell Sage Foundation.

Bullough, Vera L., and Bullough, Bonnie: The emergence of modern nursing, ed. 2, New York, 1969, The Macmillan Co.

Cafferty, Kathryn W., and Sugarman, Leone K.: Stepping stones to professional nursing, ed. 5, St. Louis, 1971, The C. V. Mosby Co.

Carroll, John B.: Problems of measurement related to the concept of learning for mastery, Educational Horizons, Spring, pp. 71-80, 1970.

Channing, Rose M.: The associate degree nurse in the health care delivery system—now and in the eighties. In Associate degree education—current issues, 1972. Papers presented at the Fifth Conference of the Council of Associate Degree Programs, Dallas, Texas, March 1-3, 1972, New York, 1972, The National League for Nursing.

Chater, Shirley: Selection of content for associate degree programs, Nursing Outlook 18:50-52, July, 1970.

Chater, Shirley, Skodol, Holly, and Waters, Verle H.: Differentiation between technical and professional nursing—an annotated bibliography, New York, 1972, The National League for Nursing, League Exchange No. 97.

Committee on the Grading of Nursing Schools: Nursing schools today and tomorrow, New York, 1937, The National League for Nursing.

"Con" debate: ladder. The concept in nursing education, "con," Nursing Outlook 19:727-730, November, 1971.

Corona, Dorothy F.: A continuous progress curriculum in nursing, Nursing Outlook 18:46-48, January, 1970.

De Lorey, Philip E.: Selecting learning experiences which encourage deviant behavior, American Journal of Nursing 69:800-803, April, 1969.

De Tornyay, Rheba: Instructional technology and nursing education, Journal of Nursing Education 9:3-8, April, 1970.

Ellerbrock, Sister Mary Coralita: About Christian commitment to education for nursing, Nursing Outlook 15:38, March, 1967.

Fagin, Claire M.: The clinical specialist as supervisor, Nursing Outlook 15:34, January, 1967.

Fritz, Edna: Baccalaureate nursing education—what is its job? American Journal of Nursing 66:1312-1316, June, 1966.

Feldman, Marvin J.: Opting for career education: emergence of the community college. In Puckinski, Roman C., and Hirsch, Sharlene, P., editors: The courage to change: new directions for career education, Englewood Cliffs, N. J., 1971, Prentice-Hall, Inc., pp. 109-120.

Goodson, Max R.: Professional education, American Journal of Nursing 66:798-801, April, 1966.

Griffin, Gerald J., and others: New dimensions for the improvement of clinical nursing, Nursing Research 15:292-302, Fall, 1966.

Griffin, Gerald J., and others: Clinical nursing instruction by television, New York, 1965, Columbia University Press.

Hallinan, Bernadene C.: The associate degree nurse in the health care delivery system—now and in the eighties. In Associate degree education—current issues, 1972. Papers presented at the Fifth Conference of the Council of Associate Degree Programs, Dallas, Texas, March 1-3, 1972, New York, 1972, The National League for Nursing.

Hassenplug, Lulu Wolf: Going on for a bachelor's degree, American Journal of Nursing 66:83-85, January, 1966.

Hassenplug, Lulu Wolf: Preparation of the nurse practitioner, Journal of Nursing Education 4: 29-37, January, 1965.

Hoexter, Joan C.: Perceptions of faculty members in nursing of their place in the academic community, unpublished doctoral thesis, Teachers College, Columbia University, New York, 1967, pp. 101-102.

Huther, John W.: The open door: how open is it? Junior College Journal 41:24-27, April, 1971.

Jennings, Frank G.: The two-year stretch, Change, March-April, 1970.

Johnson, Dorothy, Wilcox, Joan, and Moidel, Harriet: The clinical specialist as a practitioner, American Journal of Nursing 67:2298-2303, November, 1967.

Johnson, Rita B.: Self-instructional packages: good or bad? Junior College Journal 42:18-20, August-September, 1971.

Katzell, Mildred E.: Upward mobility in nursing, Nursing Outlook 18:36-39, September, 1970.

Kelly, Dorothy N.: Equating the nurse's economic rewards with the service given, American Journal of Nursing 67:1642-1645, August, 1967.

Kemp, Jerrold: Instructional design, Palo Alto, Calif., 1971, Fearon Publishers.

King, Stanley H.: Perceptions of illness and medical practice, New York, 1962, Russell Sage Foundation.

Kriegel, Julia: Are we earning our salaries? Nursing Outlook 15:60, December, 1967.

Lambertsen, Eleanor C.: No school can prepare nurses for all the hospital situations, Modern Hospital 108:127, February, 1967.

Lewis, Edith P.: Scutari, U.S.A., American Journal of Nursing 65:100, March, 1965.

Longway, Ina M.: Curriculum concepts—an historial analysis, Nursing Outlook 20:116-120, February, 1972.

MacDonald, Gwendoline: Development and accreditation in collegiate nursing education, Philadelphia, 1965, J. B. Lippincott Co.

Marshall, Helen E.: Dorothea Dix: forgotten samaritan, New York, 1967, Russell Sage Foundation.

Martin, Almeda B.: Associate degree nursing . . . are changes needed in the practice field for new graduates? Journal of Nursing Education 8:7-12, August, 1969.

Matheney, Ruth: Can nursing live with open admissions? American Journal of Nursing 70: 2561, December, 1970.

Matheney, Ruth: Pre- and post-conferences for students, American Journal of Nursing 69: 286-289, February, 1969.

Metz, Edith A., and McCleary, Carol M.: Knowing the learner, Journal of Nursing Education 9:3-9, January, 1970.

Montag, Mildred: Community college education for nursing, New York, 1959, McGraw-Hill Book Co.

Moore, Sister Anne Joachim: The ladder and the lattice, Nursing Outlook 20:330-332, May, 1972.

Moses, Evelyn: Nursing economic plight, American Journal of Nursing 65:68, January, 1965.

National Commission for the Study of Nursing and Nursing Education (Jerome P. Lysaught, director): an abstract for action, New York, 1970, McGraw-Hill Book Co.

Novotny, Dorothy R.: Suited for space life, American Journal of Nursing 67:1655-1657, August, 1967.

Nuckolis, Katherine B.: Tenderness and technique via TV, American Journal of Nursing 66: 2690, December, 1966.

Nursing and nursing education in the United States, Report of the Rockefeller Committee for the Study of Nursing Education, New York, 1923, The Macmillan Co.

Ogden, Gordon L.: Upward mobility of licensed vocational nurses, Junior College Journal 40: 45-47, April, 1970.

Olson, Edith V.: Education—for what? American Journal of Nursing 70:1508, July, 1970.

Operating room nursing—is it professional nursing? American Journal of Nursing 65:58, August, 1965.

Pope, Irene: Medicare—impetus for change, Nursing Outlook 16:34, January, 1968.

Porth, Carol, and May, Katherine E.: The mobile library cart—practical aid to learning, Nursing Outlook 19:602-603, September, 1971.

Price, Elimina: Data processing: present and potential, American Journal of Nursing 67: 2558-2564, December, 1967.

Rasmussen, Sandra, editor: Technical nursing—dimensions and dynamics, Philadelphia, 1972, F. A. Davis Co.

Reiter, Frances: The nurse clinician, American Journal of Nursing 66:274-280, February, 1966.

Roberts, Mary M.: American nursing history and interpretation, New York, 1961, The Macmillan Co.

Rogers, Martha E.: Educational revolution in nursing, New York, 1961, The Macmillan Co., p. 10.

Rothberg, June S.: Why nursing diagnosis? American Journal of Nursing 67:1040-1042, May, 1967.

Rutherford, Ruby: What bothers staff nurses, American Journal of Nursing **67:**315-318, February, 1967.

Schmidt, Mildred S.: Factors affecting the establishment of associate degree programs in nursing, New York, 1966, The National League for Nursing, League Exchange No. 77.

Selden, William K.: Implications of SASHEP for AAJC and NLN. In Associate degree education —current issues, 1972. Papers presented at the Fifth Conference of the Council of Associate Degree Programs, Dallas, Texas, March 1-3, 1972, New York, 1972, The National League for Nursing.

Sheahan, Sister Dorothy: The game of the name: nurse professional and nurse technician, Nursing Outlook **20:**440-444, July, 1972.

Silver, Henry, and Ford, Loretta: The pediatric nurse practitioner at Colorado, American Journal of Nursing **67:**1443-1444, July, 1967.

Smith, Dorothy W.: Some problems of baccalaureate programs, American Journal of Nursing **70:**120, January, 1970.

Society in crisis: Nursing Outlook **18:**44, June, 1970.

Spalding, Eugenia K., and Notter, Lucille E.: Professional nursing, ed. 8, Philadelphia, 1970, J. B. Lippincott Co.

Spencer, Tom: Is our integrity above reproach? Junior College Journal **41:**20-23, June-July, 1971.

Steinbaum, Barbara H., and O'Neil, Grace J.: Part-time evening nursing program, Nursing Outlook **20:**124-125, February, 1972.

Stokes, Joseph: More physicians, more highly trained nurses, or a new health worker? American Journal of Nursing **67:**1441-1442, July, 1967.

Tate, Barbara, and Knopf, Lucille: Nursing students—who are they? American Journal of Nursing **65:**99, September, 1965.

The Surgeon General looks at nursing, American Journal of Nursing **67:**64-67, January, 1967.

Transition in nursing education, American Journal of Nursing **67:**1211-1223, June, 1967.

Two-organization structure, American Journal of Nursing **50:**741, 1950.

Walsh, Margaret E.: N.L.N. faces the seventies (editorial), Nursing Outlook **18:**27, March, 1970.

Walsh, Margaret E.: The role of NLN in continuing education in nursing, Journal of Continuing Education in Nursing **3** (3):44-48, 1972.

Western Interstate Commission for Higher Education: Continuing education in nursing, Boulder, Colo., 1969, The Commission.

Whitaker, Judith G.: The nurse as a professional person, Nursing Outlook **9:**217-219, April, 1961.

White, Dorothy T.: Abilities needed by teachers of nursing in community colleges, New York, 1961, The National League for Nursing, League Exchange No. 56.

Wittmeyer, Alma: Teaching by audiotape, Nursing Outlook **19:**162-163, March, 1971.

Woolley, Alma S.: The "now" generation in nursing, Nursing Outlook **16:**26, March, 1968.

Zimmerman, Esther D.: The associate degree program graduate in nursing service, Journal of Nursing Education **5:**11-16, 39-41, April, 1966.

UNIT SEVEN
An overview of
nursing from 1914 to 1945

Wars have always accelerated the need for nurses and emphasized the necessity of better nursing service, and in nursing, the
years between World Wars I and II were anything but quiet.
The type of nursing education prevalent before World War I
was no longer adequate to meet the demands placed upon it.
Increased specialization in nursing service developed rapidly,
and the need for a better basic nursing education as well as for
the development of postgraduate education was evident. The
years between wars were characterized by study and research.
Nursing owes much to the branches of the service for the continuous upgrading of nursing care.

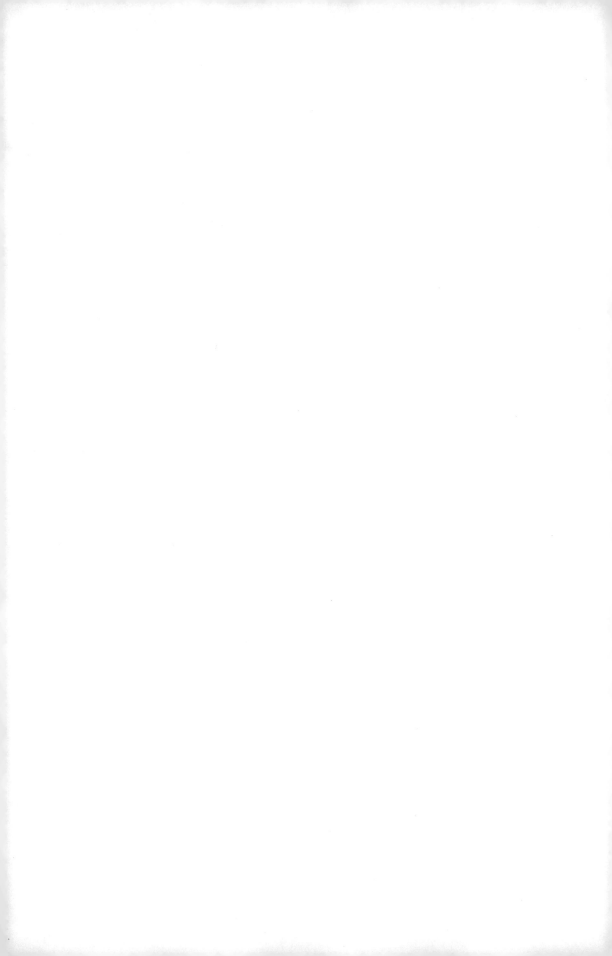

CHAPTER 25 NURSING DURING WORLD WAR I

■ At the beginning of World War I there were only about 400 nurses in the Army Nurse Corps. During the next year and a half, aided by reserves from the American National Red Cross Nursing Service, the number was increased to over 21,000. A total of 10,000 served overseas. Even during World War I, army nurses, although members of the army, had no definite military rank as officers or commissioned personnel. They were, however, subject to military law and had some military privileges. Mainly in recognition for outstanding professional service during the war, relative rank was given to them in 1920.

Although European countries were involved in World War I from 1914 to 1918, American participation in the war was from 1917 to 1918. American doctors and nurses as well as many other professional and technical individuals and services served with European countries, particularly with Great Britain and France. The British medical and nursing services were much better prepared and much larger than the American as far as their military personnel were concerned. Before America entered the war her medical personnel learned much from contact with Great Britain and France.

At the outbreak of World War I in 1914, the American navy had no hospitals in Europe, but some navy nurses were temporarily enlisted to serve in France with the American Red Cross. In 1916 the United States Naval Reserve Force was created, including a provision for reserve nurses. The total number was small. By 1917 regular and reserve force nurses totaled only 466. Nurses began to be sent to the Navy's base hospitals in England, Ireland, Scotland, and France. During this same year schools of nursing were established by the navy nurses at St. Croix and St. Thomas in the Virgin Islands, and one of these nurses was assigned to the Richmond Insane and Leper Asylum as a supervisor.

By 1918 the total number of navy nurses had increased to 1,386. It was not until 1918 that the base pay was increased to $60 per month.

It was fortunate that Jane Delano was head of nursing in the American Red Cross when the United States entered World War I. She was an experienced nurse administrator and former superintendent of the Army Nurse Corps. The nursing service of the Red Cross immediately became a recognized reserve of the Army Nurse Corps.

In addition to recruiting army nurses the Red Cross Nursing Service staffed many American Red Cross installations overseas and recruited nurses for the Navy Nurse Corps and for the United States Public Health Service.

In all the Red Cross recruited over 20,000 professional nurses during World War I. This was about four fifths of the total number of professional nurses who served in the World War. During this same period the Red Cross recruited and trained over 2,000

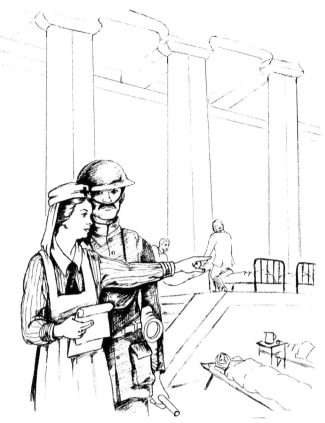

During World War I the wounded were withdrawn from field stations to temporary hospitals
set up in large commandeered buildings such as chateaux.

nurses' aides. Of these about 250 were sent overseas.

The increased importance of home-nursing instruction was evident as the war continued and was emphasized during the influenza epidemic of 1918 and 1919.

ARMY SCHOOL OF NURSING

With the general enthusiasm for the army created by the war, a move was launched to create an army school of nursing. It was organized and opened its doors in 1918 with Annie W. Goodrich as dean. The course was three years with a special credit of nine months to college graduates. These students were trained in army hospitals and affiliated with civilian hospitals for such ser-

vices as pediatrics and public health. In 1921 it graduated its first class of 500 students, probably the largest class of nurses ever graduated. After this the classes grew smaller, and the school was closed in 1932 as one of the general economy measures of the time.

VASSAR TRAINING CAMP

In answer to an appeal for college women to assist in the war, Vassar College offered its facilities for the training of college women in the summer of 1918. A 12-week preclinical course in the basic sciences and elementary nursing was offered as part of a two-year course in nursing for college women. When the summer courses had been satisfactorily completed, students were assigned to selected general hospitals as regular students for the remainder of the nurse program. In all, 430 young women from 115 colleges and universities, representing 41 states, enrolled for the Vassar Training Camp Program. These young women were from many professional fields and created a great interest in nursing in colleges and universities throughout the country.

CONCLUSION

At the end of World War I, Julia Stimson, the first woman major in the United States Army, was superintendent of the Nurse Corps. She headed the corps from 1920 to 1937, when she was succeeded by Colonel Julia Flikke. Major Stimson felt strongly the anomaly of the nurses' being part of the army organization and yet being without rank. This was further emphasized by conditions in the British army in which nurses did have military rank. The defect was remedied in 1920 when the superintendent of the corps was created a major, and all nurses below her were given appropriate rank.

Shortly after the Armistice, Jane Delano went to Europe for a tour of inspection of nursing in military hospitals. While there she contracted an ear infection and died of mastoiditis in France in 1919. She was succeeded in her work with the Red Cross by Clara D. Noyes, who had acted as her assistant for several years. In 1929 the League of Red Cross Societies, an international organization, was created to continue the work of the Red Cross in peacetime.

CHAPTER 26 NURSING BETWEEN WORLD WAR I AND WORLD WAR II

■ We now come to a period in the evolution of nursing that future historians may call the armistice between World War I and World War II. For nursing these were important years, for while in the preceding period nursing had been established as a profession, in this period nurses became aware of the fact that they were a potent social power. Nursing was recognized as something far more comprehensive than taking care of the sick; an equal emphasis was to be placed upon the preservation of health, and out of the feeble beginning of visiting nurses of the past developed the entire field of public health nursing.

In realizing their importance, the nurses also became critical of themselves. It was not enough to have established high aims and standards—the time had now come to formulate and enforce them. Two great investigations of the nursing field as a whole occurred in this period. Many recommendations resulting from the investigations were put into action.

During World War I nursing was shaken out of any complacency it may have developed. Weaknesses in the form of a poor selection of students and poor training became apparent, in addition to the great scarcity of well-trained personnel. Because of more constructive future planning the public health movement made great advances during and after the war, prevention was emphasized, and more nurses specialized in public health nursing than ever before.

A greater interest in nursing was developed by the community during and after World War I. Professional nurses began to work more closely with educational institutions in solving common problems in education. All these activities needed financial support, and endowments from private funds and grants from public sources began to be available.

SPECIALIZATION

Traditionally nursing had offered three main fields of endeavor: hospital nursing (including teaching and administration), public health nursing, and private duty nursing. After World War I, nursing in each of the first two areas developed and created a tremendous need for nurses with advanced preparation for special jobs in hospitals, health agencies, schools, and industries. To meet the great need for specialization many courses were worked out, mainly in connection with colleges and universities, to give special preparation.

It is necessary to follow the further development of some of the movements that had started before the war, notably the establishment of school of nursing within universities. Following the success of Dr. Richard Beard's Minnesota experiment, other schools adopted the idea, and by the year 1920 there were 180 nursing schools with academic standing, and by 1938 there were 45 universities sponsoring complete courses in nursing. They did not all follow the same pattern, nor did they all endeavor to serve the same purpose. So vast had the field of nursing become that many schools could afford to emphasize certain aspects thereof to the neglect of others. Often the schools at the same time achieved the endowment that had been envisioned by Miss Nightingale as a necessity, without which the best work could not be done unless funds were contributed by the university. Some of these endowed schools resulted from the reports we are about to discuss, but they are also the logical consequences of the movement that we have under consideration.

During the years that followed, many schools of nursing were reorganized on a university basis; some courses were four and some were five years in length. At the end of the course students received both a baccalaureate degree and a diploma in nursing.

ENDOWED SCHOOLS

The outstanding attempt at an endowed university school admitting only students with a college degree was the Yale University School of Nursing, which in its organization followed many of the recommendations made by the Committee for the Study of Nursing Education. Its endowment was granted by the Rockefeller Foundation. In this school the balance between the needs of the hospital and the needs of the students was struck entirely in favor of the students. All theoretical and practical work was planned to fit their requirements. Patients allotted to each student were assigned on this basis, and the case method was worked out in nursing. The staff, too, was chosen for its teaching ability. Annie W. Goodrich was the first dean of this school.

The experiment proved eminently successful, and in 1929 the school was established on a permanent basis with a large foundation grant. The Rockefeller Foundation was particularly interested because this school was in line with the trend of placing an increasing emphasis on the public health aspects of nursing. However, because of

changing needs in nurse education, the corporation of Yale University in 1956 voted to discontinue the basic program and to concentrate on graduate nurse education.

The School of Nursing of Western Reserve University came into prominence in the early twenties; it was made financially independent by the Frances Payne Bolton Foundation. Since then other endowed nursing schools have been established along the same general lines, placing emphasis on education and public health. Some have been established abroad, such as the School of Nursing at Toronto University, Canada.

In addition to endowed schools of nursing state universities now have well-developed schools of nursing, and some have departments of nursing education. The first of these was, as we have seen, that of the University of Minnesota.

The work in these schools has amply proved that superior nursing education is worthwhile. Although the number of endowed schools is still pitifully small, in the future, unquestionably, a number of schools of nursing will be established on a sound financial footing for the purpose of furnishing highly educated nurses for all the positions that are rapidly becoming available for persons capable of filling them. Educational standards are rapidly increasing throughout the country. The doctors, hospital administrators, and business executives with whom modern nurses must deal have increasingly better educational backgrounds and will, more than formerly, expect their nurses to have an adequate educational background.

THE ASSOCIATION OF COLLEGIATE SCHOOLS OF NURSING*

The development of some form of association between nursing schools and colleges

---

*In 1952 this association merged with other nursing organizations to form the National League for Nursing.

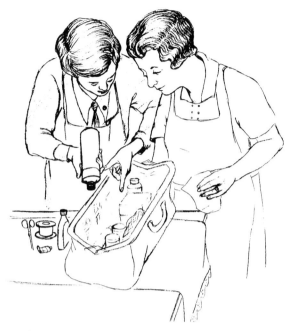

Among the long-standing and still important duties of the visiting nurse is instructing the family and friends in the care of a bedridden patient. The modern nurse still finds this most rewarding, as did the nurse pictured here in the 1930's.

or universities continued. This relationship varied from a loose, nonacademic tie, in which the school was called a university school merely because the supporting hospital was attached to a medical school, to the establishment of the nursing school as a professional school meeting academic standards set up by the college or university. This situation in university schools of nursing and the variety of standards were studied for several years before the establishment of The Association of Collegiate Schools of Nursing. A first conference held at Teachers College, Columbia, in January, 1933, was formed of 21 institutions whose representatives agreed to formulate standards and to set up machinery for the permanent organization, which took place in 1935. The objectives of the association as stated in the constitution were these:

1. To develop nursing education on a professional and collegiate level.
2. To promote and strengthen relationships between schools of nursing and institutions of higher education.

3. To promote study and experimentation in nursing service and nursing education.

Membership in the association was restricted to schools or departments on a collegiate and professional level or part of the system of higher education.

It provided for two classes of membership, as follows:

Active membership shall be open to an accredited school of nursing definitely established as a constituent part of an accredited college or university which offers a combined academic and basic professional program leading to a baccalaureate degree. The organization of the school shall accord with that of other professional schools in the university or college.

Associate membership shall be open to an accredited school of nursing whose professional curriculum meets the standards set by the ACSN, provided that the school (1) is definitely established as a constituent part of an accredited college or university or one of the divisions thereof or (2) maintains a close educational and organizational relationship with an accredited college or university or one of the divisions thereof which makes its resources and facilities available to the school of nursing.

SPECIALIZATION IN PUBLIC HEALTH NURSING

We have noted that as the field of public health nursing expanded, many branches became so sharply defined that they appeared almost like small fields in themselves. Nurses who engaged in them found themselves limited in their activities; school nursing, tuberculosis control, and venereal disease control are examples of such fields. For a while it was argued that nurses seeking special preparation in public health should be able to train themselves and to gain recognition in only one of these specialties. Fortunately this view did not prevail. Actually it was as absurd as to suggest that nurses in their postgraduate training should restrict themselves to dietetics, operating room work, or nursing of contagious disease. Nothing increases the value of a specialized training as much as a broad educational foundation. This is the tendency of modern public health nursing; the undergraduate nurse should receive a taste of it to know what it is about. The graduate nurse who decides to make public health nursing a lifework should have a thorough grounding in the entire field before limiting this work to a special branch. Besides, when working for a big organization like a municipality, the nurse may be shifted from one agency to another. Furthermore, unless a public health agency is established for a specific purpose, as for instance in compliance with a grant for the elimination of trachoma in a certain region, the broader its scope, the more useful it is likely to be, for one public health problem rarely exists alone. Most of them are born out of poverty, squalor, and ignorance, which generally will produce more than one plague at a time. Although much specialization may be found abroad in public health nursing, in the United States it is less emphasized except for the purpose of facilitating organization.

Cooperation between the Red Cross and public health nurses did not stop with World War I. When it was over, thousands of nurses, freed from war service, thronged to participate in the rapidly expanding public health activities. Again the task of the cooperating societies was twofold: organization of the field and an endeavor to fill the posts with properly qualified nurses, which in many cases meant that the nurses had to be prepared in this field before they could be appointed. One thing was in their favor; the trend of the times was to give to worthy causes, so that financing was relatively easy. The Red Cross could finance scholarships through which nurses could properly equip themselves. Generally the county was considered the unit suitable for such a project. Child welfare, tuberculosis prevention, and other similar endeavors have prospered under the joint auspices, often in cooperation with special national associations such as the National Tuberculosis Association.

One practical expression of cooperation is the Delano Red Cross Nursing Service es-

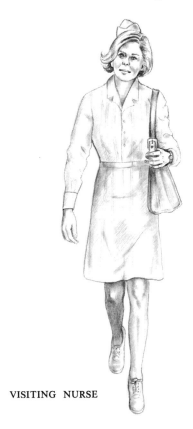

VISITING NURSE

tablished by a bequest from the will of Jane Delano. It provides one or more public health nurses to go into regions in which such work would otherwise not be financially possible. Under its provisions nurses have gone into the mountains of North Carolina, the cold of Alaska, and the islands off the coast of Maine.

The cooperation became international in scope when the Red Cross sponsored public health efforts in war-torn Europe, especially child welfare, and still more so when the above-mentioned courses were established in London under the international auspices of the League of Red Cross Societies. This was an effort that was far more than technical in scope, for it is through such association of young persons from all countries that a foundation can be laid, which perhaps some day may render armed international conflicts not only impossible but unthinkable and relegate them to the dark ages where they rightfully belong. Wars, like squalor and poverty, are largely the children of ignorance. Modern wars may have discouraged such efforts for a time, but there is in them a sterling value that will survive all vicissitudes, and it may be hoped that, when wars are over, friend and foe may again meet to further the common cause of health for all mankind.

INDUSTRIAL NURSING

As children grow up and leave school the majority of them, at least in urban areas, go into industry and business. The logical extension of health service has been to place nurses also in these areas to carry the load, along with the medical service that is now almost universal in large concerns. Here, however, the emphasis is not entirely upon health, for first aid and attention to minor ailments occupy a larger share of the nurse's time. Industrial nursing had its origin at the end of the last century, when some manufacturers employed nurses to visit sick employees. Soon it was discovered that the use-

fulness of nurses could be greatly expanded within the industrial plant, and by the time of World War I the employment of nurses in industry was quite general. However, in this case the nursing profession found itself closely tied to the economic cycle. When unemployment followed in the postwar period, industrial nursing shared in the retrenchment, and only in the last few years before World War II did industry again make a great demand on nursing. However, with the rising tide of better working conditions and obvious advantage of early health measures, this field may be considered as having been barely explored. It is still in its early stages of organization; some special preparation for it is available at a few universities, and it will undoubtedly prove attractive in the future. In April, 1942, the American Association of Industrial Nursing was organized from a nucleus of several industrial nurses' clubs, which had existed for several years to stimulate interest in the special problems of the industrial nurse and to provide a means for the discussion of these problems.

NURSING SERVICE IN THE FEDERAL GOVERNMENT

Nursing in the federal services has become extremely varied. Nurses are employed in many branches of the federal government, all of the positions being classified by the United States Civil Service Commission except those in the Navy Nurse Corps and, since January, 1946, the Veterans Administration. Through the years, positions in these agencies have followed the general lines of specialization existing elsewhere in the wide field of nursing and range from general duty or staff nursing to top administrative jobs.

It was not until 1920 that the first navy nurses were assigned to serve aboard a hospital ship. This first assignment was on the *U.S.S. Relief*. In 1922 J. Beatrice Bowman was appointed to succeed Mrs. Higbee.

During 1920 the Navy Nurse Corps was reduced, in keeping with the total program of disarmament. Educational programs in dietetics, laboratory technic, anesthesia, and tuberculosis nursing were instituted. Salaries gradually increased, gratuity for uniforms was provided, and legislation was passed providing for retirement with pay for members incurring physical disability in the line of duty.

Nursing in the United States Indian Service

The Office of Indian Affairs has had a nursing service for a long time. However, in 1924 with the appointment of Elinor Gregg as supervisor of nurses for the Bureau of Indian Affairs, many important and lasting improvements were made; she laid the foundation for the modern program of health work with the American Indian in our states, including Alaska. Nurses are assigned to hospitals on Indian reservations and to other medical stations. Those in the field positions must be public health nurses. In Alaska a physician and from two to six nurses are employed in each of the government hospitals, and, in addition, public health nurses do rural nursing. Medical care for the Indian has recently been placed under the United States Public Health Service of the Department of Health, Education and Welfare.

Nursing in the Children's Bureau

The nursing division of the Children's Bureau has been greatly expanded in recent years as the federal government through grants-in-aid has been reaching into the states to help them plan and put into effect programs for handicapped children as well as maternal and infant welfare services. The Children's Bureau was first proposed by Lillian Wald, a public health nurse. Public health nursing consultants were employed by the bureau, especially after the Sheppard-Towner Act in 1921. In 1935 when the Social Security Act was passed, there was renewed stimulus for improvement of maternal and health services. The Children's Bureau was to administer three types of services as provided for in the act: (1) maternal and child health services, (2) services for crippled children, and (3) child welfare services.

In 1935 a unit of public health nursing with a director, Naomi Deutsch, was set up.

THE LEAGUE OF RED CROSS SOCIETIES

During and immediately after World War I it became clear that the Red Cross could be an instrument of the greatest social service also in peace. The president of the War Council of the American Red Cross, H. P. Davison, therefore, proposed in 1919 that a "league" of Red Cross societies be formed for the general relief of suffering humanity, the prevention of disease, and the improvement of health—a greatly expanded program. The league is ruled by a board of governors, one from each component society. The secretariat of the league, originally in Geneva, with the international committee was in 1922 transferred to Paris. By thus enlarging and extending its purpose, the Red Cross now found it easy to extend into South America, which had been less friendly as long as the organization's activities were concerned only with war. The establishment of the league resulted within a few years in the accession of 23 new societies and a great increase in its membership.

To encourage international cooperation and to exchange experiences, the league has sponsored world international and regional international congresses, and museums have been established for collections of Red Cross material in order that technical improvements in one area can be readily available to other societies.

For disaster relief the local chapters of the Red Cross are primarily responsible. Each chapter is organized with a group of volunteers ready to respond to any call. Dressings and other relief material are stored in readily accessible places. The various chapters are coordinated to meet an emergency of any magnitude, even on a national scale, such as the great earthquakes in Iran and Japan. Some of the volunteers are lay persons with varying amounts of training in first aid; others are trained nurses and doctors.

Work in public health has been conducted as an educational campaign, more specifically in maternal and child welfare. Close cooperation has been established with other international societies with related purposes, such as The International Union Against Tuberculosis and societies for better working conditions of seamen. It will be noted that much of this work is in the nature of social service.

Nursing and the League of Red Cross Societies

Of greatest interest for our purpose is the work of the league in the field of nursing. Under its auspices an international nursing center was established in London in 1920 under a graduate nurse. The chief purposes in the field of nursing were to encourage the highest standards of nurses' training—especially in backward countries (in some countries this was done by actually sponsoring schools of nursing) by emphasizing the opportunities in public health and preventive medicine for specially trained nurses—and to improve international relationships by offering postgraduate courses to nurses from various countries. This last was done at Bedford College for Women and at the College of Nursing in London. The British Red Cross provided the league with a house in London for the students. By thus acting as a stimulus and by coordinating the field of nursing with all its other activities, the League of Red Cross Societies has tremendously furthered the cause of nursing and has helped to increase the opportunities in the field.

Finally it must be mentioned that by establishing the Junior Red Cross the league has strengthened itself by extending its activities to boys and girls who, thus trained in first aid and relief, have become a valuable recruiting ground for the organization.

CHAPTER *27* NURSING DURING WORLD WAR II

■ In the continuing world struggle between dictatorship and democracy, it is important to study and to reevaluate the lessons that have been learned in periods of national emergency. One of these is that democracies are able to mobilize their resources to achieve a mission in which all citizens are united.

"The nurses of this country—and those who worked with them in planning, organizing, and directing their voluntary mobilization in World War II—may well be proud that the unprecedented needs for nursing services both in the war theaters and at home were met. Contributing in a major way to this achievement was the United States Cadet Nurse Corps."*

Nursing in World War II differed from nursing in any other war, as did all activities of war. Tremendous advances in medical science and the widespread activities of a great variety of fighting men presented a challenge and a great responsibility to the Army and Navy Nurse Corps. In World War II the army and navy nurses served in every part of the world. World War II has often been described as a total war, and for that reason the nurse had to be trained under combat conditions and had to know how to adapt her technics to meet changing situa-

tions. The medical department worked as a team so successfully that 97% of all casualties were saved, and the death rate from diseases was reduced to one-twentieth of what it had been in World War I. In 1944 full military recognition was given to the nurses of World War II, and they became a permanent part of the regular military force. Colonel Julia O. Flikke, superintendent of the Army Nurse Corps from 1937 to 1942, was the first woman to be a colonel in the United States Army. In 1942 she was succeeded by Colonel Florence A. Blanchfield. Training for all military nursing personnel was the responsibility of the Office of the Surgeon General. Direction of the Navy Nurse Corps was under the chief of the bureau of Medicine and Surgery.

With the outbreak of World War II, members of the Navy Nurse Corps found themselves in the center of initial activity. When the Japanese attacked and took Guam in December, 1941, five nurses were taken prisoner. Just about one year later they were returned to the United States aboard the exchange ship *Gripsholm*. At Manila 11 nurses were captured in 1942 and were held as prisoners of war for 37 months.

By July, 1942, a total of 1,778 nurses were on duty with the Navy; 827 were United States Navy, and 951 were United States Naval Reserve. In that year legislation was passed giving navy nurses relative rank, from ensign through lieutenant commander. The base pay for an ensign was in-

---

*United States Cadet Nurse Corps, 1943-1948, Federal Security Agency, United States Public Health Service, Washington, D. C., 1950, Government Printing Office, p. v.

creased from $90 to $150 a month. Sue Dauser was superintendent of the Navy Nurse Corps at that time and took the oath as its first captain. She was the first woman captain of the American navy.

Early in 1944 student nurses under the cadet program reported to naval hospitals to begin a six months' practice period during their senior year. By 1945 the Navy Nurse Corps had increased to over 11,000, including both regular and reserve corps members on active duty. In the United States they served in 40 naval hospitals, 176 dispensaries, and six hospital corps schools. They served aboard 12 hospital ships and at land base establishments in many foreign countries.

In 1944 the destroyer *U.S.S. Higbee* was launched. This was the first combat ship to be named for a woman of the service.

When the surrender was signed aboard the *U.S.S. Missouri,* navy nurses were stationed aboard three hospital ships of the Third Fleet, waiting to go ashore to Allied prisoners and to help evacuate them from Japan.

In line with other military developments, training for the air evacuation of casualties became increasingly important, and the first naval school for the instruction of nurses in the air evacuation of casualties was opened. Instruction and developments during World War II were rapid and followed developments in general naval science as indicated by the overall military plans and programs.

All during the war basic training or indoctrination courses were given to nurses in the army and navy. Education in various nursing specialties, particularly in such areas as psychiatric nursing, was provided as needed. It was not until April, 1947, through Public Law 36, that a permanent nurse corps for the army and navy was established by the government.

This act has removed the need for the Red Cross to maintain a roster of reserve nurses for the army and navy. The Red Cross nursing program has been organized since the end of the war. At present the Red Cross program has the following objectives: continuing development of nursing service for times of epidemic disease or other national emergency, voluntary community service such as teaching home nursing courses, and the development of the National Blood Bank Program of the American Red Cross.

RECRUITMENT PROBLEMS

In the period immediately before the outbreak of war there had been discussion among nursing leaders and the surgeon general of the advisability of having either an army school of nursing or a summer training camp for nurses similar to the Vassar Training Camp of World War I. Neither of these ideas seemed to be completely satisfactory, although in the summer of 1941, Bryn Mawr College contributed its campus and plant to this project, in cooperation with the Red Cross. However, only 30 students instead of an anticipated 200 registered for the course. This country was not yet at war, and enthusiasm for such activities had not developed.

In the summer of 1941 some American nurses went overseas with the American Red Cross–Harvard Field Hospital Unit. This unit was intended primarily to function in England as a research center in communicable disease; when fully staffed it included 63 nurses. In crossing to England five nurses and a house mother were lost because of German submarine activity. The bombing of England had increased during 1941, and many of these American nurses worked in British hospitals and air-raid shelters.

The Red Cross, in cooperation with the Office of Civilian Defense, developed a program for training nurses' aides. This program was actually carried out by Red Cross chapters all over the country and greatly relieved the pressure in civilian hospitals. During World War II the Red Cross certified almost all of the over 77,000 nurses who served with the armed forces. The need for extending the nurses' aide program during World War II was evident. The Red Cross Volunteer Special Service, in cooperation with the Office of Civilian Defense, recruited and trained more than 200,000 nurses' aides. This training course supplied the country with a large group of volunteer nurses' aides who gave invaluable service in relieving the shortages in hospitals and health programs that resulted from the large numbers of nurses serving in the armed forces.

Instruction was given in two home nursing programs: the Home Care of the Sick, and Mother and Baby Care. Many of the teaching technics that were being used successfully in industry to teach skills safely and quickly were used in this instruction.

The nursing service of the Red Cross during World War II also recruited nurses to serve in the blood collection centers, which had been established to procure blood to meet both military and civilian needs.

After Pearl Harbor the number of professional nurses enrolling with the Red Cross for work with the armed forces increased

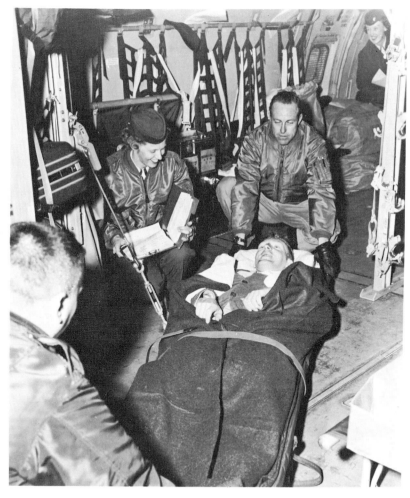

NURSES OF THE AIR FORCE CORPS "ON DUTY."
(Courtesy U. S. Air Force; from Morison, Luella J.: Steppingstones to professional nursing, ed. 4, St. Louis, 1965, The C. V. Mosby Co.)

rapidly. At times there was some resentment on the part of nurses who did not understand the background about why they had to enter the armed forces through the Red Cross. The surgeon general's office had stated repeatedly that it did not want to assume the responsibility of recruiting nurses; the situation was clarified a great deal in 1942 when the surgeon general's office made an announcement that the Red Cross was the official recruiting agency of the Army Nurse Corps. The Navy Nurse Corps did not work so closely with the Red Cross as the Army Nurse Corps did, and by the end of 1946 the Navy Nurse Corps had taken over the processing of its own applicants. In spite of all these activities the number of nurses actually in service lagged behind the number needed. Although in the spring of 1944 the goal of 40,000 nurses for the army had been reached, the surgeon general was already requesting 10,000 more. The critical situation on the battlefields was acknowledged by the leaders of this country as never before, and in January, 1945, when he gave his annual message to Congress, the President requested a draft of nurses. Three days later a draft bill was introduced into the House of Representatives. The nursing or-

ganizations at once took a stand in favor of a national service act for all men and women, not only for nurses. The bill was discussed for three months, during which time the Red Cross nursing organizations and others made a supreme effort to recruit an adequate number of nurses. Fortunately the war in Europe came to an end, and in May, two weeks after V-E Day, action on the bill was dropped.

CONCLUSION

During World War II, nursing in every branch of the armed forces matured, and the army, the navy, and the air force found that more and more nurses were proving themselves in the medical and health areas of their respective military programs.

It was not until April, 1947, through Public Law 36, that a permanent nurse corps for the army, navy, and air force was established by the government. This removed the need for the Red Cross's maintaining a roster of reserve nurses for the armed forces. Therefore, since May, 1947, the Red Cross nursing program has not been so extensive as in previous years.

CHAPTER 28 THE NATIONAL NURSING COUNCIL

■ The United States was not actively engaged in World War II until the end of 1941. However, by the middle of 1940 the Nursing Council of National Defense (forerunner of the National Nursing Council for War Service, Inc.) was organized by the six national nursing organizations. Julia C. Stimson was president, and Alma Scott was secretary. These six national nursing organizations were the American Nurses' Association, the National League of Nursing Education, the Association of Collegiate Schools of Nursing, the National Organization for Public Health Nursing, the American Red Cross Nursing Service, and the National Association of Colored Graduate Nurses. One of the main purposes of this council was to serve as a coordinating agency made up of representatives from professional nursing organizations and later representatives from hospital and medical groups and the general public. The major activities that began at once included recruitment of student nurses and the classification of all graduate nurses in the country as to their availability for military service. Under the direction of the Nursing Division, Procurement and Assignment Service, War Manpower Commission, considerations of whether the nurses were essential on the home front were made. The council cooperated with the Red Cross in recruiting nurses for the Army and Navy Nurse Corps.

INVENTORY OF NURSES

The national inventory of nursing personnel showed that there were about 100,000 nurses under 40 years of age and unmarried who were potential recruits for the Red Cross Nursing Service, first reserve. This national survey also revealed an acute shortage of nurses. In July, 1941, through the efforts of the National Nursing Council and the Committee on Educational Policies and Resources and with the cooperation of the United States Public Health Service, under the sponsorship of Representative Frances Payne Bolton of Ohio, Public Law 146 was passed by Congress. This provided for the first government funds for the education of nurses for national defense, and under the terms of the act, 1,000 graduate nurses were given postgraduate preparation and 2,500 inactive nurses were given refresher courses. Over 200 basic schools of nursing were given financial assistance, which enabled them to increase their facilities and their enrollment. During 1942 the council worked in cooperation with the armed forces trying to meet the demand. Recruitment was stimulated by advertising, and schools were helped in adopting an accelerated program. State and local councils were given assistance in recruiting graduate and student nurses. During this period the council's main financial support came from the Kellogg Foundation. The Milbank Memorial Foundation also

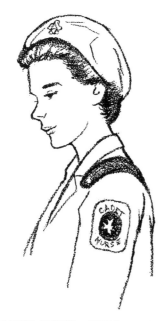

CADET NURSE—WORLD WAR II

helped, as did the professional nursing organizations.

Early in 1942 the plan that eventually produced the United States Cadet Nurse Corps was discussed, and in July the bill that has become known as the Bolton Act became a law. The main purpose of this act was to prepare nurses in adequate numbers for the armed forces, government and civilian hospitals, health services, and war industries, through appropriations to institutions qualified to give such preparation. The program was carried out by a newly created Department of Nursing Education in the United States Public Health Service, with Miss Lucile Petry as chief director, responsible to Surgeon General Parran.

LOCAL NURSING COUNCILS

The National Nursing Council for War Service, Inc., stimulated the organization of local nursing councils for war service. District and state nursing associations assumed leadership of these councils and provided a channel for better distribution of professional nurses and auxiliary help for military and civilian nursing needs. Through these councils the needs and resources of communities all over the country were studied, in many instances for the first time. A great deal of help was given to the local groups by the National League of Nursing Education and by the Nursing Division of the United States Public Health Service. The National Council had given a great deal of attention to the training and use of practical nurses and to the training of nurses' aides. Working with the Red Cross Nursing Service, more than 100,000 nurses were actually certified during the war, and more than 200,000 nurses' aides were recruited and trained all over the country. As the war went on, the National Nursing Council for War Service, Inc., had representatives from the six national nursing organizations already mentioned and in addition included representatives from the Council of Federal Nurse Services; the Division of Nursing Education, United States Public Health Service; Nursing Division, Procurement and Assignment Service, War Manpower Commission; Subcommittee on Nursing, Health, and Medical Committee; International Council of Nurses; the American Hospital Association; and members-at-large. All during the war the national council provided a splendid way of integrating and coordinating the programs of organized nursing and of fulfilling the war needs, both civilian and military.

CONCLUSION

In 1943 when the federal nursing programs were established, the national council members voted to keep the council incorporated and active for the duration of the war and six months thereafter. Soon after V-J Day the Kellogg Foundation guaranteed to finance the national council programs through the middle of 1946. The name was changed to the National Nursing Council.

QUESTIONS AND STUDY PROJECTS FOR UNIT SEVEN

1. Discuss the National Nursing Council for War Service, Inc. Why was it organized, what were its achievements, and what did it lead on to?
2. Discuss the association of the Red Cross with the Army and Navy Nurse Corps during World War II.
3. How did the National Nursing Council for War Services, Inc., function?
4. Discuss the activities of the nurse in World War II and compare these activities, both civilian and military, with nursing during other wars. Why was World War II different?
5. What has been the development of endowed schools of nursing in this country?
6. Make an annotated bibliography of recent articles appearing in *The American Journal of Nursing, Nursing Outlook, Nursing Research,* and any other journals available in your library relating to the discussion in this unit.

REFERENCES FOR UNIT SEVEN

Archard, Theresa: G. I. Nightingale, New York, 1945, W. W. Norton & Co., Inc.

Army Nurse, United States Army Nurse Corps, Washington, D. C., 1944.

Baehr, George: Mobilization of the nursing profession for war. Proceedings of the thirty-third convention of the American Nurses' Association, New York, 1942, American Nurses' Association, p. 153.

Bolton Bill, American Journal of Nursing **43**:617, July, 1943.

Bradley, LaVerne: Women in uniform. Insignia and decorations of the United States Armed Forces, revised edition, Washington, D. C., 1944, National Geographic Society, pp. 159-198.

Connelly, Ellen H.: Shipmates in white, American Journal of Nursing **49**:204, April, 1949.

Cooper, Page: Navy nurse, New York, 1946, McGraw-Hill Book Co., Inc.

Flikke, Julia O.: Nurses in action, Philadelphia, 1943, J. B. Lippincott Co.

Marsh, Penny, and Lee, Ginger: Wartime nurses, New York, 1943, Dodd, Mead & Co., Inc.

Miller, Jean Dupont: Shipmates in white, New York, 1944, Dodd, Mead & Co., Inc.

National Nursing Planning Committee, American Journal of Nursing **45**:513, 1945.

Newell, Hope: The History of the National Nursing Council, New York, 1951, National Organization for Public Health Nursing.

Nurse Draft Bill passed by the House, American Journal of Nursing **45**:255, 1945.

Nurses United for War Services, Public Health Nursing **36**:340, 1944.

Nursing needs and nursing resources, American Journal of Nursing **44**:1044, 1944.

Nursing in War Manpower Commission (with organization chart), American Journal of Nursing **43**:741, 1943.

Redmond, Juanita: I served on Bataan, Philadelphia, 1943, J. B. Lippincott Co.

Schaffter, Dorothy: What comes of training women for war, Washington, D. C., 1948, American Council on Education.

United States Cadet Nurse Corps, and other Federal nurse training programs, United States Public Health Service Publication No. 38, Washington, D. C., 1950, United States Government Printing Office.

War Manpower Commission; Classification, clearance and appeals procedure, American Journal of Nursing **43**:885, 1943.

UNIT EIGHT
Contemporary developments and trends

"The leaders of the nursing profession were faced with a serious dilemma. Since the days of Florence Nightingale, they had insisted that nurses, and nurses alone, must determine how to discharge their responsibilities to society. Although every profession has the ultimate responsibility and autonomy for determining its own role, the leadership in nursing was becoming increasingly aware that many problems with which they had to grapple were only in part professional and not subject to assessment and solution by nurses alone. Because many crucial issues had major ramifications in medicine, government, education, administration, and economics, it seemed wise to elicit the assistance of experts in these other fields."*

---

*The Committee on the Function of Nursing. Eli Ginzberg, and others. A program for the nursing profession, New York, 1941, The Macmillan Co., pp. vii, viii.

CHAPTER 29 A SURVEY OF NURSING PRACTICE

■ Demands for nursing services are constantly increasing, and specilization has entered the wide field of nursing. Opportunities in nursing are greater today than ever before and seem to be increasing constantly. Not only is there a need for many more nurses than are now available, but many nurses are needed in such clinical specialties as, medical-surgical nursing, maternal and child nursing, psychiatric nursing, rehabilitative nursing, and community or public health nursing. In addition there are such specialized fields as the military, government health field research, the Peace Corps, and international organizations like the World Health Organization, which require nurses who can function as supervisors or educators.

Traditionally nurses have worked in hospitals or other institutions, in private homes, or with the military in giving care to patients. As the field of health services developed, expanded, and became specialized, variations and job combinations extended far beyond the relatively simple nursing situations of 50 years ago.

CLINICAL SPECIALISTS

One of the newest and most exciting developments within nursing today is the development of the nurse clinician, or clinical nursing specialist. This evolving functional role, which is being established on an equal basis with the teacher and supervisor, re-

quires postgraduate educational preparation, usually on the master's level or beyond. Education at this level is financially available to almost any qualified applicant because of the large numbers of scholarships, fellowships, and educational grants and loans. An extensive list of these is available from the Committee on Careers, a joint ANA-NLN committee.

SPECIAL FIELDS OF NURSING PRACTICE
Anesthesia

Since the 1880's nurses have been administering anesthetics in America, and postgraduate instruction of nurses in anesthesiology was instituted about the same time. The first schools for teaching this specialty for nurses, however, were not organized until about 1910. Membership in the American Association of Nurse Anesthetists is open to all qualified nurse anesthetists.

Many states by law allow the administration of anesthetic by nurses. A case in the Supreme Court of California in 1946 decided that administration of anesthetic by a nurse was not contrary to the Medical Practice Act of that state. In no other state has the legality of nurse anesthetists been tested. As in other specialties in nursing, there is great need for nurse anesthetists, not only in civilian but also in military hospitals. The professional organization of this group is the American Association of Nurse An-

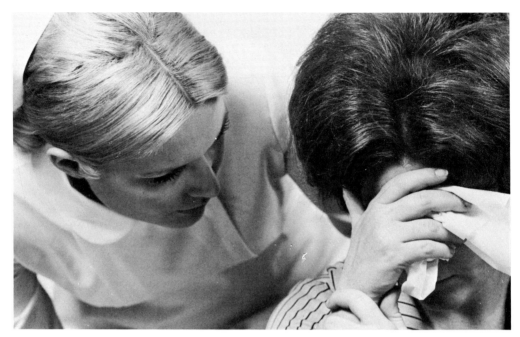

The nurse strives to understand the problems of the depressed patient. (From Mereness, Dorothy: Essentials of psychiatric nursing, ed. 8, St. Louis, 1970, The C. V. Mosby Co.)

esthetists, which publishes a quarterly journal, *Journal of the American Association of Nurse Anesthetists.*

Industrial nursing

Industrial nursing has expanded, as has industrial medicine, from first-aid stations to a complicated practice of industrial health. This field has been given great impetus since World War II. It is estimated that there are over 12,000 industrial nurses in this country. The industrial nurse needs technical skill to deal with diagnostic and treatment situations. She must come in close contact with all workers and their health problems. Knowledge of the health problems of the worker and his family combined with a knowledge of community resources helps industry to maintain health and individual productivity on as high a level as possible.

Requirements in this field are that the person be a registered nurse with a foundation of nursing skill in modern health work. Current state registration is necessary. In industrial work the nurse must like people, be able to work effectively on the health

team, and be able to work well with patients' families. Industrial nursing is extremely varied; for example, the industrial nurse may work in an industrial hospital or in an industry in which the services are comparable to those in outpatient departments.

Nurse-midwifery

The first school for nurse-midwifery in the United States was opened in 1932 by the Association for the Promotion and Standardization of Midwifery, Inc., in cooperation with the Maternity Center of New York. In 1935 the Lobenstein Midwifery Clinic was consolidated with the Maternity Center Association. During the first 20 years this school graduated 231 nurse-midwives, but with the growing recognition of the place of this professional worker, the demand for graduates has always far exceeded the supply.

At present several universities offer courses in nurse-midwifery. The one at the Johns Hopkins University School of Medicine and the one under the Faculty of Medi-

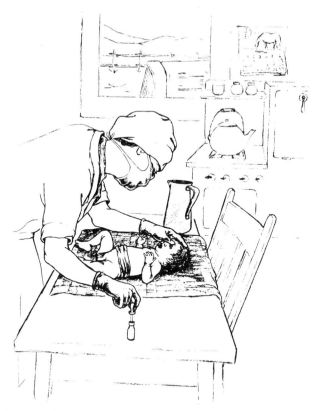

In certain rural areas of the United States where medical care is scarce, the nurse midwife often performs home deliveries.

cine of Columbia University have been developed in cooperation with the Maternity Center Association of New York. A third program is part of the facilities of the Yale Medical Center.

Schools preparing for the practice of nurse-midwifery are also operated by the Frontier Nursing Service in Lexington, Kentucky, and in Santa Fe, New Mexico. Historically, practice of this specialty has been in rural areas where there was inadequate prenatal care. A fascinating account of the development of the Frontier Nursing Service is found in *Nurse on Horse Back,* by Mary Breckinridge, founder of the service.

Nursing in the Department of Health, Education and Welfare

Under the Department of Health, Education and Welfare a nurse may work in one of the public health service hospitals serving seamen, personnel of the United States Coast Guard, officers of the Coast and Geodetic Survey, federal employees injured at work, and public health officers. The nurse may also work with the American Indian in one of the 56 Indian hospitals and clinics scattered through our states. Since 1956 the responsibility of the health of the Indian has been placed in the Department of Health, Education and Welfare.

In 1953 the Clinic Center opened in Bethesda, Maryland, as part of the National Institutes of Health of the United States Public Health Service. The National Institutes of Health include several institutes: heart, cancer, mental health, arthritis and metabolic diseases, neurological diseases and stroke, and allergies and infectious diseases. In the large 500-bed hospital, research and clinical care of patients are closely integrated. The nurse is a member not only of

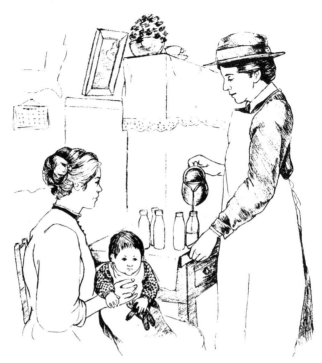

In the early 1900's the baby welfare nurse played an important role in starting a baby off on a long and healthy life.

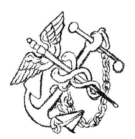

UNITED STATES
PUBLIC HEALTH SERVICE INSIGNIA

the patient care team but also of the research team.

Members of the United States Public Health Service do valuable work in the field of public health nursing by participating in studies, working on health teams in various control programs, and, when qualified, by serving as nurse consultants.

The United States Public Health Service has expanded its overseas program since World War II. These nurses serve in many areas of Latin America, Africa, the Near East, and the Far East. In the United States Public Health Service a graduate nurse, male or female, may enter either by appointment to its commissioned corps as a regular or reserve officer or through federal civil service employment.

The Army Nurse Corps

The Army Nurse Corps is the oldest of all the women's military services and is made up entirely of registered nurses representing all fields of nursing.

The Army-Navy Nurses Act of 1947 granted to nurses permanent commission status in the United States Army. An Army Nurse Corps section was established in the Officer Reserve Corps. Colonel Florence A. Blanchfield worked hard to achieve this and was the first woman to receive permanent commissioned rank of colonel. Not only the

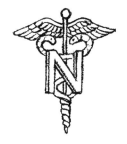

ARMY NURSE CORPS INSIGNIA

variety of service but also the security found in the military nursing fields may be attractive; for example, personnel policies, complete hospital, medical, surgical, and dental care when needed, limited health services for dependents, generous retirement benefits after 20 years of service, substantial allowance for initial purchase of officer's uniform, and, of course, pay increases for all grades, depending upon length of service.

In addition to such positions as head nurse, chief of nursing service, instructor, general duty nurse, and supervisor, many specialized positions such as an army health nurse, chief of nursing personnel, and nurse education coordinator exist. Specialists are needed in various fields and are given instruction by the army; for example, in operating room technic and management, in anesthesiology, in neuropsychiatric nursing, and in nursing and hospital administration. Through the army's information and education program, army nurses may enroll in extension and other collegiate courses at reduced rates.

Army nurses may serve in America or in any of the foreign stations in which the United States Army functions. Applicants must be registered professional nurses, citizens between the ages of 21 and 45, physically and professionally qualified, and graduates of schools acceptable to the Surgeon General. Married nurses are accepted for reserve appointments or extended active duty if they do not have dependent children under 18 year of age. Applicants must pass a physical examination conducted at an army or air force medical center or by a civilian physician at no expense to the government. For appointment as a second lieutentant, the nurse must be a high school graduate, have graduated from a basic nursing program, and meet citizenship and physical qualifications and moral requirements specified. As a first lieutenant the young nurse must meet the above requirements, be registered in the United States or United States territory, and have 15 semester hours in an accredited college or university, and three years' professional experience. A nurse currently certified by the American Association of Nurse Anesthetists with three years' professional experience in anesthesiology or experience within 24 months prior to the appointment may also be appointed as first lieutenant. For appointment as a captain the basic requirements for first lieutenant are needed plus a bachelor's degree from an accredited college or university, with the major field in nursing and seven years' experience including two years' teaching, supervising, or administration; or a master's degree from an accredited college or university, with the major field in nursing, allied medical science, or personnel field, and six years' experience, including two years' supervision or administration; or current certification by the American Association of Nurse Anesthetists and seven years of anesthesia practice, terminating not more than 24 months prior to the appointment.*

The Navy Nurse Corps

Today, navy nurses serve in the United States and abroad. Nurses in this military branch have an opportunity to practice all phases of nursing care for men and women of the navy and marine corps and their families. All initial appointments are made

*Young people interested in army nurse experience and information should apply to the Army Nurse Corps Counselor's Office, Headquarters Fifth Avenue, 1660 East Hyde Park Blvd., Chicago, Illinois 60615, or the Surgeon General, Department of the Army, Washington, D. C. 20315.

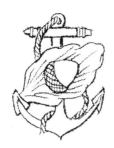

NAVY NURSE CORPS INSIGNIA

by the Nurse Corps, United States Naval Reserve. The basic qualifications for commission are that the individuals be graduates of schools of nursing whose educational and professional standards are approved by the surgeon general, United States Navy; currently registered at least in one state or the District of Columbia; high school graduate; a native-born or naturalized citizen of the United States; between the ages of 21 and 40 years; either single or married, but with no dependents under the age of 18 years; and physically qualified by the standards set up by the naval officers. Appointments are made in grades of ensign through lieutenant, senior grade, depending upon age and qualifications.

The functions of the navy nurse are to give bedside care to patients, to instruct hospital corpsmen, and to help in the management and supervision of wards and clinics. In addition to the officers the men and women of the armed forces and the families of the armed forces are also given care. As in the army, there is an extensive in-service educational program in all navy hospitals. Members of the Nurse corps may be assigned to attend educational programs in colleges and universities. All nurses are encouraged to continue their education.

In keeping with the development of educational programs, both in civilian and in military groups, the navy nurse postwar educational program was established in 1946. Navy nurses were assigned to schools for training in physiotherapy, anesthesiology, occupational therapy, dietetics, and ward ad-

ministration. In 1947 the Army Nurse Act established the nurse corps as a permanent staff corps of the United States Navy. Captian DeWitt became the first director of the permanent corps.

The Korean emergency of 1950 necessitated a recall of reserve nurses to help care for Korean casualties. In 1955 continued education for the navy nurse was stimulated by Public Law 20, called The Career Incentive Act, which provided incentives in increased pay and allowances. Later in the same year an educational program was instituted that allowed a limited number of hospital corps waves to enroll in approved collegiate schools of nursing with the expenses borne by the navy. Upon the satisfactory completion of this program these students are commissioned as ensigns in the Navy Nurse Corps Reserve.

During 1957 and 1958 educational programs were continued, and increases in salary and promotions resulted. In 1957 the Navy Nurse Corps Cadet Program permitted qualified students in approved collegiate schools of nursing to enlist during their final year in the school of nursing. Educational expenses are paid by the navy, and upon graduation from the school of nursing the nurses are commissioned as ensigns in the Navy Nurse Corps Reserve.

In May of 1958 the nurse corps proudly celebrated its golden anniversary, having established for itself, as other branches of the military have, an honored place in the military history of America.

The Air Force Nurse Corps

Until 1949 army medical personnel had been assigned to duty with the air force. Since that date, however, the Air Force Medical Service has become an entity distinct from the Army Medical Service. Since World War I, air force medicine had been concerned with such problems as lack of oxygen at high altitude, the forces and strains to which the human being is subjected because of great rates of speed, quick changes in temperature, and other areas now included in aviation medicine.

The United States Air Force Medical Service is composed of six groups of medical personnel: medical, veterinary, medical service, dental, women's medical specialist corp (dietitians, physiotherapists, and occupational therapists), and the Air Force Nurse Corps, which includes both the flight nurses and the air force nurses serving on the ground in air force hospitals.

During World War II official air evacuation was begun in 1942 when an Air Ambulance Battalion was organized at Fort Benning, Georgia. This was moved to Beaumont Field, Kentucky, later in the year, and training for flight nurses in air evacuation squadrons began. Flight teams consisting of one flight medical technician and one flight nurse were organized. The Flight Nurse School is now located at the Gunter branch of the Aviation School of Medicine, Gunter Air Force Base, Montgomery, Alabama.

Nurses entering the Air Force Nurse Corps today must be graduates of a nursing school acceptable to the Surgeon General, United States Air Force; have active registration in any state, territory, or the District of Columbia, and be physically and professionally qualified; be between the ages of 21 and 45 years, either married or single; and be citizens of the United States with high moral standards. Appointments are made from second lieutenant to major, depending upon age, professional experience, and educational equipment. The minimum tour of active duty is two years. Training programs and in-service education are an important part of the program.

The course of study includes such subjects as aviation physiology, psychology, nursing procedures for the in-flight care of patients, and the newest development in therapeutics. The course is difficult, but responsibilities as a flight nurse are great. Satisfactory completion of the course entitles the nurse to wear silver wings with an "N" superimposed upon them.

In addition to bedside nursing and the instruction and supervision of nonprofessional workers, a nurse may be assigned to many clinical specialties such as head nurse, supervisor, chief nurse, or administrative director. She may also go into one of the specialized fields—operating room supervision, nurse anesthetist, psychiatric nursing, or flight nursing. Personnel policies make it possible for both regular air force and reserve nurses to become eligible for retirement benefits. Regular air force nurses may retire after 20 years; retirement pay is determined by length of service and grade held. Reserve air force nurses may apply for retirement benefits after the age of 60 years, having completed 20 years of satisfactory active and/or reserve service. A number of regular and reserve air force personnel nurses are given university education leading to a degree, during which time they receive full pay and allowances. Other educational opportunities are made available through the United States Armed Forces Institute and the United States Air Force Extension Institute. The Air Force Nurse Corps, as true of other military branches, provides for health supervision and medical care. Physical examination is given at the time of appointment and repeated annually. Nurses receive immunization regularly, and hospitalization and sick leave are provided when required.

Aerospace nursing

A relatively new specialty developing within the Air Force Nurse Corps is aerospace nursing. An intensive 52-week course was initiated in 1965 at Patrick Air Force Base, Cape Kennedy, to equip nurses to function as part of the Bioastronautic Operational Support Unit. BOSU is engaged in intensive research on the effects of all forms of stress on healthy human beings. This research reveals new knowledge that can be applied here on earth as well as in space. Nurses working in BOSU are concerned not only with the care of the astronauts but also

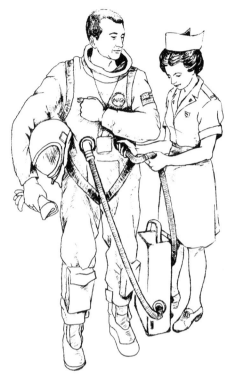

One of the most exciting fields in modern life, the space program, presents new opportunities for the nurse and her special skills.

with preparation for disaster on the test range.

Nursing service in the Veterans Administration

The history of the present nursing service of the Veterans Administration has a multiple origin, stemming principally from developments after World War I.

On May 1, 1922, as the result of an executive order signed by the President, 46 hospitals of the United States Public Health Service were transferred to the jurisdiction of the Veterans' Bureau. This resulted in the transfer to the Veterans' Bureau of 12,069 World War I veterans and 10,251 hospital personnel, including 1,420 professional nurses. Also 755 commissioned medical officers in the Public Health Service were detailed to the Veterans' Bureau. All personnel other than physicians were converted to civil service status. Thus for the first time a superintendent of nurses and an assistant superintendent were assigned to the Veterans' Bureau in Washington, D. C.

The passage of Public Law 293 by the Seventy-ninth Congress, January 3, 1946, raised the status of the nursing service immeasurably. Shortly before this the Civil Service Commission had changed the classification of nurses from subprofessional to professional. While this was a step forward, Public Law 293 removed them from civil service, making them members of the Department of Medicine and Surgery of the Veterans Administration, along with doctors and dentists. Salaries were made commensurate with their professional qualifications, regardless of duties performed. Many highly qualified nurses were attracted to the new department. The Veterans Administration has been a leader among the federal nursing services in the utilization of the services of men nurses. Currently 500 men nurses are employed within the hospital system.

The Veterans Administration is the third largest federal agency, serving some 28 million veterans. The nursing service is the largest service of its kind in the United States and offers unusual career opportunities to nurses with varied professional interests. It employs 50,519 persons, including 18,863 professional nurses. They staff 168 hospitals, besides having 202 clinics and 63 nursing homes.

In 1972 the number of inpatients totaled 855,000, and the outpatient service facilities extended to over 8 million.

The present director of nursing service (1973) is Virginia B. Longest, and her deputy director is Gloria S. Hope.

The Peace Corps

The Peace Corps presents that great opportunity for "people to help people" directly in providing economic, social, or educational assistance. The cause of peace is thus advanced through mutual understand-

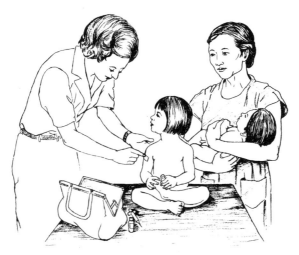

The Peace Corps volunteer is called upon to practice a wide range of nursing skills.

ing, personal love and affection, and by sharing.

The corps came into being on March 1, 1961, when President Kennedy issued an executive order establishing the corps on a provisional basis. Congress established the Peace Corps permanently on September 21, 1961. Objectives defined by the act for the Peace Corps are to promote world peace and friendship by making available to interested countries Americans who will do the following:

1. Help the people of these countries meet their needs for trained manpower
2. Help promote a better understanding of the American people on the part of the peoples served
3. Help promote a better understanding of other peoples on the part of the American people

Registered nurses are in demand by the Peace Corps, and any registered nurse or student nurse in her last year of nursing school, regardless of age, who is a United States citizen may apply for service as a Peace Corps volunteer. Volunteers must be in excellent physical and mental health. After an intensive Peace Corps training designed to prepare volunteers for effective service overseas, a nurse will be sent to any one of 20 countries in Latin America, Africa, the Near East, South East Asia, or South West Asia.*

MEN IN NURSING

According to the 1958-1960 census figures there were 440,355 nurses in the United States. Of this total, men nurses comprised 1%; this made them the smallest subprofessional group in the health field in the United States. The history of men in nursing extends back through the history of the Christian Era. It reached its height during the time of the Crusades when the flowering of European manhood were members of the various military religious orders whose essential work was nursing and hospital administration. Their many hospitals and holdings dotted the countryside of Europe. Some remnants of these orders still remain, but for the most part, the role of men in modern nursing in the United States began about 1888 when the first school of nursing for men was established at Bellevue Hospital in New York City. It was named the Mills School, after Ogden Mills who had en-

---

*To apply, write to the Professional and Technical Division, Peace Corps, Washington, D. C. 20325.

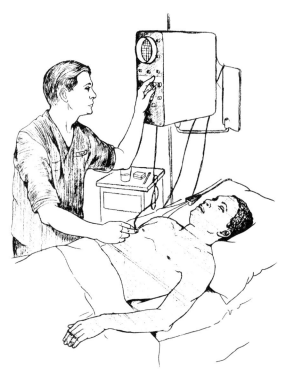

Nursing is becoming an increasingly popular occupation for men as it expands in scope, especially in the associate degree programs.

dowed the school. Except for the war years, this school has been in operation continuously. Many other schools of nursing for men have since developed. It is, however, only recently that men have been admitted into regular schools of nursing in any large numbers. The percentage of men in nursing schools, particularly in the associate degree programs, is much higher than the 1% of nursing practitioners from this group would indicate.

ECONOMIC SECURITY

The years 1964 through 1973 were ones of ferment and turmoil for nursing. All over the country, courageous nurses banded together for the first time in history to act as a cohesive social force in a battle to win improved working conditions and increased economic security.

The first major victory, which received national attention from the public, was won by over 3,500 nurses employed in the New York City Department of Hospitals. Negotiations begun in May, 1965, were concluded one year later, just five days before the nurses' resignations would have become effective. National news was also made by nurses who resigned, or threatened to resign, in Chicago, San Francisco, and Los Angeles. It was not just in the giant metropolises that these actions occurred, however. The ANA Economic Security Unit reported over 140 "situations" all over the country in the first six months of 1966.

The public's support was behind nursing when they learned that the resignations, "slow downs," and "strikes" were not only over salaries but also because of hospital conditions that made adequate patient care impossible. Major contractual concessions included establishment of committees to examine nursing and non-nursing duties and released time and reimbursement for attending professional meetings and workshops.

The most significant gain, however, has been substantial salary increases across the country. At the biennial convention of the American Nurses' Association in 1966 the House of Delegates adopted a resolution calling for a minimum base salary of $6,500. In a nationwide press conference about this salary goal, Jo Eleanor Elliott, ANA President, said, "If quality care is to be assured to all persons, salaries of nurses must be more attractive. Today's salaries discourage the recruitment of qualified young people. We know, too, that many married nurses with young children cannot afford to practice their profession; the salaries they can earn are not enough to compensate them for costs of child care. Substantial increases in salaries are required to regain the services of many nurses."

CONCLUSION

In a dynamic society any fundamental function such as nursing is bound to change if it is to meet the needs of the society. Nursing functions today range from uncomplicated activities such as those dealing mainly with personal hygiene or assisting with and carrying out relatively simple procedures to complex ones demanding not only expert skill, judgment, and technical experience but also knowledge in such fields as sociology, psychology, social work, and other health, social, and welfare areas.

The very nature of nursing and the wide range of functions from the relatively simple to the complex have resulted in the need for more than one kind of nurse.

The educational programs for preparation of nurses today are changing to meet the changing demands made on the profession. Conditions are progressing so rapidly that changes may be made in the program during a student's own experience in school.

In such fields as industrial nursing, anesthesiology, office nursing, nursing in vari-

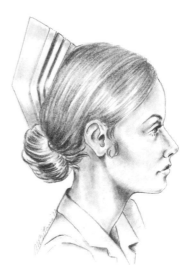

UNIVERSITY HOSPITAL OF
GOOD SHEPHERD GRADUATE NURSE

ous health agencies, and such administrative positions as those with state and national nursing organizations, we find ever-growing specialization, resulting in constantly increasing job opportunities.

Many married nurses continue nursing, either part or full time. Although there was a traditional attitude against married nurses, and particularly against any student's getting married, during World War II and the following years this attitude has changed as has the situation: the number of married women in all industries has increased steadily.

It is becoming more and more important for nurses to take an active part in community activities, in addition to belonging to professional organizations. Until relatively recent times all professional nurses except the few in public health nursing lived highly institutionalized lives and even after graduation continued to live in the nurses' residence, with little opportunity or wish for outside activities.

The demand for nurses continues to outrun the supply. Increasing demands from hospitals and expanding community health services, industry, military services, and international programs have all contributed to this shortage. It is important for young people to know that opportunities in nursing are likely to continue and to expand in the coming years.

Since World War II new hospitals have been built in many communities and old hospitals have increased their facilities. It has not been uncommon to find that many institutions have not been able to expand as rapidly as needed because of the scarcity of nurses and other health personnel. Many agencies, both civilian and military, yearly report shortages. It must be remembered that the problem of nursing shortage is one of quality as well as quantity.

There are demands for nurses with the broad training that can be obtained in collegiate programs. Graduate programs equip individuals for leadership, particularly in administrative, supervisory, teaching, and clinical specializations. Because of the development of specialization in functional areas as well as in the clinical areas, great demands are placed upon nurses for additional education and experience. Thus the young person wishing to function effectively today in any clinical area finds that he or she must take postgraduate work. It is an era of specialization, and the great wealth of information that must be mastered by anyone practicing in a special field necessitates education beyond what it is possible to give to any undergraduate nursing student. The effective nurse today must know a great deal more than the nurse of 25 years ago.

Newly discovered drugs and treatments, the implementation of the concept of the relationship betweeen emotions and physical illness, and new knowledge about people and disease have necessitated programs of continuing education for all workers in the health fields.

To better utilize all professional workers, studies are being made to discover more effective ways of using all personnel to meet health needs. Practical nurses, hospital aides, clerical workers, and other professional workers, such as dietitians, social workers, and occupational therapists, can often work on a team basis with the nurse and the doctor to provide better care than we have been accustomed to in the past.

The nurse shortage in 1953 was attributed to five major factors.

1. The shortage of young women in the population.
2. The increase among young women with home responsibilities.
3. Nurses' salaries and the cost of education.
4. Higher professional requirements.
5. The present utilization of professional nursing personnel.*

These factors were valid because of the maturation of the decreased number of "depression babies" from the early 1930's. However, at this time, although there is no shortage of young women in the population, nursing is not attracting a proportionate number of young people.

In February, 1963, the surgeon general's report identified the following as problems and reasons for the continuing shortage:

Too few schools are providing adequate education for nursing.

Not enough capable young people are being recruited to meet the demand.

Too few college-bound students are entering the nursing field.

More nursing schools are needed within colleges and universities.

The continuing lag in the social and economic status of nurses discourages people from entering the field and remaining active in it.

Available nursing personnel are not being fully utilized for effective patient care, including supervision and teaching as well as clinical care.

Too little research is being conducted on the advancement of nursing practice.†

---

*Professional nursing occupations, Medical Services Series, Bulletin No. 203-3, revised, United States Department of Labor, Women's Bureau, Washington, D. C., 1953, Government Printing Office, pp. 20 ff.

†Report of the Surgeon General's Consultant Group on Nursing, United States Department of Health, Education and Welfare, Public Health Service, Public Health Publication No. 992, Feb., 1963.

The increase in the number of nurses has been almost double that of the population increase in the past decade, and there is still a decided shortage. To add further complications, every prediction indicates a continuing population explosion that will demand more nursing care. Even the modest proposed goal of 300 nurses per 100,000 population in 1960 reached only 282 per 100,000 by 1970.

CHAPTER 30 MAJOR TRENDS AFFECTING HEALTH CARE

■ The community's interest in matters of health has always been accelerated by war; even when the acute war need is past, that interest is found to be at a higher level in all matters of health at the end of a war than at the beginning. Since World War II the field of public health has expanded in many directions. Many communities have increased the size and scope of existing health facilities or have built additional ones with the aid of funds from both voluntary and governmental sources. Most middle-class Americans are covered by some form of health insurance either to pay possible hospitalization expenses or to provide for payment of other medical expenses. Mass media bombard us with information and misinformation about health and illness. All these factors contribute to an increase in the utilization of existing health facilities and a public demand for quality.

MAJOR TRENDS

Among major factors influencing health care and the provisions of health services are the following:

1. There has been a surge of knowledge within the health sciences concerning people and diseases. This increased knowledge has led to technological development which refines the quality of care that can be provided for people but makes the administration of that care far more complex than it was 10 or 15 years ago.

2. A true revolutionary change has taken place in diagnosis and treatment, resulting from the numbers of people outside the medical field who have contributed to scientific discoveries of biochemistry, technological equipment, and the psychosocial aspects of medicine. This is particularly true of many of the newer drugs, beginning with the discovery of penicillin by Sir Alexander Fleming, a biologist. Renal dialysis, the heart-lung machine, various monitoring devices, closed-circuit television, computers, and radioactive isotopes are only a sampling of the complex treatments and equipment invented or perfected by nonmedical workers and used in present-day hospitals.

3. The provision of health services has changed radically as a result of increased knowledge and the use of newer technological devices. Knowledge and management of the machines require rigorous scientific training of responsible health personnel.

4. A recent basic change in the way in which Americans view health has exerted a profound change on the provision of health services. When health is seen as a right, rather than a privilege, then society assumes an obligation to provide this service to its

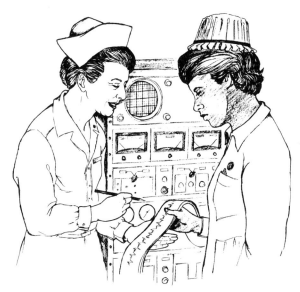

The nurse plays a vital role in those aspects dealing with patient care as the use of technological equipment increases.

members, regardless of their ability to pay for it. The British Health Service exemplifies one form of this. In the United States, Medicare on the federal level provides financial access to this right for all our citizens over age 65. There has been discussion of proposing legislation which would provide similar facilities for dependent children as well. These forms of health insurance not only make care available to the particular citizens for whom it is designed, but also serve to upgrade the quality of the facilities of care in many regions. Indirectly, therefore, all people are benefited through these official governmental actions.

5. Because of the nurse shortage, more and more schools of practical nursing have been established and continue to grow at an accelerated rate. These have been encouraged and supported by federal funds. A whole corps of auxiliary personnel, such as aides and volunteers, has been added to the staff of hospital wards.

6. The pattern of incidence of patient illness has undergone vast change in the last generation. The emphasis in hospitals is upon early discharge. The patient's condition is followed up by health workers, including the public health nurse. The treatment of long-term illness is through outpatient and extended-care facilities.

7. The patients' expectations have also changed. Because of effective means of communication, patients know more about particular diseases. The World Health Organization's concept of health has become operational; we no longer think of health in terms of the absence of disease but as a state of physical, mental, and social well-being.

8. More people now receive direct medical supervision. In other words, more people are being cared for constantly. Almost all industrial plants have nurses educated to follow the entire work force. Colleges, for the most part, now have a medical officer. Grade school children are placed under supervision at the time they enter school, and their health records are kept for them through elementary school, high school, college, and at work. In the larger cities

these children have already been registered at well-baby clinics shortly after birth. Medicare now assures retired workers of the financial ability to continue to receive competent health supervision.

9. The continued emancipation of women has had its effect upon health care. Although more and more women enter the labor market, the opportunities for employment in service occupations are increasing. Unfortunately the predominantly female occupation of nursing no longer has the first claim on young women it previously enjoyed. The percentage of eligible young women electing nursing as a career has steadily declined over the past decades from 7% in the 1950's to 5% in the 1960's. The Bureau of Labor Statistics of the Department of Labor projects an increase in the demand for workers in the health service industries of about 45% between 1966 and 1975 (from 3.7 to 5.35 million).

10. The phenomenon of the "college-bound" youth in America probably accounts for the tremendous growth of the junior/community colleges. By 1970, nursing programs within these institutions had increased 445%. Besides nursing, many other health careers have established educational programs under the aegis of the junior/community college. The Department of Health, Education and Welfare lists 27 categories of health workers, both professional and technical.

11. The population explosion that occurred after World War II gave great impetus to development of the family planning movement. Contraceptive technics had been available for a selected segment of the population prior to this time. As the number of babies being born increased, the desire on the part of society to limit the population explosion as well as the choice on the part of

parents to space their children spurred the development of more effective technics as well as more universal dispersal of information about these technics.

These trends all demonstrate the dynamism of health care and the internal and external pressures upon nursing and other health services to change. What is true today most certainly will not be valid ten years from now. This compounds the existing internal struggle in nursing to identify its unique role within the health team and to differentiate the preparation and function of its various practitioners.

CONTEMPORARY SOCIAL AND HEALTH PROBLEMS

Between 1900 and 1952 the nation's population doubled. The birth rate continued to increase until 1973, when the population birth rate was reduced to zero, primarily through education, the new social status of women, and more effective methods of birth control. People are living longer. Statistics show that the number of individuals 65 years of age or over had grown from 3 to 11½ million and by 1960 had reached 15½ million. Hospital admissions in 1966 totaled over 29 million. In addition there were more than 100 million visits to outpatient and emergency departments.

This utilization of health agencies has been the result of health education, the growing confidence in hospitals by all people, the complicated medical and health treatments that necessitate a hospital environment in which to operate, and insurance and hospital plans that enable individuals to pay for hospital care. New medical technics and drugs have helped to shorten the average patient's stay in the hospital from 18 to 8 days. While in the hospital most patients need skilled nursing care.

Public health services have been extended in all communities; industrial nursing, school nursing, and bedside nursing in the home have increased as rapidly as trained personnel and institutions are available. The requirements of the military and the Veterans Administration continue to increase and make demands upon professional and nonprofessional nursing personnel.

Life expectancy in the United States has increased. With more individuals living to be over 60 years of age, the incidence of degenerative diseases is on the increase. The development of communicable disease control and better child welfare programs have resulted in a great decrease in contagious diseases. Such conditions as smallpox, diphtheria, and typhoid fever have been almost eliminated in many communities. Heart disease, cancer, and kidney disease rank high as the causes of death. Chronic illnesses associated with degenerative diseases are more frequent.

Changes in morbidity and mortality patterns mean that the nurse needs a different type of preparation now than was needed 25 or 50 years ago. Prevention and better treatment are slowly taking the place of custodial care of the mentally ill. However, many states are still so hampered by the lack of finances, trained personnel, and adequate institutions that custodial care for the mentally ill and for patients with chronic illnesses still prevails. There has been a real reduction in maternal and infant mortality as well as improvement in the diagnosis and treatment of many heretofore incurable conditions. Chemotherapy has revolutionized the treatment of many severe illnesses.

The effects of President Truman's commission to study the health needs of the nation are still being felt. A great deal of this report dealt with health personnel, that is, physicians, dentists, nurses, and paramedical technicians. This report emphasized the concept of the medical team with doctors and nurses serving as leaders of teams with other auxiliary medical workers and technicians. As medicine has become more specialized, a need has been created for workers with special education in many fields closely allied to medicine. With the expansion of preventive, psychiatric, and rehabilitative services has come a demand for auxiliary workers in these fields. As a result there are more than 30 paramedical specialists, such as medical laboratory technicians, x-ray technicians, dietitians, physical

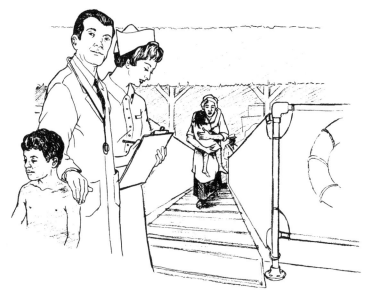

Health teams, such as those provided by project HOPE, expand good will and provide much needed medical care in less fortunate areas of the world.

therapists, speech therapists, medical record librarians, social workers, clinical psychologists, hospital administrators, and many others whose education ranges from one year after high school to several years after college. Such education is invariably expensive and often beyond the financial ability of an average student. The federal government has assumed an increasing share of the costs of both professional and technical education in the health fields through direct scholarship aid as well as through indirect subsidization of both students and schools via project and construction grants and loans. Much of this federal assistance has been provided through the Bureau of Health Manpower under the Health Professions Educational Assistance Act of 1963, the Nurse Training Act of 1964, the Allied Health Professions Personnel Training Act of 1966, the Nurse Training Act amendments of 1968, and the Nurse Training Act of 1971.

One problem in all communities is that of providing adequate facilities and educating adequate personnel to use the facilities and to provide the type of medical health care we now know individuals and communities need.

Changes in the patterns of illness have created the need for not only a different kind of education but also a different type of hospital construction; for example, instead of hospitals for communicable diseases, more facilities are needed for extended care of the mentally and physically disabled and chronic custodial care.

One of the great difficulties in providing adequate care for everyone in the United States is that health workers and health facilities are located in the urban centers. A better distribution of health institutions and health personnel is a problem that is being studied by medical, health, and nursing organizations—state, regional, and federal. To study this problem the Hill-Burton Act, 1946, provided assistance to the states to plan and provide modern hospitals and public health facilities. States, with the help of the federal government, made studies, and Congress authorized an appropriation for the construction of hospital and allied facilities.

Not too long ago nurses, graduate and student, did all the nursing necessary in both hospital and community. Nursing was relatively simple and usually included personal hygiene measures and technics to make the patient comfortable, such as bathing, changing his position, and giving a few medications, usually by mouth. Nursing has increased in complexity as nurses have assumed such functions as the administration of parenteral medication, collection of specimens, and participation in the performance of complicated diagnostic tests as well as therapeutic procedures, all of which require increased vigilance and careful observation of the patient.

To carry out the increased number and variety of activities, more personnel are needed to help at the less technical level. Therefore the practical nurse and the nurses' aide, the ward clerk, the unit manager, and the messenger have been added to the team. Until quite recently there was some resistance to the practical nurse. At first the practical nurse was an untrained person who, because of her aptitude for nursing and her interest in it, became a useful person in the hospital and community. As the duties given to the practical nurse increased, it became apparent that a formal course of education must be worked out and that this group should be licensed.

Since World War II the number of approved schools of practical nursing has increased nationally. Most of these have developed in the vocational department of the board of education. Many obtain funds from the federal government, as well as from the state, to develop a program. All this instruction in approved schools for practical nursing is under the direction of professional nurses. Today all states have some type of licensure for nurses.

INFLUENCE OF HOSPITALS AS MAJOR HEALTH FACILITIES

In most public health work the hospital looms in the background either for diagnosis and treatment or for the care of specialized conditions. Even now most active nurses spend their lives in close contact with the hospital.

In the evolution of the hospital several influences operate with varying force at different periods.

1. The community has always found it expedient to isolate its members if they suffer from loathsome or contagious diseases; thus pesthouses, leper houses, and lunatic asylums developed. To this day the motive of the isolation hospital is quite as much protection of society as it is care of the patient.

2. The second important motive is charity toward the sick, particularly the sick poor. This was an important motive as early as in the ancient Indian hospitals. It was all-important in the hospitals of the Middle Ages under the auspices of the church and was strongly emphasized when nursing was "born" again a hundred years ago. It was important to Miss Nightingale and those she inspired. In the modern hospital, personal charity is most apparent in the strictly denominational hospital; in the others, nondenominational, university, or government (city, state, or federal) hospitals, the directly charitable relation has yielded to an impersonal acknowledgment that the community must look after its citizens when they are sick and cannot take care of themselves. It is a twentieth century version of altruism, which, although less personal, may be more acceptable to the patient who receives it.

3. The third motive is the facilities for instruction that the hospital offers. Although doctors were not necessarily a part of the primitive hospital, they became increasingly important in it. The modern hospital is unthinkable without a medical staff. The establishment of medical schools within, or closely allied to, hospitals greatly stimulated the growth of hospitals. As medical training became more complicated, the demands on the hospital grew; today almost every outstanding hospital is committed to the training of doctors. A similar relationship of nursing schools to hospitals developed much later. Until recently, organized nursing education had been financed by hospitals.

4. The hospital is essential for expansion of medical knowledge. Originally a doctor grew wiser from personal experience supplemented by books. Thus wisdom is acquired; however, the validity of clinical impressions must be tested before they can be accepted. It became necessary to rely not on individual scattered clinical impressions but on large numbers of cases observed under more or less similar conditions. The modern hospital has facilities for carrying out investigative procedures that would be impractical or impossible at home.

5. Finally, in recent years the best practice of medicine has required a large number of technical procedures that necessitate a specially constructed plant. It is difficult to arrange outside the hospital a substitute for the modern operating room, x-ray department, clinical laboratory with all its branches, and the nutrition department. Although these department have reached their present high state of development within the memory of living man, they have, nevertheless, grown to become one of the most important reasons for the existence of the modern hospital.

With all this the hospital is an expensive business. Three billion dollars are invested in American hospitals, and the cost per patient has escalated with the economy. This increased cost of medical care has created a new problem, which has

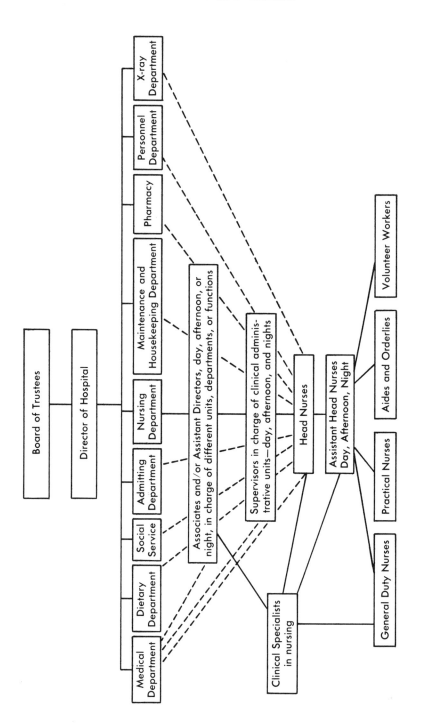

Simplified chart showing organization of a hospital without a school of nursing.

been subjected to repeated analysis. The old voluntary hospital, run entirely on gifts, is almost obsolete. Increasing costs threaten to exceed voluntary contributions, and increasing taxes prevent the accumulation of wealth from which gifts can be made. The hospital financed by local or federal government has generally been restricted to providing care for the indigent; yet most people who become sick cannot pay the entire cost of the medical aid that they receive. The financial structure of hospitals is constantly changing to meet these difficulties; public funds are more available to fill the gap between the amount patients can pay and the cost of their care. The hospital is becoming a public service. On the other hand, attempts are being made to spread the cost over large groups of persons by group hospital insurance schemes. When each person pays a little each month, funds can be accumulated to carry the load for the individual when he is least able to shoulder it. During World War II and in the postwar period a great increase in community interest called attention to the need for volunteer workers. Individuals for the first time in history began to learn about their hospitals by working in them. Individuals who are asked to support hospitals naturally have become interested. They want to know how the hospital is being administered and believe they should have a share in knowing how their money, whether tax or voluntary contributions, is being spent.

Hospitals may be classified in two general ways—first by type of service offered and second by ownership or control. In 1951 the American Medical Association found that nongovernment or private hospitals comprise almost 70% of the hospitals in this country and government hospitals, 30%. Church and religious groups have from pioneer days controlled and administered many of our hospitals. This is reflected by the national hospital organizations: the American Hospital Association, the Catholic Hospital Association, and the American Protestant Hospital Association. The mod-

ern hospital is a diagnostic, therapeutic, preventive, rehabilitative, and educational institution, as well as one carrying on the traditional functions of providing health facilities and services. With medical progress, specialization within the hospital has revolutionized hospital administration and construction. The chart on p. 206 shows the many different departments necessary in the modern hospital. All this has added tremendously to the cost of hospital care. So much money has been invested in the modern hospital that, unless hospitals are carefully and skillfully administered, the cost of medical care could be exorbitant.

The patient today knows about many new diagnostic and therapeutic aids and demands them; therefore the modern hospital has to be equipped to give such service. The hospital has to meet standards set by the state, by the American Hospital Association, and by the American College of Surgeons. One of the most outstanding achievements of the American College of Surgeons has been hospital standardization. This movement, begun in 1918, was aimed at giving the patient the best professional, scientific, and humanitarian care possible. A survey made by the American College of Surgeons in 1944 showed that 80.6% surveyed met the high standards. The Catholic Hospital Association and the American Protestant Hospital Association cooperate in maintaining these standards. Because of advances in transportation, modern medical centers are usually located in large cities where not only professional personnel but also scientific and technical equipment are concentrated. Today the large modern hospitals are usually situated in urban centers, with smaller hospitals in outlying towns, from which patients are brought for the more complicated treatments and surgical operations.

The educational and community functions of the modern hospital have been well expressed by a leading hospital administrator in the following statements:

1. Develop public understanding and appreciation of hospital service.

2. Foster an attitude of genuine good will on the part of the public toward the hospital.
3. Stimulate a more accurate analysis of community needs and institutional resources so that the hospital may assume its rightful place in the life of the community.
4. Promote a greater desire on the part of the personnel to understand the work of the hospital and to effect closer contact between the personnel and the public.
5. Cooperate with other health agencies in the community so as to meet more adequately the health and welfare needs of the community.
6. Clarify to the public and to governmental bodies the status of voluntary hospitals so that the many economic problems now being controversially discussed may be solved in the most desirable manner.
7. Effect a thorough understanding as to the legitimate reasons for hospital construction, make known the disadvantages of overhospitalization, and stimulate the greater use of existing hospital facilities.
8. Remove the influence of politics from governmentally owned and controlled institutions.
9. Explain the reasons for hospital standards—what they are, how they protect human life and promote safer and more adequate care of the sick and injured.
10. Encourage the public to look to national organizations cooperating with hospitals for information and guidance in problems of health and welfare.
11. Clarify to the public the position of the hospital as the principal source of skilled and continuous nursing so that it may be generally understood that this service is available to the community.
12. Improve the health and welfare conditions of the community by encouraging the use of hos-

pital facilities in the periodic health examination.
13. Promote closer cooperation and integration of all hospitals in each community and entirely eliminate any spirit of competition.
14. Encourage the use of the hospital by people previously fearful of institutional care.
15. Stimulate voluntary contributions and public and private endowments.*

CONCLUSION

A dynamic society and a period when rapid change is taking place result in strain on existing institutions and professions. This is noted particularly in such traditional institutions as the hospital and such traditional professions as medicine and nursing. No longer is the old method of treating disease adequate and no longer is the old method of educating doctors and nurses satisfactory to meet the demands placed on these workers by society. Hospitals, health agencies, and professional organizations are striving hard to change in constructive ways in order to meet these needs. National and state medical, nursing, and health professions are constantly studying the activities of their workers and striving to adjust the educational qualifications so that they will be able to function more effectively in contemporary society.

---

*MacEachern, Malcolm T.: Hospital organization and management, Chicago, 1940, Physicians' Record Co., pp. 796-797.

CHAPTER 31 THE NURSE PRACTITIONER

■ The role of nurse practitioner is sometimes described as the expanded role of the nurse and is rapidly developing because of the need for a new system of health care delivery. Another reason for the expansion is the expenditure of federal funds under the Nurse Training Act of 1971. The American Nurses' Association's definition of the term follows:

A nurse practitioner is a licensed professional nurse who provides direct care to individuals, families and other groups in a variety of settings including homes, institutions, offices, industry, schools and other community agencies. The service provided by the nurse practitioner is aimed at the delivery of primary, acute or chronic care which focuses on the achievement, maintenance or restoration of optimal functions in the population. The nurse practitioner engages in independent decision making about the nursing care needs of clients and collaborates with other health professionals, such as physicians, social workers and nutritionists, in making decisions about other health care needs. The nurse practitioner plans and institutes health care programs as a member of the health care team.

The acquisition of knowledge in depth and competence in skill performance in a particular field of practice enables this practitioner to:
1. Assess the physical and psychosocial health-illness status of individuals and families by health and developmental history taking and physical examinations.
2. Evaluate and interpret data in order to plan and execute appropriate nursing intervention.
3. Engage in decision making and implementation of therapeutic actions cooperatively with other members of the health care team.

This practitioner institutes and provides health care to patients within established regimens such as supervising and managing normal pregnancy and delivery, pediatric health supervision and diagnostic screening. The nurse practitioner provides counseling, health teaching and support to individuals and families.

The nurse practitioner is directly accountable and responsible to the recipient for the quality of care rendered.

For the purposes of interpreting the Nurse Training Act of 1971 the term "nurse practitioner" refers to one who has completed a program of study leading to competence as a registered nurse in an expanded role whose responsibility encompasses:

1. Obtaining a health history.
2. Assessing health-illness status.
3. Entering a person into the health care system.
4. Sustaining and supporting persons who are impaired, infirm, ill and during programs of diagnosis and therapy.
5. Managing a medical care regimen for acute and chronically ill patients within established standing orders.
6. Aiding in restoring persons to wellness and maximum function.
7. Teaching and counseling persons about health and illness.
8. Supervising and managing care regimens of normal pregnant women.
9. Helping parents in guidance of children with a view to their optimal physical and emotional development.
10. Counseling and supporting persons with regard to the aging process.
11. Aiding people and their survivors during the dying process.
12. Supervising assistants to nurses.

More than $6 million in contracts has been awarded by the Department of Health, Education and Welfare to train registered nurses for new and expanded responsibilities as nurse practitioners since the Nurse Training Act of 1971 authorized such training.

In making these awards the Division of Nursing director, Jessie M. Scott, said, "By preparing nurses in all areas of practice for expanded roles in the primary care and teaching of patients we can reduce gaps in medical services and bring quality health care to greater numbers of people. In these contracts we are focusing on improving care both in hospitals and out in the community, for entire families as well as individual patients."

The type of training includes the following:

1. Pediatric nurse practitioner
2. Pediatric and maternal nurse practitioner
3. Nurse midwifery
4. Medical nurse practitioner
5. Family nurse practitioner

Independent nurse practitioner

Whether nurses setting up an independent practice will become a trend in nursing is not certain. However, after 25 years in nursing, Lucille Kinlein, assistant professor, Georgetown University School of Nursing, Washington, D. C., established an independent practice in 1971 and set up her office in a residential section of College Park, Maryland. Her ultimate purpose is to provide and improve health care for persons somewhat lost in the present health care delivery system.

REFERENCES

A conceptual model of organized primary care and comprehensive community health services, Rockville, Maryland, Public Health Service, Health Services and Mental Health Administration, Community Health Service, Division of Health Care Services, United States Department of Health, Education and Welfare, 1970.

American Nurses' Association and American Academy of Pediatrics: Guidelines on short-term continuing education programs for pediatric nurse associates, American Journal of Nursing 71:509-512, March, 1971.

Andrews, P., Yankauer, A., and Connelly, J. P.: Changing the patterns of ambulatory pediatric caretaking: an action-oriented training program for nurses, American Journal of Public Health 60:870-879, 1970.

Bates, B.: Doctor and nurse: changing roles and relations, New England Journal of Medicine 283:129, 1970.

Birk, Peter, Ward, Thomas, and Dutton, Cynthia: Problem oriented analysis of medical care episodes—a new evaluation model, Presented before American Public Health Association Ninty-ninth Annual Meeting, Minneapolis, Minn., Medical Care Section, 1971.

Carnegie Commission on the Future of Higher Education: Higher education and the nation's health, policies for medical and dental education; a special report and recommendations, New York, 1970, McGraw-Hill Book Co.

Collins, M. C., and Bonnyman, G. G.: Physician's assistants and nurse associates: a review, Washington, D. C., 1971, The Institute for the Study of Health and Society.

Committee on Nursing: Medicine and nursing in the 1970s—a position statement, Jounral of the American Medical Association 213:1881, 1970.

Driscoll, Veronica: Liberating nursing practice, Nursing Outlook 20:24-28, January, 1972.

Health resources statistics, health manpower and health facilities, 1970, Public Health Service Publication No. 1509, Rockville, Maryland, Public Health Service, Health Services and Mental Health Administration, National Center for Health Statistics, United States Department of Health, Education and Welfare, 1971, p. 139.

Kinlein, M. Lucille: Independent nurse practitioner, Nursing Outlook 20:22-24, January, 1972.

Lambertsen, Eleanor C.: Perspective on the physician's assistant, Nursing Outlook 20:32-36, January, 1972.

Murray, B. Louise: A case for independent group nursing practice, Nursing Outlook 20:60-63, January, 1972.

National Commission for the Study of Nursing and Nursing Education: An abstract for action, New York, 1970, McGraw-Hill Book Co.

New members of the physician's health team: physician's assistants, report of the Ad Hoc Panel on New Members of the Physician's Health Team of the Board on Medicine of the National Academy of Sciences, 1970.

Rogers, Martha E.: Nursing: to be or not to be? Nursing Outlook 20:42-46, January, 1972.

Selected training programs for physician support personnel, Bethesda, Maryland, National Institutes of Health, Bureau of Health Professions Education and Manpower Training, United States Department of Health, Education and Welfare, 1970.

Shetland, Margaret L.: An approach to role expansion—the elaborate network, American Journal of Public Health **61:**41-46, October, 1971.

Silver, H. K., and Hecker, J. A.: The child health advocate: University of Colorado trains a new type of health professional, Hospitals **44:**47-49, 1970.

Silver, H. K., and Hecker, J. A.: The pediatric nurse practitioner and the child health associate: new types of health professionals, Journal of Medical Education **45:**171-176, 1970.

Walker, A. Elizabeth: PRIMEX—the family nurse practitioner program, Nursing Outlook **20:**28-31, January, 1972.

Weed, Lawrence L.: Medical records. Medical education and patient care, Cleveland Ohio, 1970, The Press of Case Western Reserve University.

Young, Lucie S.: Physician's assistants and the law, Nursing Outlook **20:**36-41, January, 1972.

CHAPTER 32 CONTINUING EDUCATION

■ Because of the explosion of knowledge and new techniques in medicine and health care, continuing education for the health care worker is actually being made mandatory by the legislatures in some states, which are encouraged by the national organizations, federal government, and many state nurses' associations.

The Special Committee on Continuing Education of the New York State Student Nurses' Association approved the following recommendations for New York State in the fall of 1971:

a. That New York State Student Nurses' Association sponsor legislation in the 1973 legislative session to require participation in continuing education approved by the professional association as a condition for re-registration of the license to practice as a registered professional nurse.

b. That the effective date of the above legislative proposal be 1975 in preparation for the 1977 biennial registration period.

c. That the Board of Directors establish at the earliest possible date, a permanent body within the Association to be known as the Committee to Approve Continuing Education Programs. This body is charged with the ongoing responsibility for establishing requirements for mandatory continuing education, and for approving continuing education programs and experiences applicable toward such requirements.

d. That the Board of Directors adopt in principle, the Committee's protocol for use in interpreting the essence of the Association's proposal for mandatory continuing education and that this protocol be referred to the permanent Committee to Approve Continuing Education Programs.

e. That the Committee be authorized to present its proposals for review and recommendation to the nurses in attendance at the 1972 New York State Student Nurses' Association Convention and at other NYSSNA programs prior to and during the 1973 legislative session.

f. That the life of the Committee be extended in order that it may address itself to the task of proposing a system for certification of nursing practitioners through the professional association.

As an example of legislative action, parts of the Assembly Bill No. 449 of the California legislature, approved by the Governor November 15, 1971, filed with the Secretary of State November 18, 1971, reads as follows:

Chapter 1.5. Continuing Education

900. In its concern for the health of the people of California, the Legislature intends to establish in this chapter a framework for the continuing education of those persons licensed in the healing arts who are subject to this chapter. It is the purpose of this chapter to provide a system for assuring that such healing arts professionals are fully informed of current technical knowledge in their professions, thereby providing to the citizens of California the best possible health services. It is the intent of the Legislature that the Council on Continuing Education for Health Occupations established by this chapter assume primary responsibility for the implementation of all statutory continuing education requirements for those health professions licensed in California which are subject to this chapter.

901. There is established in the Department of Consumer Affairs, to be transferred to the De-

partment of Health whenever the healing arts licensing agencies are transferred to the Department of Health in accordance with the Governor's Reorganization Plan No. 1 of 1970, a Council on Continuing Education for Health Occupations, consisting of the director or his designee, who shall serve as chairman of the council, and four additional members, appointed by the director, as follows:

(a) One administrator of a licensed hospital.

(b) One registered nurse.

(c) One licensed vocational nurse.

(d) One public member.

902. The council shall be appointed and begin its meetings by July 1, 1972.

903. The Council on Continuing Education for the Health Occupations, by regulation, shall establish standards for the continuing education in each of the fields covered by this chapter which will assure reasonable currency of knowledge as a basis for safe practice by licensees in each such field. The standards shall be established in a manner to assure that a variety of alternatives is available to licensees to comply with the continuing education requirements for renewal of licenses and taking cognizance of specialized areas of practice. Such alternatives include, but are not limited to, academic studies, inservice education, institutes, seminars, lectures, conferences, workshops, extension studies, and home-study programs. The council may organize committees from its membership to formulate proposed standards in each occupational field, and shall, in addition, invite and consider recommendations from each of the affected licensing agencies or boards concerning such standards. The occupations subject to this chapter are those of licensed vocational nurse and registered nurse.

CHAPTER 33 LADDER CONCEPT

■ The "ladder concept" in nursing has grown with the continued development and expansion of both the licensed practical nurse and associate degree nursing programs.

Great impetus has been given this idea because in many areas promotion in the hospital setting is based on the achievement of a bachelor of science degree.

Many colleges, some very prestigious, are now once more giving blanket credit to both diploma and associate degree graduates with the promise of a bachelor of science degree with no upper division major in nursing but courses "that will enhance the basic education of the new graduate." The new baccalaureate program is generally one year and perhaps a summer session in length.

The practice became so widespread that the Board of Directors of the National League for Nursing in 1970 and 1971 issued the following two statements:

A STATEMENT OF CONCERN ABOUT DEGREE PROGRAMS FOR NURSING STUDENTS THAT HAVE NO MAJOR IN NURSING*

The National League for Nursing notes with concern the growth in the number of collegiate programs that have no major in nursing but are designed to appeal specifically to potential and enrolled nursing students and registered nurses. Publicity about these programs leads students to believe that they offer preparation for advanced positions in nursing or provide the base needed for further education in nursing when this is not the case.

The programs in question lead to associate or baccalaureate degrees in such fields as applied science, biology, education, health science, occupational therapy, psychology, and sociology. Large blocks of credit are promised the student for nursing education obtained outside the college. The collegiate programs may provide the student with increased knowledge in the specified area of the major, but they do not offer additional preparation in nursing.

The National League for Nursing believes the misguidance of the students occurs because of publicity about these programs which:

1. Implies that a major in another field is the equal of the major in nursing as preparation for nursing practice—when it is not.
2. Implies that they are acceptable as a base for further education in nursing—when they are not.
3. Implies that they lead to advancement in employment—which in many instances they do not.
4. Implies that because only graduates of NLN-accredited nursing programs are awarded credit, the degree programs are therefore approved by NLN—which they are not.

All too frequently it is only after a considerable investment of time and money that students in these programs discover how limited the programs are as preparation for nursing practice and a career in nursing. The National League for Nursing therefore believes that colleges that offer these special degree programs have an obligation to interpret them accurately in all promotional and decriptive materials.

THE OPEN CURRICULUM IN NURSING EDUCATION*

An open curriculum in nursing education is a system which takes into account the different pur-

*Statement approved by the Board of Directors, National League for Nursing, October, 1971.

*Statement approved by the Board of Directors, National League for Nursing, February, 1970.

poses of the various types of programs but recognizes common areas of achievement. Such a system permits student mobility in the light of ability, changing career goals, and changing aspirations. It also requires clear delineation of the achievement expectations of nursing programs, from practical nursing through graduate education. It recognizes the possibility of mobility from other health related fields. It is an interrelated system of achievement in nursing education with open doors rather than quantitative serial steps.

The National League for Nursing believes that:

1. Individuals who wish to change career goals should have the opportunity to do so.
2. Educational opportunities should be provided for those who are interested in upward mobility without lowering standards.
3. In any type of nursing program opportunity should be provided to validate previous education and experience.
4. Sound educational plans must be developed to avoid unsound projects and programs.
5. More effective guidance is urgently needed at all stages of student development.
6. If projects and endeavors in this area are to be successful, nursing must accept the above concept of the open curriculum.

The concept has several names—"ladder," "lattice," "career mobility," "upward mobility," and "articulation." The recent nursing literature is filled with references and articles, both pro and con, referring to the concept. It is truly one of the most discussed issues in nursing at the present time.

Possibly the ultimate in this concept is exemplified by the Regents External Degree of the University of the State of New York.

Commissioner Nyquist of the University of the State of New York has put it succinctly when he states, "If attendance at a college is the only road to college credentials, those who cannot, or have not, availed themselves of this route, but have acquired knowledge and skills through other sources, will be denied the recognition to which they are entitled. Neither the State nor the Nation can afford such waste, nor should they tolerate such inequity. The costs of traditionalism are too high."

The first candidates for the nursing program were admitted in September, 1973.

Requirements for the associate in applied science in nursing degree include the cognitive and clinical aspects of the nursing sciences and general education. The widely accepted college proficiency examinations in the nursing sciences provide a useful point of departure.

Part of the proposal for legislation in California is an example of how far this concept extends.

The people of the State of California do enact as follows:

Section 1. In its concern for the quality and availability of health care services in California, the Legislature finds that a number of factors prevent the full utilization of the service capabilities of nursing personnel, as well as preventing full career development for nurses. First, the ability of a licensed vocational nurse has been hampered because responsibility for licensing these two occupations was divided between two licensing boards. Second, basic differences in the content and duration of various training programs for registered nurses prevent development of a nursing "career ladder," and is particularly discouraging to minorities who wish to become registered nurses. Third, the legal status of nurses performing certain procedures or acting in certain roles is ambiguous at this time, despite the demonstrated competence of many nurses to perform them. Fourth, the lack of any legal standards for nurses aides prevents them from receiving credit for their knowledge and skill in attempting to advance to a licensed category of nursing, as well as failing to provide adequate standards for public protection. Fifth, the full development of career opportunities and service utilization of psychiatric technicians is limited because they are licensed by the same licensing board as licensed vocational nurses.

It is the purpose of the Legislature in enacting this act that:

(a) Responsibility for licensing vocational and registered nurses be combined under one licensing board, with a view of nursing education as a continuous process for training nurses to perform at successively higher levels of responsibility.

(b) Training programs for registered nurses are encouraged to offer courses enabling students to become licensed as vocational nurses after the first year of training, to give vocational nurses maximum opportunity for advancing to the registered nursing field.

(c) Licensing requirements for categories of nurses should not include graduation from an educational program if the courses required for graduation do not relate to the capability of graduates to perform as nurses.

(d) Nursing education programs offering a baccalaureate degree are encouraged to offer licensure-related courses first, as lower division courses, so that registered nurses who are graduated from other types of nursing programs can transfer to these schools for advanced training without loss of credit.

(e) The licensing board for nursing personnel should develop a standard equivalency test for licensure as a vocational nurse, and for licensure as a registered nurse, to eliminate the problems that have occurred by delegating this function to schools. The parts of these tests should relate to the educational qualifications for licensure, so that an individual should not have to take courses for licensure if he demonstrates his proficiency by passing that part, or parts, of the equivalency examination.

(f) The state should issue a state associate of science degree to every nurse who is a graduate of a diploma nursing education program and does not already possess a degree. This associate degree will be equivalent to associate degrees issued by community colleges to nursing graduates for purposes of matriculating to schools offering a baccalaureate in nursing and shall be accepted by all universities and colleges in California with a nursing program.

(g) Responsibility for licensing psychiatric technicians should be separated from the agency licensing nurses, and phased into an appropriate licensing body.

(h) Training programs for nurses aides should be certified to allow graduates to achieve recognition for their capabilities in advancing to higher levels of nursing.*

---

*California legislature Assembly Bill No. 1495, amended in assembly April 27, 1972.

CHAPTER 34 NURSING PUBLICATIONS

■ As long as nursing remained in the apprenticeship stage and before it began to develop as a profession, there was little use for publications to express its needs, activities, and progress and to interpret its work to members of its own group, to other professions, and to the community. Florence Nightingale was the first nurse to contribute significantly to professional literature.

Today there are many publications in the nursing world. They can be classified as official and nonofficial organs or publications. The official publications of the professional nursing organizations in this country are *The American Journal of Nursing, Nursing Outlook* (with which is combined *Public Health Nursing*), and *Nursing Research*.

A magazine which is controlled, and this usually implies ownership, by the nursing organization which sponsors it, is known as the "official organ" of that association. It is the voice of the association and of the profession, or those branches of it which the association was organized to promote. Like the association itself, the publication is based upon an ideal of service to nurses and through them to the public which they serve. The primary function of a professional publication is to encourage the members to exceed their own best efforts and thus to increase their professional stature.

Professional nursing publications are not published primarily for financial profit. However, if there are earnings, they are used to extend the work of the professional group which the publication represents. No individual receives personal financial profit from any earnings of the *American Journal, Public Health Nursing,* or the official bulletins of the state and district nurses associations.*

There are several other nursing organizations that have their own official publications described later in this chapter.

THE AMERICAN JOURNAL OF NURSING

During the history of professional nursing in this country *The American Journal of Nursing* has been its official mouthpiece. As soon as the early leaders began to meet and discuss the need for national organizations, the need for a representative nursing journal was appreciated. In fact the American Society of Superintendents of Training Schools had considered it, but because they knew the limitations of their scope they thought this project should be delayed until the alumnae association had become a national organization and truly representative of American nurses. One of the first activities of the Associated Alumnae was to appoint a committee to investigate how a journal could be started. The first committee failed, but a second was appointed in 1899. Among its members were both Isabel Hampton Robb and Mary Adelaide Nutting; only the records of their courage can explain why

---

*Editorial: What are professional nursing periodicals? American Journal of Nursing 37:1369, December, 1937.

these women set out on such a journalistic adventure without experience or outside financial assistance. The *Journal* was started as a joint stock company, the shares were $100 each, to be sold only to nurses—Linda Richards held share No. 1, Mrs. Robb No. 4, and Miss Nutting No. 6. As the *Journal* grew, it used its savings to buy back the stock, and finally in 1912 it owned all of it so that it is now truly the property of the American nurses, controlled by their association, and its official organ. It states that it has three functions: (1) to be a continuous record of nursing events, (2) to be a means of communication between nurses, and (3) to be a means of "interpreting nursing to the public." It particularly backs legislative efforts to regulate nursing, sponsors the cause of nursing education, and has many other functions of interest to the nursing profession. Sophie Palmer was editor-in-chief of the *Journal* from its first issue in October, 1900, until her death in 1920. Katherine DeWitt came to assist her in 1906 and remained until her retirement in 1932. She held the position of assistant editor, editor pro tem, coeditor, and finally managing editor.

In 1921 Mary Roberts was appointed to succeed Miss Palmer as editor; she retained that position until her resignation in 1949, when she was appointed editor emeritus. Nell Beeby was editor from 1949 until her death in 1957. Thelma M. Schorr is the present editor. As developments in the profession demanded it, the *Journal* has increased both in content and in variety of subjects discussed. Assistants have been added to the staff as this work increased.

The story of the organizational development of nursing can be traced through the *Journal* from 1900 until the present day. During its early days, nurses were very much concerned about registration and the development of adequate nurse practice acts. In one of the early *Journals* there is an article by Lavinia Dock, "What We May Expect of the Law." Accounts of the development of the Army and Navy Nurse Corps,

nursing in the Veterans Administration, and nursing during the wars and in times of disaster appear regularly in this magazine, in addition to the continuous story of what nurses and their organizations are doing.

The *Journal* makes available to nurses all over the country authentic material on new and approved methods of diagnosis, therapy, or prevention, including nursing care. Circulation has now grown to over 250,000 annual subscriptions. To help its readers the *Journal* has a field representative on its staff who meets with nursing groups all over the country, interpreting its activities and program. In addition an annual index is published during January of each year. A cumulative index in five volumes, the first covering the years 1900 to 1920, the second, 1921 to 1930, the third, 1931 to 1940, the fourth, 1941 to 1950, and the fifth, 1951 to 1960, is another valuable help in using this magazine.

AMERICAN JOURNAL OF NURSING COMPANY

The American Journal of Nursing Company is an incorporated body with its own board of directors elected annually by the board of directors of the American Nurses' Association. It is the publishing corporation for the professional jounrals.

The American Journal of Nursing Company stock is wholly owned by the American Nurses' Association, and the board of directors of the ANA serve as sole stockholders for the American Journal of Nursing Company. This company also publishes the two other official professional nursing magazines, *Nursing Outlook* and *Nursing Research*.

NURSING OUTLOOK

When the National League for Nursing was formed in 1952, it asked the American Journal of Nursing Company to publish its new official organ, *Nursing Outlook*. Until 1912 articles of interest to public health nurses had been presented in *The American Journal of Nursing.* Since 1909 the Cleveland Visiting Nurses' Association had been editing their own *Visiting Nurses' Quarterly.* When the National Organization for Public Health Nursing was formed in 1912, the owners of the *Visiting Nurses' Quarterly* gave this magazine to the new organization and endowed it liberally so that it would not become an economic liability for the new organization. This periodical was a success; in 1918 the name was changed to the *Public Health Nurse,* and it was known by that title until its last issue in December, 1952. The magazine became the nucleus for *Nursing Outlook,* whose first issue was January, 1953. Hedwig Cohen was the last editor of *Public Health Nurse* and then joined the staff of NLN as associate director of public health nursing and later headed the department. Upon her retirement in 1969, the Hedwig Cohen Fund was established to index the articles in *Public Health Nurse.* *Nursing Outlook,* then, like *The American Journal of Nursing,* is owned and published by the American Journal of Nursing Company. The board of directors determines the overall policy of the magazine. NLN representatives are on the board of directors. Mildred Hall was the first editor of this new magazine; the editorial staff is made up of professional nurses. Mildred Gaynor was the second editor; she retired in 1966. The present editor is Edith P. Lewis.

Since the NLN is interested in the development and improvement of nursing service, as well as nursing education, many articles are devoted to the two broad fields of nursing service and nursing education. It will be remembered that the National Organization for Public Health Nursing and the Association of Collegiate Schools of Nursing had non-nurse members as well as agency membership, as does the NLN. The official organ of this new organization, *Nursing Outlook,* therefore includes articles about nursing in relation to the community as well as articles in the field of public health in general and public health nursing in particular.

NURSING RESEARCH

Nursing Research, also published by the American Journal of Nursing Company, appears four times a year. Lucille E. Notter is the present editor. The first issue was published in June, 1952. This magazine actually was started before the NLN was organized, as an activity of the Association of Collegiate Schools of Nursing. Early in 1952 the ACSN asked the American Journal of Nursing Company to publish a magazine that would be devoted to research in nursing. Its stated purposes were (1) to inform members of the nursing and allied professions of the results of scientific study in nursing and (2) to stimulate research in nursing. It was designed to serve nurses in all fields and branches of the profession and represents the first concerted effort for the establishment of a magazine that had as its primary purpose the reporting of studies. The sponsoring organization was the Association of Collegiate Schools of Nursing; the publisher, the American Journal of Nursing Company. The editorial board consisted of 20 persons representing different branches of nursing and education and coming from different parts of the country.

To finance this project the ACSN gave $900, and the ANA, $500; individual contributions amounted to another $500. When the National League for Nursing was formed in 1952, into which the Association of Collegiate Schools of Nursing merged, it took over this new magazine. The NLN nominates members for the editorial board, and the American Journal of Nursing Company appoints them. Helen H. Bunge was the first chairman of the editorial board. Members of the editorial board are nurses, educators, or research workers in colleges, universities, or agencies interested in nursing research.

INTERNATIONAL NURSING INDEX

The *International Nursing Index* is the latest publication to join the official family of the American Journal of Nursing Company. It was first published in 1966 in co-operation with the National Library of Medicine. Over 160 nursing journals received from all over the world are indexed. It is divided by a subject section and a name section.

Before concluding this discussion of official nursing publications, it may be interesting to know that other literature is available from the nursing organizations; for example, *The American Journal of Nursing* publishes an annual index and a cumulative index at the end of every ten-year period. The ANA and the NLN publish bibliographies from time to time. *Facts About Nursing,* a statistical summary, published annually by the ANA, began in 1935 as the *Yearbook on Nursing.* These professional organizations also publish bulletins and books from time to time on subjects of interest to nurses. Various bulletins have been published by the different organizations that came together to form the NLN. These publications are revised quite frequently.

There are many other magazines and journals of interest to nurses. Some of them are directed to people with a major clinical interest, such as: *The Journal of the American Association of Nurse Anesthetists, Bulletin of the American College of Nurse-Midwifery, Journal of Psychiatric Nursing,* and *Perspectives in Psychiatric Care.* Others have an audience that consists of people with a particular functional orientation, as: *American Association of Industrial Nurses' Journal* and the *Journal of Nursing Education.* Still others are directed toward nurses with a particular religious affiliation: *The Catholic Nurse* and *News for Nurses. R.N.* and *Nursing Forum* have a broader appeal to nurses who are employed in a variety of positions.

BOOKS

When instruction for nurses became organized and particularly when the first schools modeled on the Nightingale plan were started, books became a necessity. Miss Nightingale's *Notes on Nursing, What It Is and What It Is Not,* appeared and became the textbook not only for nurses at the St. Thomas's School for Nursing but also for other schools, both in England and in America, and was translated into foreign languages. Many of the early schools of nursing used medical texts. In this country the first manual for nurses, the *New Haven Manual of Nursing,* was published by the Connecticut Training School in 1879. Other schools, including Bellevue, worked out manuals for nursing. They were what we would now call books in nursing arts. As nursing became organized, as leaders became more sure of nursing needs, and as more leaders appeared, they became articulate in print. One of the early books to obtain wide circulation, believed to be the first nursing text in America, was *Textbook of Nursing* written by a nurse, Clara Weeks Shaw, and published in 1885. It was a standard nursing text for many years. Another early text, written by Diane Kimber particularly for nurses, concerned the fields of anatomy and physiology. Succeeding editions of that book have continued to be published, and it is now known as Kimber and Gray's *Anatomy* and *Physiology.* Other well-known texts were Lavinia Dock's *Materia Medica,* Mary Reed's *Bacteriology,* and Harriet Camp's *Ethics.* Isabel Hampton Robb wrote two texts, *Nursing Ethics* and *Nursing, Its Principles and Practice for Hospital and Private Use.*

Before World War I, books on clinical subjects written particularly for nurses began to appear. These were usually written by doctors, occasionally by a nurse in collaboration with a doctor. Few were written by nurses alone. Since World War I, a more dynamic approach to nursing texts and reference books has been noticed. One of the early books giving the new look to texts for nurses was Bertha Harmer's *Principles and Practice of Nursing,* which appeared in 1923. Since then, in nursing as in all other fields, the amount of literature available is tremendous, with an increasiing amount being written by nurses.

CONCLUSION

The last two paragraphs of Barbara Schutt's editorial in the January, 1972, issue of the *American Journal of Nursing,* commenting on Lillian Wald's being elected to the Hall of Fame for Great Americans, seems a fittting conclusion for this section of the book.

The kind of health care Lillian Wald began preaching and practicing in 1893 is the kind the people of this country are still crying for. She demonstrated with no need to rest on formal research that nursing could serve as the entry point —not only for health care, but for dealing with many other social ills of which sickness is only a part. She felt that nurses should go to the sick, instead of expecting the sick to come to them (and waiting for physicians to refer them!); that

care of persons in the home, especially children, was far more effective and much less expensive except perhaps for those needing, to use her own word, "intensive" care; that the nurse was also a teacher, who respected the **capacity of the dis**advantaged to learn, just as she always respected their right to human dignity. And, as for teaching the disadvantaged, Lillian Wald went to live among them a good half century before the Peace Corps and Vista were conceived.

A frightening amount of what she said in her Henry Street books could be paraphrased to read like a book on our ghettos, our intentions in that expanded practice of nursing, our problems of health care today. Perhaps Lillian Wald's election to the Hall of Fame will force more of us to acknowledge how relevant to our times are the answers she conceived to the problems she encountered. If so, we are all as indebted to that noble institution as to this noble person it will enshrine.*

---

*Schutt, Barbara: Editorial, American Journal of Nursing, January, 1972.

QUESTIONS AND STUDY PROJECTS FOR UNIT EIGHT

1. Describe how you would function as an independent nurse practitioner.
2. Where do you think education should be held for the "nurse practitioner"?
3. What meaning does the "ladder concept" have for you?
4. What is a "terminal program" in nursing?
5. Give a detailed history of your favorite nursing publication.
6. Which publication is considered the official magazine for nurses?

REFERENCES FOR UNIT EIGHT

Alford, Harold J.: Continuing education in action, (published for the W. K. Kellogg Foundation), New York, 1968, John Wiley & Sons, Inc.

Allyn, Nathaniel C.: College credit by examination, Nursing Outlook **17:**44-46, April, 1969.

Bergeven, Paul, Morris, Dwight, and Smith, Robert M.: Adult education procedures, New York, 1963, The Seabury Press, Inc.

Bergeven, Paul, and McKinley, John: Psychiatric training for adult education, St. Louis, 1972, The Bethany Press.

Boocock, Sarane, S., and Schild, E. O.: Simulation games in learning, Beverly Hills, Calif., 1968, Sage Publications, Inc.

Bradford, Leland P., Gibb, Jack R., and Benne, Kenneth D.: T-group theory and laboratory method, New York, 1964, John Wiley & Sons, Inc.

Brodt, Dagmar E.: College bound but why, Nursing Outlook **17:**48-49, January, 1969.

Burnside, Helen: Practical nurses become associate degree graduates, Nursing Outlook **17:**47, April, 1969.

Carey, James J.: Forms and forces in university adult education, Syracuse, N.Y., 1963, Center for the Study of Liberal Education.

Carnegie Commission on the Future of Higher Education: Open-door colleges, New York, 1970, McGraw-Hill Book Co.

Cartwright, Dorwin, and Zander, Alvin: Group dynamics, research and theory, ed. 3, New York, 1968, Harper & Row, Publishers.

Curtis, Frieda, Darragh, Rita M., Fancher, Joanna E., Ingmire, Alice E., Lesnan, Verle B., Orwig,

Bernice I., Popiel, Elda S., and Shores, W. Louise: Continuing education in nursing, Boulder, Colo., 1969, Western Interstate Commission for Higher Education.

Hangartner, Carl A.: College credit for equivalency and advanced standing, Nursing Outlook **14:**30-32, May, 1966.

Helping people in groups. Six background papers from the Workshop on Group Services, April 19-23, 1965, United States Department of Health, Education and Welfare, Welfare Administration, Bureau of Family Services, Washington, D. C.

Ingles, Thelma, and Montag, Mildred: Debate: the ladder concept in nursing education. Pro . . . Thelma Ingles, Con . . . Mildred Montag, Nursing Outlook **19:**726, 1971.

Kidd, James Robbins: How adults learn, New York, 1963, Association Press.

Kidd, James Robbins: Financing continuing education, New York, 1962, Scarecrow Press, Inc.

Knowles, Malcolm S., editor: Handbook of adult education in the United States, Chicago, 1960, Adult Education Association of the U.S.A.

Knowles, Malcolm S.: The modern practice of adult education: andragogy versus pedagogy, New York, 1970, Association Press.

Kurland, Norman D.: College credit for off campus learning, Nursing Outlook **14:**33-35, May, 1966.

MacDonald, Gwendoline: Baccalaureate education for graduates of diploma and associate degree programs, Nursing Outlook **12:**52-56, June, 1964.

Malkin, Evelyn: Direction or dilemma for R.N.'s in baccalaureate education, Nursing Outlook **14:**36-38, May, 1966.

Miller, Harry L.: Teaching and learning in adult education, New York, 1967, The Macmillan Co.

Nahm, Helen: Continuity and progression in nursing education, American Journal of Nursing **58:**845-847, June, 1958.

Schmidt, Mildred S., and Lyons, William: Credit for what you know, American Journal of Nursing **69:**101-104, January, 1969.

Smith, Robert G., Jr.: The development of training objectives, The George Washington University Human Resources Research Office, Research Bulletin II, June, 1964.

Stewart, William H.: The challenge to nursing, American Protestant Hospital Association Bulletin, July, 1967.

Stewart, William H.: Surgeon general looks at nursing, American Journal of Nursing **67:**64-67, January, 1967.

UNIT NINE
Organizational changes

Nursing is attempting to keep its own house in order and at the same time meet the societal needs for accountability and representation. This is reflected in the manner the profession organized itself in the early 1950's.

The emergence of new demands and circumstances makes for almost constant changes. Nursing has always met these organizational changes but sometimes in spurts of growth. The changes have not come easily, but they have developed along with the massive change in our contemporary society.

CHAPTER 35 BEGINNING OF TWO ORGANIZATIONS

■ In planning for the future it is fitting that consideration be given to the type of organization that will function best. The organization of nurses is of vital importance if plans and programs for the future are to be carried out satisfactorily.

In 1939 the question arose of uniting more closely the three oldest nursing organizations: the National League of Nursing Education, the National Organization for Public Health Nursing, and the American Nurses' Association. World War II both helped and hindered this movement. It was not until 1944 that definite plans for these three organizations could be considered. In 1945 the National Association of Colored Graduate Nurses, the American Association of Industrial Nurses, and the Association of Collegiate Schools of Nursing were added to the committee.

THE RICH REPORT

The National Nursing Council for War Service, Inc., prepared a comprehensive program for postwar nursing, which appeared in *The American Journal of Nursing,* September, 1945, under the title "A Comprehensive Program for Nationwide Action." Many doubts were revealed about the existing structures of the national nursing organizations, and it was believed that these doubts could be resolved only by a complete study. Consequently the Raymond Rich Associates were empowered to make this study,

hereafter referred to as the Structure Study.

At the biennial convention in 1946 the Rich Report was discussed and studied. The study was continued during the greater part of 1946 and the spring and summer of 1947 through the national and state structure study committees. In September, 1947, the House of Delegates of the American Nurses' Association held a special meeting to study the Rich Report. At that session the delegates of the American Nurses' Association were given the right to express opinions and to vote on the structure committee as other delegates had from the beginning. At this time the average nurse showed more interest in the organization of the profession than ever before. The Rich Report actually gave the nurses and lay people a new interest in and knowledge about nursing. They asked, "Why is a new organization necessary?" "Why should all types of nursing care be organized under one head?" or "Should they?" "Can the industrial nurse join with the staff nurses and have specialized needs in organization recognized?" "Should the Negro nurses be given the added help that will be found in a larger organization of all nurses or will these nurses become a minority group without voice?"

In the 1947 plan, called a "tentative plan," there was to be one organization, to be known as the American Nursing Organization, with nurse members grouped into sections of interest and composing the house of delegates and the board of governors.

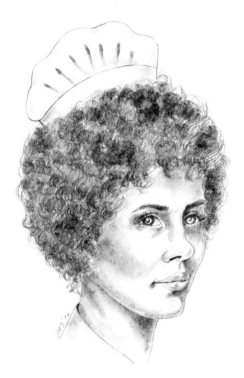

COLUMBIA, SOUTH CAROLINA,
HOSPITAL GRADUATE NURSE

In addition, this single association was to have divisions, which were to have non-nurse, agency, and school members as well as nurse members. Only nurse members of the divisions were to be eligible for election as division representatives in the house of delegates and board of governors, but all types of members were to elect the division representatives.

This organization was not considered adequate by the National Organization for Public Health Nursing and the National League of Nursing Education who, had had great support and help from their lay members. They believed that the lay members should have equal consideration in an organization if they were to continue to take an active interest in that organizaion.

Then the question of membership in the International Council of Nurses arose. Could an organization with active lay participation still remain a member of the International Council of Nurses? The International Council of Nurses' rules state that the member organization from any country must be of and controlled by nurses. After extensive study there seemed no way to have a single organization with free lay participation and continued membership in the International Council of Nurses.

Revised plans in 1949 provided for the establishment of two organizations. This plan was based upon an effort to increase more democratic participation in the work of the organization, both by every registered graduate nurse and by the lay public interested in nursing service. The inclusion of the lay member in a professional nurses' organization is a controversial subject. If a nurse believes that active lay participation is necessary for the furtherance of nursing service, this nurse will believe that it should be provided for in the organization. However, there are nurses who have never worked with cooperative lay members and who fear the idea of the lay persons' taking an active voting part in the organization's work.

Basically the Structure Study was an effort of the six national nursing organizations to coordinate their work and to make it more effective in service to nurses as they tried to meet the nation's constantly increasing demand for nursing services.

It was the Structure Study committee's assigned task to bring to the profession a recommendation of the organizational structure most favorable to the best development of nursing. In pursuing this primary objective, more has been learned about organizational life of professional nursing than ever before.

At the biennial convention in Atlantic City in 1952, nurses voted to have two national organizations: the American Nurses' Association and the National League for Nursing.

The original joint statement of purposes and functions is given on pages 229 to 231.

During the 20 years since nursing voted for two national groups many organizational difficulties have arisen between the two

THE AMERICAN NURSES' ASSOCIATION AND
THE NATIONAL LEAGUE FOR NURSING

A JOINT STATEMENT ON PURPOSES AND FUNCTIONS*

The American Nurses' Association and the National League for Nursing are separate organizations with a common objective—to provide the best possible nursing care for the American people.

Each organization has distinct purposes and functions.

PURPOSES

Through ANA, nurses work for the continuing improvement of professional practice, the economic and general welfare of nurses and the health needs of the American public.

In the NLN, nurses and friends of nursing of all races, creeds and national origins act together to provide the people of their communities with the best possible nursing services and to assure good nursing education.

FUNCTIONS AND SERVICES

ANA	NLN
Defines functions and promotes standards of professional nurse practice	Defines standards for organized nursing services and education
Defines qualifications for practitioners of nursing, including those in various nursing specialties	Stimulates and assists communities, nursing services and educational institutions in achieving these standards through effective distribution, organization, administration and utilization of personnel
Promotes legislation and speaks for nurses regarding legislative action for general health and welfare programs	Promotes continual study and adjustments in nursing services and educational curricula to meet changing needs
Surveys periodically the nurse resources of the nation	Assists with or conducts community nursing surveys
Promotes the economic and general welfare of nurses and works to eliminate discrimination against minority-group nurses in job opportunities	Provides consultation, publications, cost analysis methods and data, and other services to individuals, nursing services, schools and communities
Provides professional counseling service to individual nurses and to employers in regard to employment opportunities and available personnel	Conducts a national student nurse recruitment program cosponsored by the ANA, the American Hospital Association, the American Medical Association
Finances studies on nursing functions	Carries out and promotes studies and research related to organized nursing services and educational programs
Represents and serves as national spokesman for nurses with allied professional and governmental groups and with the public	Represents nursing services and nursing education units with allied professional, governmental and international groups and with the public
Implements the international exchange of nurses program and assists displaced persons who are nurses	Accredits educational programs in nursing
Serves as the official representative of American nurses in the International Council of Nurses	Offers comprehensive testing and guidance services to institutions with practical, basic or advanced nursing education programs
Works closely with the various State Boards of Nursing in the interpretation of nurse practice acts and the facilitation of interstate licensure by endorsement.	Provides, in cooperation with state licensing authorities, examinations and related services for use in licensing professional and practical nurses

*Pamphlet published by the American Nurses' Association and the National League for Nursing, 10 Columbus Circle, New York, N. Y.

MEMBERSHIP

All ANA members are professional registered nurses, representing every occupational field of nursing. There are two types of members: Active and Associate (retired or inactive nurses).

NLN members are professional and practical nurses, men and women in allied professions, other people interested in good nursing, nursing service agencies—hospitals and public health —and institutions offering educational programs in nursing.

CONSTITUENT GROUPS

The ANA is a federation of 53 constituent associations including the [48] states, the District of Columbia, Puerto Rico, the Panama Canal Zone, Alaska and Hawaii. State Nurses Associations, in turn, usually are composed of constituent District Associations. ANA membership also is divided into district, state and national sections according to occupational specialties within nursing.

As of April, 1954, NLN counted as affiliates 45 state Leagues for Nursing, the District of Columbia, Hawaii, and Puerto Rico. Many state Leagues are organizing constituents known as local Leagues for Nursing. A Council of State Leagues for Nursing, comprised of the president or alternate of each state League, NLN's officers and the ANA's president, coordinates state programs and purposes with those of the National League for Nursing.

OPERATING PLAN

Members of state sections elect representatives to the ANA House of Delegates who, in turn, vote for the Board of Directors. ANA section executive committees are elected by section members attending the biennial conventions. Programs and policies of ANA are determined by the House of Delegates. The work of the ANA between conventions is furthered through the activities of standing and special committees and the Board of Directors. A national headquarters with an administrative staff is maintained.

Every NLN member has a voice in the organization's policies and programs. The Board of Directors is elected by direct vote of all members. Four departments represent major fields of interest in nursing service and education. A steering committee, elected by department members, guides the staff in carrying out each department's program. Each department also has a Council of its Member Agencies. Interdivisional councils and committees represent cross-sections of special interest groups.

HISTORY

ANA

ANA was organized in 1896 as the Nurses' Associated Alumnae of the United States and Canada. When the Association was incorporated in New York in 1901, it was no longer possible for Canadian nurses to be affiliated. The present name was adopted ten years later. In 1951 the National Association of Colored Graduate Nurses became integrated with ANA. A year later, in the structure reorganization of nursing groups, ANA took over some of the work (definition of functions and qualifications by individual practitioners) formerly carried by the National League of Nursing Education and the National Organization for Public Health Nursing, which were combined into NLN.

NLN

The NLN was formed in 1952 when three national nursing organizations and four national committees combined their programs and resources. National League of Nursing education (founded 1893), National Organization for Public Health Nursing (1912), Association of Collegiate Schools of Nursing (1933), Joint Committee on Practical Nurses and Auxiliary Workers in Nursing Services (1945), Joint Committee on Careers in Nursing (1948), National Committee for the Improvement of Nursing Services (1949), and National Nursing Accrediting Service (1949)

MAGAZINES

The American Journal of Nursing, founded in 1900, is the official magazine of the ANA. NLN's official magazine is *Nursing Outlook,* founded in 1953. NLN also sponsors *Nursing Research.*

(These magazines are published by the American Journal of Nursing Company, 10 Columbus Circle, New York, N. Y. 10019.)

COORDINATING COUNCIL

The ANA and the NLN coordinate programs of common concern, and keep in touch with each other's work and wth the activities of the National Student Nurse Association through a Coordinating Council, composed of their combined Boards of Directors.

STUDENT ORGANIZATION

The National Student Nurse Association was organized in 1953 by students from 43 states and the District of Columbia, under the guidance of ANA and NLN. One member each from the Boards of ANA and NLN serves on the Advisory Council of the student association.

---

structures. Perhaps the grand ideals embodied in the original concepts were too global, too complex. Perhaps the professional organization felt it had relinquished some of its vital prerogatives to a "lay" group. Thus in 1958 the ANA House of Delegates called for one national organization. This call proved to be unobtainable for a variety of reasons. However, since this action the two organizations have improved relationships noticeably and have issued joint statements clarifying their functions. A similar motion calling for one organization was presented to the ANA Convention in 1972 and was almost unanimously tabled immediately; thus indirectly once more supporting and reaffirming the concept of two national nursing organizations. Two of the joint statements follow:

WORKING RELATIONSHIPS BETWEEN
THE AMERICAN NURSES' ASSOCIATION AND
NATIONAL LEAGUE FOR NURSING*

The American Nurses' Association and the National League for Nursing as cooperating organizations in the field of nursing have the need to

---

*Statement approved by ANA and NLN boards of directors, January, 1966.

---

examine periodically the fundamental premises on which they will work together and serve society. While they are totally different organizations in both responsibilities and structure, they are complementary in purpose and function.

The American Nurses' Association, as the professional organization, is moving to fulfill those functions of standard setting for education, practice and organized services traditionally carried by professional organizations. In the development and modification of such standards, ANA secures consultation and advice from NLN and elsewhere, but retains responsibility for deciding the final content. Normally, standards are in advance of current practice. They are authoritative, based on the expertise of the profession. ANA works through its members and its constituencies, with NLN and with a variety of organizations and governmental bodies to implement these standards.

The National League for Nursing, composed of individuals, educational institutions, and nursing service agencies, is the organization to which the profession and the public look for services to promote and to improve nursing education programs and organized nursing services. These activities of NLN include among others accreditation, consultation, and involvement of educational programs and service agencies in programs of self-improvement. In planning and conducting such services, NLN involves its appropriate membership in the development of criteria for the purpose of evaluation. Such criteria and related guides must reflect the broad standards enunciated by ANA and their goals of the profession. NLN studies the application of criteria and their implications for standards and practice for education and for organized nursing services. These findings are shared with ANA. In these ways the two organizations are complementary, each with distinctive responsibilities and both necessary in meeting society's needs for nursing service.

The needs of the profession and the needs of the public for nursing service are different in 1966 from those of 1952 when a design for function and structure of both organizations was adopted. Change in the demands upon both organizations has caused each to examine its own functions and structure, and its relationship with the other. It is essential that ANA and NLN work cooperatively in areas of common concern as each builds its program in full recognition of the role of the other.

THE AMERICAN NURSES' ASSOCIATION AND THE NATIONAL LEAGUE FOR NURSING JOINT STATEMENT ON COMMUNITY PLANNING FOR NURSING EDUCATION

In recognition of the many changes taking place in the health field and the need for appropriate education for nursing personnel to meet present and future requirements, both in quantity and quality of nursing services, the American Nurses' Association and the National League for Nursing believe that sound community planning for nursing education is essential and should be begun or accelerated promptly.

The overriding concern of both organizations is that the nation receive the best possible nursing care. This will require increasing numbers of nursing personnel with quality preparation to meet the changing health care needs of the community and to fill the needs of institutions and agencies providing nursing services.

Both organizations have recently taken official positions on the future of nursing education. The American Nurses' Association in December 1965 issued a position paper stating that all nursing personnel should be prepared with the general system of education. The statement advocates baccalaureate preparation as the minimum education for professional nursing practice, associate degree preparation as the minimum for technical nursing practice, and vocational school preparation for nursing assistants. The National League for Nursing in May 1965 passed a resolution advocating community planning to implement the orderly transition of nursing education into institutions of higher education in such a way that the flow of nurses into the community will not be interrupted.

As was pointed out in the Report of the Surgeon General's Consultant Group on Nursing, "If new and expanded programs of nursing education are to be established in places where they are needed and in educational settings where they will thrive, it is essential that they be intelligently planned. Such planning . . . must consider needs for cooperation among adjoining geographic areas. . . . Cooperation within and among states in the planning of nursing education programs is desirable both to prevent needless duplication of effort and as a basis for pooling of . . . resources."

Today when major changes are taking place in the type and placement of nursing education programs, it cannot be left to chance that the right number of nurses with the appropriate level of education can and will be produced.

The ANA and NLN both believe that guaranteeing the continuity and character of the nursing supply transcends the nursing profession itself. Educational, health, and welfare authorities, professional and volunteer groups in the health field and community planning bodies must plan and work cooperatively with nursing to insure an adequate nursing supply. Careful planning on the community level must precede any action to transfer or to develop new or different programs. Depending upon the social and demographic complexion of the area, planning may be undertaken for a local community, for several communities together, for a state, or for a region.

Communities are urged to base their decision as to the types of nursing education programs to be retained, revised, or newly developed taking into account:
1. What are the nursing care needs of the community? What kinds of nursing personnel are required to meet these needs?
2. What are the physical resources now available or planned in the community for educating nursing personnel? What junior and senior colleges, universities and clinical laboratory facilities are available for educational excellence?
3. Are qualified faculty available?
4. What financial resources are available which can be utilized for nursing education?
5. How can available resources be channelled into a new design of education for nursing personnel to meet the current and anticipated needs of the community?

Only through such planning and studying of the total situation is it possible to assure that nurses will be prepared in accordance with the needs of society and to assure the most effective use of available resources.

CONCLUSION

One of the achievements of professional nursing after World War II was the completion of the plans for the reorganization of the structure of professional nursing, which resulted in two major national organizations. One organization of, by, and for professional nurses, to have the full responsibility for those functions which the members of any profession should perform for themselves, is the American Nurses' Association. The second organization, the National League for Nursing brought together the National League of Nursing Education, the American Association of Collegiate Schools of Nursing, and the National Organization for Public Health Nursing. It provided, for the first time in nursing history, that all nurses from every occupational field would be able to plan jointly with allied professional workers and agencies for the best utilization, distribution, and financial support of nursing services and nursing education.

Miss McIver* in her article "Nursing Moves Forward" stated the principles that influence nursing development even today.

1. The supply of womanpower is limited; therefore, nursing personnel must be utilized for those functions that require nursing skill and judgment. Functions that do not require nursing skill or knowledge should be delegated to other types of workers trained for these functions. Auxiliary workers can be trained on the job, the professional nurse being by education and experience a team leader.

*McIver, Pearl: Nursing moves forward, Fifty-eighth Annual Report of the NLN, New York, 1953, pp. 181-187.

2. A second important principle is that because womanpower is limited, all schools must select students carefully. Educational programs and conditions of undergraduate experience should be such that desirable students not only come to the school but also stay there.
3. Another basic principle is that nursing schools in organization, administration, and support become integral parts of the total educational program and that the administration of nursing education be vested in educational institutions.
4. The fourth principle is based on the theory that demands for nursing services are likely to increase more rapidly than supply. Thus, demands for nursing are increasing as the types of fields expand tremendously, and the type of work and responsibility change rapidly as general medicine, science, and health change.
5. Every qualified member of a profession has the right and responsibility to participate in such professional activities as (a) defining the functions of a particular occupational group, (b) determining desirable qualifications for practice, (c) establishing employment standards, (d) conducting studies that will improve individual practice, and (e) promoting legislative action that will improve nursing standards and benefit nursing.

The American Nurses' Association is the organization through which the nurse will carry out these responsibilities. The National League for Nursing, on the other hand, provides the opportunity for nurses and allied professional personnel and the public to work together to provide the amount and kind of nursing service and education needed in this country.

CHAPTER 36 THE AMERICAN NURSES' ASSOCIATION

■ The American Nurses' Association has continued its twofold purpose of providing better nursing service and of helping the graduate nurse in every way possible. Through its programs, better personnel policies have been worked out through state and local nursing organizations, and much closer contact is developing between local and national groups as representatives from national headquarters go into local areas to help with special problems in nursing.

Since 1950 the ANA has been actively sponsoring a research program. Nurses have supported this program both through voluntary subscription and through dues. The ANA now has a technical committee on studies of nursing functions and a research and statistics unit. Studies are being made in the changing role of the professional nurse, and a fact-finding and research service is available for ANA members. In addition to compiling *Facts About Nursing* annually, and the inventories of professional nurses periodically, these committees help staff members and other committees conduct research.

The ANA special groups section was organized in 1952. The main purpose of this section is to bring together nurses whose occupations place them in specialized groups too small to qualify for section status. Some of the interests represented are the executive secretaries of the American Nurses' Association and district nurse associations, recruitment, nurses in the armed services, registrars, some Red Cross nurses, nurses in public relations, nurse editors, nurse anesthetists, physical therapists, and occupational therapists. The second purpose for this section is to give these groups a place to discuss their problems until the groups are large enough to form new sections. The ANA bylaws at present provide that a new national section may be established if at least one third of the state nurses' associations have such a section.

During the 1962 convention in Detroit two new conference groups were organized: one on geriatric nursing practice with 67 nurses from 27 states as members, and one on medical-surgical nursing with 144 nurses as members.

After years of study, discussion, and deliberation by the study committee on the functions of ANA, the house of delegates in San Francisco voted for sweeping organizational changes in the structure.

Nursing expertise was regrouped into divisions on practice and commissions. The divisions on practice that held their organizational meetings at the 1968 ANA Convention in Dallas are community health nursing, geriatric nursing, maternal and child health nursing, medical-surgical nursing, and psychiatric and mental health nursing.

The new commissions are economic security and general welfare, education, and nursing services.

To encourage constant improvement for the practitioner, the new structure provides

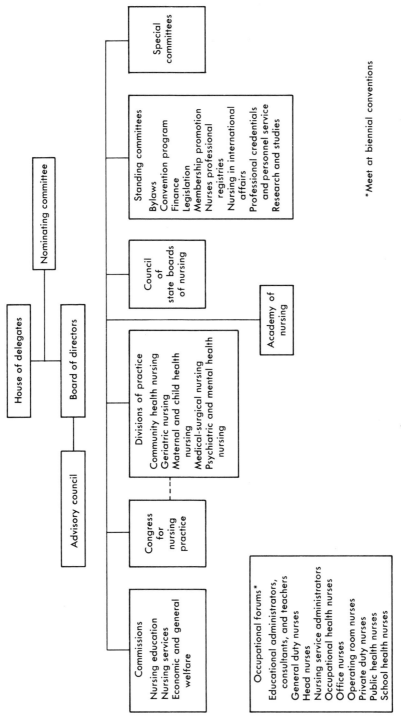

House of delegates

Nominating committee

Board of directors

Advisory council

Commissions
Nursing education
Nursing services
Economic and general welfare

Congress for nursing practice

Divisions of practice
Community health nursing
Geriatric nursing
Maternal and child health nursing
Medical-surgical nursing
Psychiatric and mental health nursing

Council of state boards of nursing

Standing committees
Bylaws
Convention program
Finance
Legislation
Membership promotion
Nurses professional registries
Nursing in international affairs
Professional credentials and personnel service
Research and studies

Special committees

Academy of nursing

Occupational forums*
Educational administrators, consultants, and teachers
General duty nurses
Head nurses
Nursing service administrators
Occupational health nurses
Office nurses
Operating room nurses
Private duty nurses
Public health nurses
School health nurses

*Meet at biennial conventions

AMERICAN NURSES' ASSOCIATION ORGANIZATION CHART.

the mechanism for the recognition of excellence by the profession—an Academy of Nursing.

In 1970 the national organization had financial difficulties and made an appeal directly to its membership for extra contributions to maintain the organization until the convenion in 1970 when long overdue adjustments for membership were passed by the house of delegates.

In 1970 the executive committee also contemplated moving the national headquarters out of New York City. A search committee was established; after it reported, the executive committee decided that the headquarters should be moved to Kansas City. This was done September 1, 1972. The Washington office was expanded, but the main part of the organization left the familiar address of 10 Columbus Circle and is now at 2420 Pershing Road, Kansas City, Missouri.

The American Journal of Nursing Company now occupies much of the space formerly occupied by the organization.

The library also remained in New York City.

AMERICAN NURSES' ASSOCIATION PROFESSIONAL COUNSELING AND PLACEMENT SERVICE, INC.

The American Nurses' Association Professional Counseling and Placement Service, Inc., is one of the important activities of the American Nurses' Association and has developed as a nonprofit activity that provides counseling and placement service without charge. Service is given to American Nurses' Association members. The Professional Counseling and Placement Service was established in 1945. It is owned by the American Nurses' Association, and 23 of the state associations now have established counseling and placement services also. More than 120,000 nurses had their professional records on file as of December, 1972. Counseling and placement are given through some of the state nurses' associations.

Counseling assists nurses to evaluate their aptitudes and skills, to learn about the types of positions for which they are best suited, and to make long-range plans. For this purpose the PC&PS keeps confidential credentials on file and will forward them to any other professional counseling and placement service office or to an employer at the request of the nurse. This organization operates only on a national basis.

CHAPTER 37 NATIONAL LEAGUE FOR NURSING

■ The National League for Nursing maintains close relationships with such allied organizations as the American Association of Junior and Community Colleges, the American Hospital Association, the American Medical Association, the American Public Health Association, the National Association for Practical Nurse Education, and the National Federation of Licensed Practical Nurses. The NLN carries out its work through extensive correspondence, national and regional conferences, workshops and institutes, consultation services, staff visits to local communities, manuals and handbooks, tests and guides, printed bulletins, and leaflets. Vital problems for the National League for Nursing are better utilization of all nursing personnel, professional and nonprofessional; better and more extensive in-service education; and the development of teamwork among all nursing personnel, and with medical and nonprofessional nursing groups in the hospital and in the community.

Through the Council of Home Health Agencies and Community Health Services and the Assembly of Constituent Leagues for Nursing, communities are helped to meet expanding needs for nursing service in the home.

This year (1973) marks the twenty-first year of the new organization.

In the continuing studies of structure of the National League for Nursing, the committee on constitutions and bylaws presented the following major amendment, which was adopted at the 1963 convention, held in Atlantic City.

ARTICLE V. OFFICERS

Section 2. Qualifications for Officers. Any individual member except honorary members shall be eligible to hold any of the elected positions specified in Section 1 of this article. The treasurer shall be an individual who is especially skilled and experienced in handling financial matters. No person shall be eligible for position as an elected officer and as a member of the Board of Directors of the American Nurses' Association.*

This important amendment removed the restriction that the president and first vice president of the National League for Nursing must be registered professional nurses as a qualification for those offices.

During the NLN convention in New York City in 1967, following several years of study, the membership voted for an entirely new structure giving more flexibility, freedom, and voice to the local membership.

The league continues to have both individual and agency members. In 1971 its individual members are professional and practical nurses, nursing aides, doctors, hospital administrators, educators, social workers, therapists, and interested citizens. Agency members, numbering more than 1,800, include hospitals and other institutions providing nursing services, public health nursing agencies, and schools and colleges offering educational programs in nursing.

---

*Nursing Outlook **11**:272, April, 1963. Reprinted with permission.

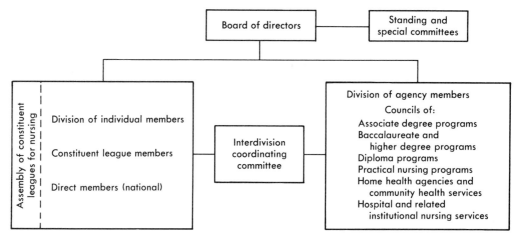

NATIONAL LEAGUE FOR NURSING ORGANIZATION CHART.

Today one of the main functions of the National League for Nursing is the accrediting services for the various types of educational programs in nursing. They are administered and conducted through four departmental units of the organization's national headquarters: The Department of Baccalaureate and Higher Degree Programs, the Department of Associate Degree Programs, the Department of Diploma Programs, and the Department of Practical Nursing Programs.

PURPOSES OF ACCREDITATION

The purposes of accrediting programs in nursing education have been stated by the NLN as follows:

1. To stimulate continuous improvement of nursing education throughout the United States and thus to promote improvement of nursing services.
2. To offer assistance to educational units in nursing in the continuous process of self-evaluation and self-improvement of their programs.
3. To describe the essential and distinctive characteristics that each type of education program should have in order to make its appropriate contribution to society.
4. To publish periodically lists of programs cur-

rently accredited as meeting the accepted criteria for the designated type of program.*

The lists that are published serve as guides for prospective students in their choice of educational programs in nursing. They assist secondary schools, colleges, and universities in advising students in their choice of educational programs in nursing; assist employers of nurses in judging the qualifications of candidates for various types of positions; and aid interinstitutional relationships such as transfer of students and admission to graduate programs.

Accreditation is conducted under the principles adopted in 1956 for the league's total program of accrediting.

1. Accreditation in nursing is conceived as a program in which the educational units themselves play a vital part. In the process, every effort is made to involve as large a number as possible of the administrative and teaching staff of each educational unit in nursing in its own self-evaluation and thus to encourage self-development.
2. Criteria for accreditation must change as the profession itself evolves and as the society which it serves makes changing demands. The

---

*Policies and procedures of accreditation of the Department of Associate Degree Programs, NLN, New York, 1967.

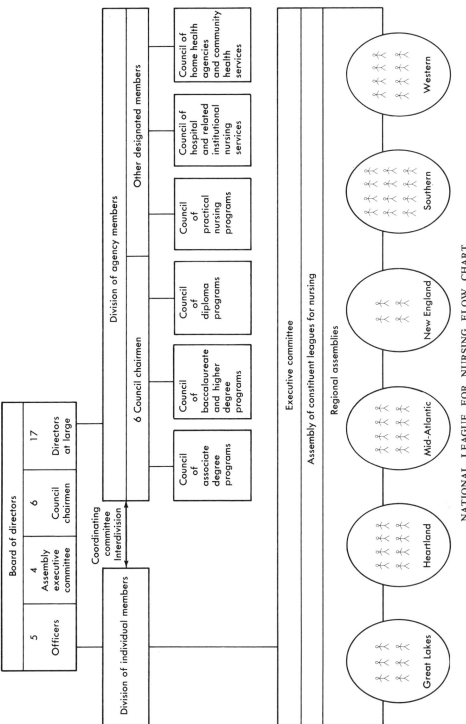

NATIONAL LEAGUE FOR NURSING FLOW CHART.

continuing development of these criteria is a responsibility of the NLN agency members. The function rests with the appropriate councils. (For associate degree programs, this is the Council of Associate Degree Programs.)

3. The individuality of institutions and their special contributions are of paramount importance. Therefore, provided that there is basic conformity to the standards generally accepted by the profession and by society as essential for the functioning of the graduate of an institution at the level and in the field for which the institution purports to train, emphasis is placed upon the evaluation of the total program and its general excellence as well as upon its achievement with regard to particular aspects. Furthermore, the dynamic quality of a program and the rapidity with which it is moving toward clearly defined and desirable goals are recognized. This implies that there will be flexibility in accrediting procedures.*

The National League for Nursing is recognized by the National Commission on Accrediting for the accreditation of baccalaureate and higher degree programs in professional nursing, and as an auxiliary accrediting association at the associate degree level.

A second major function of the National League for Nursing is helping the various constituent leagues with community planning. In 1971 the bylaws were once more changed to eliminate the division of individual members and confine this to constituent league membership for even more flexibility and ability to help.

COMMUNITY PLANNING

The constituent leagues are grouped in six regional assemblies—New England, Mid-Atlantic, Great Lakes, Heartland, Southern, and Western—for comprehensive sectional planning. Representatives of the 44 groups meet annually in regional or national assembly meetings for an avenue of exchange of

ideas and coordinated planning toward national and local goals.

Constituent league programs are tailored to meet local needs. The leagues do such things as alert communities to nursing needs; stimulate service, education, and research programs and put together recommendations for expansion of nursing services in an area; initiate retraining courses to bring retired nurses back to work; administer nursing scholarships; sponsor continuing education workshops; and work for new health facilities or special training programs.

TESTING SERVICES

The volume of the testing service had become so great that a regular department of the National League of Nursing Education was created in 1946. In addition to the state board examinations, a national test for prenursing and guidance was worked out. State Board Pool tests are now used in all of the states, District of Columbia, and several provinces in Canada.

R. Louise McManus, chairman and director of the Division of Nursing Education, Teachers College, Columbia University, was responsible for setting up the State Board Pool, which became a source for examinations and for the scoring of tests for state Boards throughout the country. To a certain extent this was a development of World War II when state boards of nurse examiners were being swamped with the work of testing and scoring state board tests; many graduates were being delayed because they could not obtain results from their examinations quickly enough. After two years Louise McManus had acquired a staff of 30 full-time workers in her testing service, and after the war the old system of state boards was not resumed, but the National League for Nursing continued this testing service.

Staff workers are constantly developing better technics in testing and are closely associated with nurse educators from different parts of the United States representing both

---

*Policies and procedures of accreditation of the Department of Associate Degree Programs, NLN, New York, 1967.

diploma and degree programs. The plan now worked out is that two nurse teachers in each of the major clinical areas of the basic programs spend one week at headquarters, deciding the general scope of material and developing test questions to be included in the examinations. In addition, the Evaluation and Guidance Service creates qualifying examinations for the graduate nurse. This examination is used by many colleges and universities.

NATIONAL COMMITTEE FOR THE IMPROVEMENT OF NURSING SERVICE

In 1951 the National Committee for the Improvement of Nursing Service was enlarged to include 40 members, representing education, medicine, and general citizen groups. At this time a *Newsletter* was published to keep the state nursing organizations informed and to help them organize state committees for the improvement of nursing service. Also published was the book *Nursing Schools at the Mid-Century*. When the interim classification of schools of nursing was made, schools were promised that the second study would be made within two years. However, it developed that a program of temporary accreditation seemed to be more helpful to schools in working toward full accreditation than a second classification would be. Funds were granted by the Rockefeller and Commonwealth Foundation and the National Foundation for Infantile Paralysis to support the program of temporary accreditation for a three-year period. This accrediting program was carried out by the National Nursing Accrediting Service, which had been organized early in 1949 under the auspices of the six national nursing organizations.

A subcommittee on the improvement of nursing service had also been developing its program during this period. Institutes on nursing service administration for both nursing administrators and hospital administrators were held by the National Committee for the Improvement of Nursing Service and the American Hospital Association.

In June, 1952, when the structure of the six national nursing organizations changed, the work and staff of the National Committee for the Improvement of Nursing Service were absorbed into the Division of Nursing Services of the National League for Nursing.

CHAPTER 38 OTHER NATIONAL ORGANIZATIONS

NATIONAL STUDENT NURSES' ASSOCIATION

■ The National Student Nurses' Association was organized during the convention of the National League for Nursing in 1953, in Cleveland. Since 1924 student nurses had attended national nursing conventions. Now students have conventions of their own. In 1950, meetings of student nurses were scheduled and sponsored by graduate nurses. In Atlantic City in June, 1952, the students met and began to talk about forming a national organizaion. Since the next national convention was to be held in Cleveland in 1953, the job of setting up the constitution and bylaws for a national student organization was delegated to the Ohio student nurses. The bylaws were formally adopted, and the first slate of officers was elected in 1953 at the meeting held in conjunction with the NLN Convention in Cleveland. Student nurse conventions are now held in conjunction with the alternating biennial conventions of the American Nurses' Association and the National League for Nursing. Most of the time, attendance exceeds 4,000 members. In 1971 and 1973 the student nurse convention was planned and held jointly with the NLN Convention.

The National Student Nurses' Association, Inc. (NSNA) consists of individual members in the 51 constituent associations in 49 states, the District of Columbia, and Puerto Rico. There are, in addition, about 240 district or local associations.

The purpose of the student organization as defined in the bylaws is, "to aid in the preparation of student nurses for the assumption of professional responsibilities."

The organization serves as spokesman for students by taking a stand on issues of importance to nursing students. The NSNA serves as a voice for students and as a source of direction and information. NSNA has taken official action in recent years in support of economic security, changes in education for nurses, a broad range of legislation, American Nurses' Association Code for Professional Nurses, and the student's right to educational experience rather than being expected to provide nursing service.

PRACTICAL NURSES

Qualified practical nurses are eligible for membership in the NLN as voted at the National League for Nursing's first convention in 1953. After this convention it was also voted unanimously to authorize the NLN Board of Directors to provide for a Department of Practical Nurse Education if advisable before the next biennial in 1955. A council on practical nursing was created at the annual convention in 1957.

The National Association for Practical Nurse Education was organized in 1941 and is concerned chiefly with education. Membership is offered to both practical and professional nurses as well as to other persons engaged in activities to further the objects of the association. One of the most important activities of this organization has been to survey and to accredit educational programs for practical nurses. Any practical nurse is eligible for NLN membership if he or she is licensed as a practical nurse or by an equivalent title in a state that provides for such licensure, or if she is a graduate of an approved school of practical nursing if the state or states within which she practices or resides do not provide for licensing.

During the 1963 Convention of the National League for Nursing, the Department of Practical Nursing Programs' Council of Member Agencies took one more step toward the development of criteria for evaluating schools of practical nursing when they met and discussed tentative statements presented by the committee to study criteria for evaluation of practical nursing programs.

OTHER NURSING ORGANIZATIONS

When the American Nurses' Association and the National League for Nursing were reorganized in 1953, not all the existing nursing organizations were incorporated within the frameworks of these two major associations of nursing. Some of the better-known nursing organizations that have retained their identity are described.

The American Association of Industrial Nurses was organized in 1942. Their official publication is the *American Association of Industrial Nurses Journal*. The aims of the association follow:

1. To formulate and develop principles and standards of industrial nursing practice in order that the nurse in industry may more fully utilize her professional knowledge and training in her service to workers and management—and to the community.
2. To promote, by means of publications, conferences, institutes, and symposia, both formal and informal programs of education designed specifically for the nurse in industry.
3. To identify the rightful place of nursing in

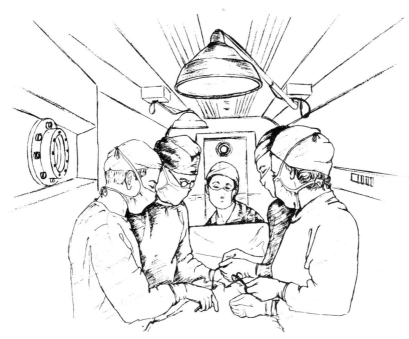

The surgical nurse is a vital part of the many exciting innovations in surgery, such as operating in a hyperbaric chamber.

the industrial health program and to encourage cooperation among all groups engaged in protecting the health and welfare of the workers.

4. To impress upon management, physicians, and allied groups the importance of integrating into the activities of industry the services of the industrial nurse.

In 1960 there were approximately 5,000 members of the American Association of Industrial Nurses.

The American College of Nurse-Midwifery was organized in 1955 since none of the existing organizations met the professional needs of this unique specialization in nursing. Representatives of the college have participated in meetings of the International Confederation of Midwives. They publish the *Bulletin of the American College of Nurse-Midwifery*.

The American Association for Nurse Anesthetists was organized in 1931 under the leadership of Agatha Hodgins. Under this association's sponsorship, minimum standards for competent practice were established, and a program of school accreditation was begun in 1952. By 1960 there were 123 accredited schools for nurse anesthetists in the United States. Their official bimonthly publication is *The Journal of the American Association of Nurse Anesthetists*.

The Association of Operating Room Nurses was organized in 1957 and currently has over 4,000 members. They hold a national four-day congress annually and sponsor two-day institutes all over the country. The official journal, *O.R. Nursing,* is published bimonthly.

As specialty groups join together to meet their specific needs, many new publications for nurses appear regularly and are too numerous to list or scrutinize.

CHAPTER 39 A NEW ORGANIZATION IS DEVELOPED

■ The American Association of Deans of College and University Schools of Nursing grew out of an ad hoc committee of deans of accredited masters programs of the Council of Baccalaureate and Higher Degree Programs of the National League for Nursing. It held its first meeting in May, 1967.

For some time the focus of the group seemed limited to concerns of deans in university medical centers. However, this focus was soon expanded but restricted to deans of educational units in nursing that offered NLN accredited programs.

The bylaws of the new organization follow:

BYLAWS OF THE AMERICAN ASSOCIATION OF NURSING COLLEGES

ARTICLE I
THE CORPORATION

Section 1 *Name*
The name of this association shall be the American Association of Nursing Colleges.

Section 2 *Purpose*
The purpose of the Association shall be to serve the public through promotion and improvement of higher education for professional nursing.

Section 3 *Membership*
(a) Membership in the Association shall be of two kinds, institutional and individual.
(b) Institutional membership is available to programs in nursing leading to a baccalaureate or higher degree and located in institutionally accredited colleges and universities.
(c) Individual membership is available to the deans or directors of the aforementioned programs.
(d) Membership is conferred upon the payment of dues.

The current president is Sister Bernadette Armiger of Niagara University.

The organization's principal function to date has been in legislative activity; the organization worked diligently to insure the passage of Public Law 92-158, which includes capitation grants to the colleges, among other benefits, and was signed into law November, 1971.

In the spring of 1973 the official name of the organization was changed to the American Association of Nursing, and a Washington, D. C., office was established.

QUESTIONS AND STUDY PROJECTS FOR UNIT NINE

1. Write a rationale for having two such large organizations in nursing.
2. Can you list at least ten other smaller nursing organizations?
3. Differentiate the functions of the ANA and NLN.
4. What is the latest nursing organization and what is its principal function?
5. What are your feelings about multiple specialized small interest groups in nursing?

REFERENCES FOR UNIT NINE

ANA: A position paper: educational preparation for nurse practitioners and assistants to nurses, New York, 1965, ANA.

Bixler, G. K., and Bixler, R. W.: The professional status of nursing, American Journal of Nursing **45**:730-735, September, 1945.

Bridgman, Margaret: On types of programs, American Journal of Nursing **60**:1465-1468, October, 1960.

Brown, Esther Lucile: Nursing as a profession, ed. 2, New York, 1940, Russell Sage Foundation.

Brown, Esther Lucile: Nursing for the future (Brown Report), New York, 1948, Russell Sage Foundation.

Brown, Esther Lucile: Newer dimensions of patient care, Part I, New York, 1961, Russell Sage Foundation.

Brown, Esther Lucile: Newer dimensions of patient care, Part II, New York, 1962, Russell Sage Foundation.

DeChow, Georgeen H.: Accreditation of associate degree nursing program, Journal of Nursing Education **4**:27-32, August, 1965.

Ginzberg, Eli: Nursing and manpower realities, Nursing Outlook **15**:26, November, 1967.

Harty, Margaret B.: Team teaching, Nursing Outlook **11**:59-61, January, 1963.

Jahoda, Marie: Nursing as a profession, American Journal of Nursing **61**:52-56, July, 1961.

Juliana, Sister: An experience in transition in nursing education, Hospital Progress **48**:67, February, 1967.

Mahoney, Anne B.: Convincing the membership, American Journal of Nursing **66**:554, March, 1966.

NLN: Department of Associate Degree Programs, criteria for the evaluation of educational programs in nursing leading to an associate degree, New York, 1973, NLN.

NLN: Policies and procedures of accreditation of the Department of Associate Degree Programs, New York, 1973, NLN.

Operating room nursing—is it professional nursing? American Journal of Nursing **65**:58, August, 1965.

UNIT TEN
Research into nursing and nursing research

Research is the framework within which new knowledge is added to any profession. The scientific method or scientific inquiry is the keystone to professionalism and further growth.

In nursing it means the development of a body of nursing science that will have an immediate effect on patient care and also will likely be the determining factor in revolutionizing the health care delivery system in the United States.

Too long much of the research has been devoted to the education of nurses only and not to nursing practice. This is rapidly changing, and much of the research is now being done to improve nursing care for the patient along with the continued research into the development of a student of nursing.

CHAPTER 40 THE AMERICAN NURSES' FOUNDATION

■ The American Nurses' Foundation was established by the American Nurses' Association in 1955 to support research and studies in nursing and to sponsor special projects. The foundation plans, guides, and coordinates nursing research and disseminates research findings. Supported in part by funds from the ANA, the foundation receives contributions from individuals and from other foundations.

During the period 1955-1971 the ANF reviewed 126 proposals, of which 59 (47%) were approved and 67 (53%) were disapproved. Of the approved proposals, 61% were developmental grants, 35% were research grants, and 4% were contracts. One half of the developmental grants were awarded to doctoral candidates for the implementation of their dissertation research projects. The developmental grants program offers the doctoral student or beginning researcher a unique opportunity to explore a researchable idea for one or two years with a funding of $3,500 per year, thus not only facilitating the completion of research for doctoral dissertations but also providing seed monies for pilot studies or the development of new tools of measurement or new mechanical instruments. A grand total of $488,000 has been awarded by ANF since 1955 for all the research projects supported.

Following is a list of projects funded by the American Nurses' Foundation from 1970 to 1972:

1970

An interdisciplinary study of care in dying patients and their families (2-70-023), Florence S. Wald, M.S.N., R.N., Yale University.

Factors affecting the appearance of secretory immunoglobulins in the external secretions of human infants (2-70-024), Camilla S. Wood, M.S., R.N., University of Utah.

The blue-collar family and family decision-making applied to health and illness behavior (2-70-025), Rosemary Johnson, M.P.H., R.N., University of California, Los Angeles.

Understanding hospitalized children through drawings (2-70-026), Juanita W. Fleming, Ph.D., R.N., University of Kentucky.

Effects of oxygen and carbon dioxide concentrations and of stimulation of sympathetic nerves on blood vessels of the pregnant sheep uterus (1-70-023), Ellen O. Fuller, Ph.D., R.N., Emory University.

A proposed study of the effect of estrogen level upon cognitive behavior (2-70-027), Effie I. Anderson, M.S., R.N., Boston University.

An investigation of the relationship between developmental factors and the presence or absence of drooling among 3- to 5-year-old mental retardates (2-70-028), Mary Jane Foster, M.S.Ed., R.N., New York University.

The effectiveness and efficiency of group and individual preoperative teaching (1-70-024), Carol Lindeman, Ph.D., R.N., Luther Hospital, Eau Claire, Wisconsin.

1971

Privacy and the hospitalization experience (2-71-029), Eleanor Schuster, M.S., R.N., University of California, San Francisco.

Relationship of adrenal cortex to ovarian function (1-71-025), Gladys A. Courtney, Ph.D.,

R.N., University of Illinois, the Medical Center.

Relationship between illness crisis and belief in personal control (1-71-026), Mary Marston, Ph.D., R.N., Case Western Reserve University.

Social process and symptom change: an epidemiological study of the relation between symptom patterning and psychiatric service (1-71-027), Helen Nakagawa, Ph.D., R.N., and Oliver H. Osborne, Ph.D., R.N., University of Washington.

1972

The role of lysosomal enzymes in the etiology of pulmonary emphysema (2-72-030), Benjamin Rosenbluth, B.S., R.N., Oklahoma Medical Center.

Speech perception in neonates (2-72-031), Veronica A. Binzley, M.A., R.N., Case Western Reserve University.

The training of alcoholism counselors: pre-training and post-training studies related to a six months' training program (2-72-032), Constance Grant Zich, M.S., R.N., Johns Hopkins University School of Hygiene & Public Health.

CHAPTER 41 NATIONAL COMMISSION FOR THE STUDY OF NURSING AND NURSING EDUCATION

■ The most recent and ongoing study of nursing and nursing education can be traced directly to the final document of the Surgeon General's Consultant Group on Nursing, "Toward Quality in Nursing."

Shortly after this report appeared, the two major organizations in nursing—the American Nurses' Association and the National League for Nursing—appropriated funds and established a joint committee to study the ways to conduct and finance such a national inquiry.

In April of 1966 W. Allen Wallis, president of the University of Rochester, agreed to head such a study if adequate financing could be obtained.

In the fall of 1966 the Board of Directors of the American Nurses' Foundation voted to grant up to $50,000 to help launch the study.

The Avalon Foundation and the Kellogg Foundation gave $100,000 each to support the investigation. Coincidentally, an anonymous benefactor contributed the sum of $300,000 to ensure the undertaking.

In January of 1967 the National Commission for the Study of Nursing and Nursing Education was officially formed.

Although the commission was a direct outgrowth of the keen interest of the ANA and NLN, it was set up as an independent agency and functioned as a self-directing group, with the power to plan and conduct its investigations as it saw fit.

At the first formal meeting of the commission in August of 1967, a director, Jerome P. Lysaught, and associate director, Charles H. Russell, were appointed to conduct the planning and actual operating of the inquiry. A headquarters was established in Rochester, New York, through the cooperation of the university, and a small staff was acquired to develop the research proposal.

The primary objective of the investigation asked: How can we improve the delivery of health care to the American people, particularly through the analysis and improvement of nursing and nursing education?

Following are the recommendations*:

1. The federal Division of Nursing, the National Center for Health Services Research and Development, other governmental agencies, and private foundations appropriate grant funds or research contracts to investigate the impact of nursing practice on the quality, effectiveness, and economy of health care.

2. The same agencies and foundations appropriate research funds and research contracts for basic and applied research into the nursing curriculum, articulation of educational systems, instructional methodologies, and facilities design so that the most functional, effective, and economic approaches are taken in the education and development of future nurses.

3. Each state have, or create, a master planning committee that will take nursing education

*From An abstract for action: report of the National Commission for the Study of Nursing and Nursing Education. Jerome P. Lysaught, editor. Copyright 1970 by McGraw-Hill Book Co. Originally published in the American Journal of Nursing 70: 286-294.

under its purview, such committees to include representatives of nursing, education, other health professions, and the public, to recommend specific guidelines, means for implementation, and deadlines to ensure that nursing education is positioned in the mainstream of American educational patterns.

4. Federal, regional, state and local governments adopt measures for the increased support of nursing research and education. Priority should be given to construction grants, institutional grants, advanced traineeships, and research grants and contracts. Further, we recommend that private funds and foundations support nursing research and educational innovations where such activities are not publicly aided. We believe that a useful guide for the beginnings of such a financial aid program would be in the amounts and distribution of funds authorized by Congress for fiscal 1970, with proportional increases from other public and private agencies.

5. A national Joint Practice Commission, with state counterpart committees, be established between Medicine and Nursing to discuss and make recommendations concerning the congruent roles of the physician and the nurse in providing quality health care, with particular attention to: the rise of the nurse clinician; the introduction of the physician's assistant; the increased activity of other professions and para-professions in areas long assumed to be the concern solely of the physician and/or the nurse.

6. Two essentially related, but differing, career patterns be developed for nursing practice:
   a. One career pattern (episodic) would emphasize nursing practice that is essentially curative and restorative, generally acute or chronic in nature, and most frequently provided in the setting of the hospital and inpatient facility.
   b. The second career pattern (distributive) would emphasize the nursing practice that is designed essentially for health maintenance and disease prevention, generally continuous in nature, seldom acute, and most frequently operative in the community or in newly developing institutional settings.

7. Continued study to be given to the use of technology, organizational practices, and specialized personnel (e.g., ward clerks and unit managers) that can release nurses from non-nursing functions which maintaining nursing control over the delivery of nursing care.

8. No less than three regional or inter-institutional committees be funded for the study and development of the nursing curriculum (similar to previous national studies in the biological, physical, and socal sciences) in order to develop objectives, universals, alternatives, and sequences for nursing instruction. These committees should specify appropriate levels of general and specialized learning for the different types of educational institutions, and should be particularly concerned with the articulation of programs between the two collegiate levels.

9. The Congress continue and expand such programs as the Health Manpower Act to provide educational loans to nurses pursuing graduate programs with provision for part or whole forgiveness based on subsequent years of teaching.

10. Federal and state funds should be provided to institutions for nursing education:
    a. For financial support proportional to the number of students enrolled, such moneys to be used to defray expenses of operation and expansion, and to provide salary increments for qualified faculty;
    b. For the building and construction of facilities including laboratories and classrooms.

11. Federal, state and private funds be utilized to implement continuing education programs on either a state-wide or broader basis (as suggested by the current inter-state compacts for higher education) in order to develop short courses, seminars, or other educational experiences. In the face of changing health roles and functions, a greater measure of continuing education programs should be planned and conducted by inter-disciplinary teams.

12. Health management and nursing administration seek to reduce turnover, increase retention, and induce a return to practice by nurses through:
    a. Building on current improvements in starting salaries to create a strong reward system by developing schedules of substantially increasing salary levels for nurses who remain in clinical practice.
    b. Establishing conditions, through organizational and staffing practices, that will give nurses an opportunity to provide optimum care to their patients, including individual planning and implementation of the care plan.
    c. Adopting personnel policies that provide for planned orientation and in-service education courses, flexible employment policies respecting part-time work, scheduling,

maternity leaves, assistance for continuing and graduate education to qualify for advancement, and leaves for educational purposes.

13. Both professional organizations and educational institutions in nursing increase counseling services and recruitment efforts directed at mature females seeking initial entries into nursing programs. These efforts should include overtures to both high school graduates and college graduates from the liberal arts and sciences.

14. A single license be retained for registered nurses. Differences in levels of nursing should be recognized through: a) designation of master clinicians by approved bodies for such purposes, presumably the Academy of Nursing; b) state licensing standards for health service units; c) qualifications regarding personnel specified in accreditation standards for health service units; d) institutional personnel policies respecting appointments, grades or ranks, and qualifications for promotion.

15. The national nursing organizations, particularly the American Nurses' Association and the National League for Nursing, press forward in their current study of functions, structures, methods for representation, and inter-relationships in order to determine: a) areas of overlap or duplication; b) areas of unmet needs; and c) areas or functions that could be transferred from one organization to another in the light of changing conditions.

To help insure the implementation of the recommendations, Dr. Lysaught received an additional grant from the Kellogg Foundation totaling $215,948.

Of the Kellogg Foundation grant, the sum of $90,948 is for support of commission activities from now through September 30, 1973, when the national commission will conclude its work. A second amount of $125,000 is provided for the support of related activities in nine designated target states being utilized as demonstration laboratories for implementation efforts.

The original commission was altered somewhat to respond to their new and continued activities. The life and activity of the commission will have a lasting effect on nursing and nursing education.

REFERENCES

An abstract for action: appendices to the report of the National Commission for the Study of Nursing and Nursing Education, New York, 1971, McGraw-Hill Book Co.

Baker, Mary: Lysaught?!! students view the National Commission for the Study of Nursing and Nursing Education, Imprint 18:18, November-December, 1971.

Baker, Mary: Lysaught?!! Part 3: students view the National Commission for the Study of Nursing and Nursing Education, Imprint 19:17, March, 1972.

Christy, Teresa E., Poulin, Muriel A., and Hover, Julie: An appraisal of an abstract for action, American Journal of Nursing 71:1574-1581, August, 1971. See also Lysaught, J. P.: Let the recommendations of the national commission be judged on their merits, not on the basis of whether nursing originated them or not, American Journal of Nursing 71:1914, October, 1971. In addition, see Letters to the Editor, American Journal of Nursing, October and November, 1971.

de Tornyay, Rheba: A Flexner report for professional nursing, California Medicine 113:81-85, September, 1970.

de Tornyay, Rheba: Today's nurses are reaching for a larger part in medical care, California's Health 28:6-10, January, 1971.

Grigg, Sherry: Lysaught?!! Part 2: students view the National Commission for the Study of Nursing and Nursing Education, Imprint 19:16, January, 1972.

Kelisch, Beatrice J.: An abstract for action, Library Journal, October 15, 1970 (a review).

Lewis, Edith P.: In perspective (editorial), Nursing Outlook 20:163, March, 1972.

Lysaught, Jerome, P., editor: An abstract for action: report of the National Commission for the Study of Nursing and Nursing Education, New York, 1970, McGraw-Hill Book Co.

Lysaught, Jerome P.: Continuing education: necessity and opportunity, Journal of Continuing Education in Nursing 1:5-10, September, 1970.

Lysaught, Jerome P.: The National Study of Nursing and Nursing Education and its relationship to the concept of the physician's assistant (Presented during the annual meeting, Federation of State Medical Boards, Chicago, February 12, 1971.), Federation Bulletin 59:107-123, March, 1972.

Lysaught, Jerome P.: From abstract into action: progress report from the National Commission for the Study of Nursing and Nursing Education, Nursing Outlook 20:173-179, March, 1972.

Lysaught, Jerome P.: Role articulation: primary

target for the future, AORN Journal **15:**109-124, 1972.

Murry, Ruth Neil: An abstract for action, Nursing Outlook **19:**380, June, 1971 (a review).

National Commission for the Study of Nursing and Nursing Education: summary report and recommendations, American Journal of Nursing **70:**279-294, February, 1970.

Russell, Charles H.: Recommendations of Commission on the Study of Nursing and Nursing Education on career development. In Novello, D., editor: Report on first state-wide institute on career development within the occupational field of nursing, June 10-12, 1970, sponsored by Committee on Education of the Pennsylvania Nurses Association, pp. 24-29.

Russell, Charles H.: The nursing service administrator and the report of the National Commission for the Study of Nursing and Nursing Education, Journal of Nursing Administration **1:**12-16, January-February, 1971.

Russell, Charles H.: Issues in continuing education for nursing. In McHenry, Ruth W., editor: End and means: the National Conference in Continuing Education in Nursing—1970, Proceedings of the Second National Conference on Continuing Education in Nursing, Sagamore, New York, October, 1970, pp. 8-20.

Smith, Kathryn M.: An abstract for action, American Journal of Nursing **71:**814-818, April, 1971 (a review).

Sorenson, Gladys: An abstract for action, Nursing Research **20:**173-174, March-April, 1971 (a review).

Statement on report of National Commission for the Study of Nursing and Nursing Education, Hospitals **45:**131, May, 1971. *See also* AHA Newsletter for the Hospital School of Nursing **4:**4, April, 1971.

Thurston, Hester I.: Education for episodic and distributive care, Nursing Outlook **20:**519-523, August, 1972.

QUESTIONS AND STUDY PROJECTS FOR UNIT TEN

1. Who funds the American Nurses' Foundation?
2. Determine if your school or community is involved in the implementation of the recommendations of the National Commission for the Study of Nursing and Nursing Education.
3. Who contributed the original "seed" monies for the lengthy study?
4. What was the impact on nursing of the National Committee for the Improvement of Nursing Service?

UNIT ELEVEN
International relationships

International code of nursing ethics*

"Professional nurses minister to the sick, assume responsibility for creating a physical, social and spiritual environment which will be conducive to recovery, and stress the prevention of illness and promotion of health by teaching and example. They render health service to the individual, the family, and the community, and coordinate their services with members of other health professions.

"Service to mankind is the primary function of nurses and the reason for the existence of the nursing profession. Need for nursing service is universal. Professional nursing service is therefore unrestricted by considerations of nationality, race, creed, color, politics, or social status.

"Inherent in the code is the fundamental concept that the nurse believes in the essential freedoms of mankind and in the preservation of human life.

"The profession recognizes that an international code cannot cover in detail all the activities and relationships of nurses, some of which are conditioned by personal philosophies and beliefs.

"1. The fundamental responsibility of the nurse is threefold: to conserve life, to alleviate suffering, and to promote health.

"2. The nurse muts maintain at all times the highest standards of nursing care and of professional conduct.

"3. The nurse must not only be well prepared to practice but must maintain her knowledge and skill at a consistently high level.

"4. The religious beliefs of a patient must be respected.

---

*Adopted by the International Council of Nurses, July, 1953; printed in American Journal of Nursing **53:**1070, September, 1953.

"5. Nurses hold in confidence all personal information entrusted to them.

"6. A nurse recognizes not only the responsibilities but the limitations of her or his professional functions; recommends or gives medical treatment without medical orders only in emergencies and reports such action to a physician at the earliest possible moment.

"7. The nurse is under an obligation to carry out the physician's orders intelligently and loyally and to refuse to participate in unethical procedures.

"8. The nurse sustains confidence in the physician and other members of the health team; incompetence or unethical conduct of associates should be exposed, but only to the proper authority.

"9. A nurse is entitled to just remuneration and accepts only such compensation as the contract, actual or implied, provides.

"10. Nurses do not permit their names to be used in connection with the advertisement of products or with any other forms of self-advertisement.

"11. The nurse cooperates with and maintains harmonious relationships with members of other professions and with her or his nursing colleagues.

"12. The nurse in private life adheres to standards of personal ethics which reflect credit upon the profession.

"13. In personal conduct nurses should not knowingly disregard the accepted patterns of behavior of the community in which they live and work.

"14. A nurse should participate and share responsibilty with other citizens and other health professions in promoting efforts to meet the health needs of the public—local, state, national, and international."

CHAPTER 42 SOME NURSING ACTIVITIES ON AN INTERNATIONAL LEVEL

■ In preceding chapters we have seen the progression of the emancipation of women toward an international movement with the increasing professionalization of nursing as an important result. We shall now see how nursing in turn has become an international development advancing first nursing, then the larger sphere of feminism, and ultimately that of internationalism and good fellowship among the peoples.

THE INTERNATIONAL COUNCIL OF NURSES

About the turn of the century the aims of the leaders of nursing, especially in Great Britain and the United States, had become very similar. In 1899 Mrs. Bedford-Fenwick placed before the Women's Council of Great Britain the proposal that the prominent nurses from many countries who were attending the International Council of Women held in London be invited to join in an International Council of Nurses. The proposal was enthusiastically accepted, and a provisional committee was promptly formed by nurses from Great Britain, the United States, Canada, New Zealand, New South Wales, Victoria, Holland, Cape Colony, and Denmark, countries that we noted in the past as being in the vanguard of nursing education. The committee promptly formulated a constitution that established the purpose of the organization: to unite and to organize nurses of all countries within one common bond in order that they may together attain complete professional freedom. Through the development of self-government they could establish the highest professional standards and serve society to the utmost of their ability. They were perfectly aware that such an organization would serve the greater cause of feminism and achieve for one group of women that which was considered at least part of the goal of all women. It was also apparent that when women from many lands met together, friendships and personal ties would be formed that could help to prevent the bloodshed of international conflict. Gradually, as we as individuals come to know personally more and more of our colleagues in other countries, we shall become less and less enthusiastic about going to war against them.

However premature the ultimate purposes may have seemed, the immediate plans met with absolute success. By 1900 the council was organized with Mrs. Bedford-Fenwick as president, Miss Lavinia Dock as honorary secretary, and Miss Snively as honorary treasurer. The first International Congress of Nurses was called during the Pan-American Exposition in Buffalo, New York, in 1901. At this time membership was individual, but it was soon decided that it should be by association. Thereby the members could better accomplish their aim, for by admitting only organizations that were controlled by nurses and had official national standing, they excluded organizations controlled by persons other than nurses, thus achieving professional self-government.

In Germany the free sisters took advantage of this. In 1903 they organized the German Nurses' Association under the able leadership of Sister Agnes Karll. In 1904 when the International Council of Women met in Berlin, they became hosts to the International Council of Nurses. The principle of admission by association was officially established, and the council was begun with three members: the National Council of Nurses of Great Britain, the American Nurses' Association, and the German Nurses' Association.

The influence of the International Council of Nurses in raising standards in many countries is on record. To become a member the national nurses' organization in a country must be self-governing. This has spurred the movement for increasing educational standards as well as obtaining recognition and support in each country.

Organization and development

Headquarters were established first in Geneva, Switzerland, later in London. At first *The American Journal of Nursing* and the *British Journal of Nursing* were the official organs for the council; later it established its own journal, the *I.C.N.*, which in 1930 became the *International Nursing Review*. It was now a most colorful and fruitful source for all information pertaining to the progress of nursing in the various countries.

Meetings were held every few years. World War I, as well as World War II, suspended such activities, but since 1922 the council has met every three or four years on both sides of the Atlantic. At each meeting more countries were admitted, so that before World War II there were 32 active members. Representatives of countries in which nursing organizations had not yet reached necessary development were admitted to associate membership, thereby

gaining the support of the greater organization in their struggle. The admittance of a new member was described by Miss Dock, who was actively associated with the movement from its beginning:

> Those who attend the congresses of the International Council of Nurses are always moved by the ceremony of initiation of member countries when, preceded by her national flag and accompanied by her national anthem, the new representative is presented by one of the older members and formally welcomed into the International sisterhood. There is something very real behind all the pageantry and symbolism of these impressive occasions. . . . The I.C.N. is a bright example of Internationalism at its best.

Much of the success of the council was due to Miss Christine Reimann, for many years its permanent secretary and editor of the *Journal*.

INTERNATIONAL POSTGRADUATE COURSES

It was soon realized that to become a potent force the council had to do more than meet and wave the flag every few years. At the meeting in Cologne in 1912 it was suggested that an educational memorial to Florence Nightingale be established. However, World War I soon broke out and temporarily stopped international activities, but when the guns were silenced, the idea was again taken up, this time by the League of Red Cross Societies. In 1920 a postgraduate nursing course in public health was established in London at King's College, later at Bedford College, where it has since remained. In 1924 a second course, in administration and teaching, was established at the College of Nursing, and nurses from many lands met under a common roof for a common purpose.

THE FLORENCE NIGHTINGALE INTERNATIONAL FOUNDATION

After about ten years of successful operation the International Council of Nurses was

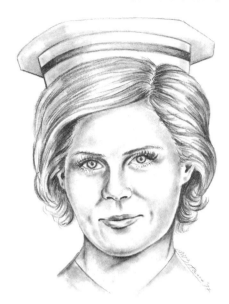

HAHNEMANN HOSPITAL GRADUATE NURSE

invited to join in the undertaking, and at the recommendation of a committee headed by Mrs. Bedford-Fenwick a partnership was established between the two bodies in July, 1934. The outcome was "The Florence Nightingale International Foundation." It was decided that its home should be in London, for it is there that "Florence Nightingale's spirit still lives in fullest radiance." The foundation is financed by an endowed trust administered by a "grand council," consisting of five representatives of the League of Red Cross Societies, five from the International Council of Nurses, and two from each component national nursing committee. The students are selected by the national committees and may pay tuition or study under a scholarship. They are selected for scholastic standing and potential leadership qualities. It is obvious that aims of the International Council of Nurses could in no way be better furthered than by bringing together a group of promising young women from different countries under a common roof where they could receive the stimulus of varied and valuable contacts. To complete the organization, the College of Nursing donated the use of the beautiful Flor-

ence Nightingale International House as a residence for the students during their stay in London.

After they finished their courses most students joined "the old internationals," which was founded in 1925 as an organization through which students could keep in touch with each other. The organization maintains a library, which should develop into a historical collection and out of which developed an International History of Nursing Society. This society was discontinued in 1939 at the outbreak of World War II. After the war the international courses in London were not reestablished.

In 1948 it was recommended that the Florence Nightingale International Foundation function within the International Council of Nurses. Through its activities the foundation is associated with the International Council of Nurses in developing wider educational programs and activities than were possible before. The invested trust fund of the Florence Nightingale International Foundation provides a small income, and the International Council of Nurses is responsible for financing the general administration and program. The overall objective of the foundation as defined by the council may be stated as improving nursing throughout the world through the stimulation and improvement of education for nursing.

Although the Florence Nightingale Foundation is the most ambitious undertaking in which the International Council of Nursing has been engaged, it is not its sole activity. Through its publications and meetings it has constantly worked for improvement of nursing standards throughout the world. By making acceptance by the council desirable, it has forced improvement in backward countries; it has constantly endeavored to better define the scope and purposes of nursing; it has encouraged research into nursing technics, and it has attempted to apply modern scientific principles to nursing and modern teaching methods to the education of nurses. The council has acted as a clearing house for the exchange of ideas and methods. In addition it has endeavored to widen the scope of nursing by applying to it the widest possible definition: "Nursing is the safeguarding and building up of life forces in the individual and in the race." The hand of the public health educator is clearly seen in this definition.

Thus it attempts, as far as possible, to recommend minimum requirements for a nursing curriculum, realizing, however, that such a guide must be influenced by the conditions of the land in which it is to be used. It does emphasize that nurses must receive a minimum of three years' consecutive training in a qualified school that is under the direction of a trained nurse and in which the curriculum comprises training in surgical, medical, and children's wards.

ACTIVITIES FOLLOWING WORLD WAR II

Headquarters of the International Council of Nurses, which had been in London and Geneva, were moved to New Haven, Connecticut, from 1939 to 1944. Miss Effie J. Taylor, dean of the School of Nursing at Yale University, had been elected president at the 1937 International Council of Nurses' meetings in London. At the end of the war, nurses in all European countries greatly needed not only books and educational tools but also uniforms, shoes, and food. A relief program was started, and the American Nurses' Association and the Canadian Nurses' Association did much to help their sister members in the International Council of Nurses. Gradually, in the years immediately after World War II, contacts were reestablished, and conferences and meetings were planned.

In 1958 the following 46 countries were members of the International Council of Nurses: Australia, Austria, Barbados, Belgium, Brazil, Canada, Ceylon, Chile, Colombia, Cuba, Denmark, Ethiopia, Finland, France, Germany, Great Britain, Greece, Haiti, Iceland, India, Iran, Ireland, Israel, Italy, Jamaica, Japan, Korea, Liberia, Luxembourg, Malaya, Netherlands, New Zealand, Northern Rhodesia, Norway, Pakistan, Panama, the Philippine Islands, South Africa, Southern Rhodesia, Sweden, Switzerland, Trinidad, Turkey, the United States of America, Uruguay, and Yugoslavia.

In 1961 the International Council of Nurses met in Melbourne, Australia. Thirteen new national nurses' associations were voted membership: Burma, British Guiana, Egypt, Ghana, Jordan, Kenya, Mexico, Nigeria, Poland, Singapore, Thailand, Venezuela, and the Republic of China. These admissions brought to 59 the number of national associations with full membership in the International Council of Nurses. At the same meeting, Mlle. Alice Clamageran of France was elected the new president of the International Council of Nurses, and Helen Nussbaum of Switzerland became the general secretary.

The International Council of Nurses has taken over the register of displaced nurses formerly maintained by the International Relief Organization and has assumed responsibility for it. In 1953 this register listed over 4,000 nurses who had had to leave their own countries for reasons beyond their control.

The International Council of Nurses is a member of the International Hospital Federation and the World Federation for Mental Health. Representatives from the International Council attend meetings of the World Medical Associaion. The council also works with the nursing bureau of the League of Red Cross Societies.

The first postwar meeting was held in 1946, in Atlantic City, when Miss Gerda Hojer was elected president. The second meeting followed in 1949 in Stockholm, Sweden. At the meeting in Stockholm in June, 1949, an important step was taken when the Florence Nightingale International Foundation was established within the International Council of Nurses as a legal entity. The foundation has benefited by having the protection and strength of an older and larger organization. The Florence Nightingale International Foundation assumed the responsibility for the overall educational activities of the International Council of Nurses. Adele Herwitz of the United States was appointed executive director of the International Council of Nurses in 1970. Prior to this appointment she had served as associate executive director of the American Nurses' Association.

ECONOMIC WELFARE OF NURSES

The Economic Welfare Committee of the International Council of Nurses was established in 1947. Its primary responsibility was outlined to be that of securing information about (1) professional recognition that has been granted to nurses and other aspects of professional and economic welfare and (2) economic conditions of nurses throughout the world in regard to salaries, pensions, and working conditions. The replies of 21 countries to a questionnaire were presented at the International Council of Nurses' conference in Brazil in 1952. Information from these questions covered such aspects as professional recognition and status, economic welfare, including machinery for the negotiation of economic conditions, salaries, pensions, hours of work, health protection, transfer, and promotion. The economic welfare committee realized that the information contained in this report should be revised, corrected, and brought up to date during the next quadrennial period and that the work of the committee should be continued through the appointment of an economic correspondent in each country.

Because of the great difference in professional status, working conditions, general economic conditions, and many other aspects peculiar to each country, much work remains to be done, but a first step has been taken to study economic conditions under which professional nurses work all over the world.

Professional nurses are finding their places as world citizens not only through the International Council of Nurses but also through such international organizations as the World Health Organization in which they are cooperating with doctors and other health workers in improving the level of health for all people.

OTHER INTERNATIONAL PROGRAMS

In striving for improvement of international health standards, the International Council of Nurses does not stand alone. The World Health Organization, the League of Red Cross Societies, and the International Health Board of the Rockefeller Foundation have similar and supplementary aims. The total enterprise of advancing public health by international cooperation continues to make marvelous progress when world politics permit.

The activities of the International Council of Nurses are by far the most important international nursing activties, but there are others that must also be mentioned.

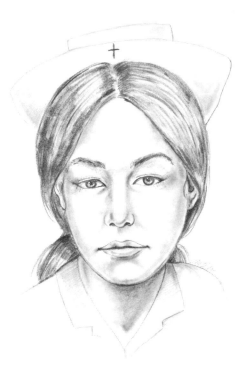

JAPANESE RED CROSS COLLEGE SCHOOL

The International Unit of the American Nurses' Association supports the International Council of Nurses and the specialized agencies of the United Nations in the promotion of better understanding between nurses of all countries. The activities of this unit center about exchange programs for graduate nurses endorsed by the International Council of Nurses. Nurses from other countries come to the United States for observation, study, and experience, and nurses from this country go abroad for similar experiences.

WORLD HEALTH ORGANIZATION

Through the International Council of Nurses the nursing profession's link with the World Health Organization has been represented at recent meetings of WHO. Over 140 American nurses have gone to 21 different countries under this organization. They have helped teach school nursing, midwifery, and dispensary work, and they have taught people of backward areas to purify water, to prepare foods, and to grow vegetables and fruits.

One hundred thirty-four nurses of 22 nationalities are employed by the World Health Organization and are engaged in nursing projects in 29 countries. The WHO publication, *Guide for National Studies of Nursing Resources,* is used by World Health Organization advisers. The assistance WHO gives in countries varies a great deal; sometimes it helps to establish good basic schools or it assists in curriculum planning or the development of regional seminars and workshops. Sometimes nurses study and observe in fields of nursing education, clinical supervision, administration, public health nursing, and midwifery. The World Health Organization has been helpful in translating nursing texts and other literature into Spanish, particularly for use in Latin America. WHO is interested in building up professional nursing in different countries capable of participating in health and nursing activities and in giving leadership in those countries. The standards of the profession set up by the International Council of Nurses are promoted in these activities.

QUESTIONS AND STUDY PROJECTS FOR UNIT ELEVEN

1. What were the social and political backgrounds out of which the International Council of Nurses developed; how have changing international conditions shaped its course?
2. What is the Florence Nightingale International Foundation, and what are its contributions to nursing?
3. What are some other international activities that affect nurses and nursing?
4. Discuss the contributions of the following persons to nursing: Lavinia Dock, Mrs. Bedford-Fenwick, Sister Agnes Karll, and Christine Reimann.
5. Discuss the development and importance of international postgraduate courses for nurses.
6. Make an annotated bibliography of recent articles appearing in *The American Journal of Nursing, Nursing Outlook, Nursing Research,* and any other journals available in your library relating to the discussion in this unit.

REFERENCES FOR UNIT ELEVEN

ANA and the United Nations, American Journal of Nursing 53:1200, October, 1953.

A Nurse's UN, American Journal of Nursing 52:1209, October, 1952.

Breay, Margaret, and Fenwick, Ethel Gordon: The history of the ICN, 1899-1925, Geneva, Switzerland, 1931, The International Council of Nurses.

Broe, Ellen: The Educational Division of the International Council of Nurses (Florence Nightingale International Foundation), International Nursing Bulletin 8:10, 1952.

Calder, Ritchie: The lamp is lit—the story of the World Health Organization (pamphlet), Geneva, 1951, World Health Organization.

Chagas, Agnes: The work of WHO in Latin America, American Journal of Nursing 53:410-411, April, 1953.

Convention report, Nursing Outlook 9:372, June, 1961.

Disbrow, Mildred A.: A foreign student or a classmate? Nursing Outlook 11:874-877, December, 1963.

Dock, Lavinia L.: Our international prospects, American Journal of Nursing 19:781-782, August, 1919.

Editorial—Internationalism in nursing, American Journal of Nursing 22:1, October, 1922.

Education and training of medical and public health personnel, Geneva, 1951, World Health Organization.

Fenwick, Ethel G.: The International Council of Nurses, American Journal of Nursing 1:785-790, August, 1901.

Garesché, Rev. Edward F.: International Catholic Guild of Nurses, American Journal of Nursing 25:188-190, March, 1925.

Goodman, Neville M.: Nursing and the World Health Organization, American Journal of Nursing 49:134-136, March, 1949.

Goodrich, Annie W.: Florence Nightingale International Foundation, National League of Nursing Education, 1936, pp. 246-251.

International aspects of nursing education (a series of mimeographed addresses provided through the Annie W. Goodrich Lectureship Fund), New York, Teachers College, Columbia University.

Nursing and the League of Nations, American Journal of Nursing 31:1283-1284, November, 1931.

Nursing on the world health front, American Journal of Nursing 50:611, 1950.

Nursing service and nursing standards throughout the world, American Journal of Nursing 53:1226-1228, October, 1953.

Patterson, Lillian B.: The Third World Health Assembly, American Journal of Nursing **50:**760, 1950.

Petry, Lucile: Nursing on the world health front, American Journal of Nursing **50:**611, October, 1950.

Petry, Lucile: WHO and nursing, American Journal of Nursing **48:**611, October, 1948.

Rice, Donald T.: International crossroads of public health, Nursing Outlook **11:**836, December, 1963.

Schwarzenberg, Anna: Activities and program of the ICN, American Journal of Nursing **45:**718, September, 1945.

Steffen, Anna M.: Fourth World Health Assembly, American Journal of Nursing **51:**747, 1951.

Taylor, Effie J.: The International Council of Nurses, American Journal of Nursing **50:**615, 1950.

Taylor, Ruth G.: Fifth World Health Assembly, American Journal of Nursing **52:**1463, 1952.

The Florence Nightingale International Foundation inaugurated, American Journal of Nursing **34:**786-792, August, 1934.

The Florence Nightingale International Foundation, American Journal of Nursing **35:**452, May, 1935.

The Florence Nightingale International Foundation, American Journal of Nursing **36:**1001-1008, October, 1936.

The Florence Nightingale International Foundation, American Journal of Nursing **38:**975-977, September, 1938.

UNIT TWELVE
Legal aspects

ROBERT G. BOWERS, B.A., J.D.

"Nursing and law are both disciplines primarily concerned with the conduct of man. Each discipline seeks to understand man's behavior. Each acknowledges a common foundation of behavioral sciences essential to comprehend his actions and the varying social means used to structure those actions."*

---

*Murchison, Irene E., and Nichols, Thomas S.: Legal foundations of nursing practice, New York, 1970, The Macmillan Co.

CHAPTER 43 INTRODUCTION TO THE LAW

■ There is no word in all the English language that takes on a wider or more varied meaning than the word "law." For example, there are laws of science, mathematics, economics, and sociology. Many papers have been written on the subject, but none have adequately defined the word. For our purposes, however, we shall define the law as a body of rules that the courts of a particular jurisdiction will uphold and enforce.

To make the study of the legal aspects of nursing even more confusing we must note that there are 51 jurisdictions within the United States, one for each state and the federal system, all having different laws.

The history of the common law can be summarized as follows: After the Battle of Hastings in England in 1066 that country was unified as a kingdom having the center of government in London, with the judges going from London into the provinces to hear and to decide the major cases of the day. Instead of purely local judges deciding local issues under local customs the judges established a rule of law that was common to the whole country.

If no adequate legal relief was available, a subject could take his plea to the king, who was not bound by precedent and who could rule on the matter as his conscience directed. However, as the country became more populous, more and more problems arose, and the king was unable or unwilling to devote sufficient time to such problems. Since the king was the head of the Church in England, and since the archbishop of Canterbury was the king's spiritual advisor and was frequently referred to as the "king's conscience," it was natural for the king to refer much matters to the archbishop of Canterbury and in time to establish the Court of Chancery. While the Court of Chancery was supposed to decide each case on its merits without being concerned for any particular rule of law, precedents were established. In time the archbishop of Canterbury was not able to handle the pleas, himself; and he delegated the chancery jurisdiction to others. There were then two court systems: one called the Court of Law and the other called the Court of Chancery or the Court of Equity. The Court of Law could award damages in money and declare ownership in property; the Court of Equity could direct special remedies such as directing a person to do or not to do a particular act.

Through the years a body of law was developed from the court decisions which we now call the *common law* or the "unwritten" law. Also, during this same time rules of law were established by the king and Parliament that were reduced to writing and that became known as the "written" law or *statutory law*.

When our country was settled by the English, they brought with them such law books as were available. Other settlers came from the main continent of Europe and brought with them many of the rules or laws that had been established in their native lands and that differed greatly from the English laws. The backgrounds of our citizens being so diverse, the various colonies established different rules so that today the law differs from state to state.

After the American Revolution it became apparent that a stable form of government would have to be established based on the will and welfare of the people.

" . . . (I)n order to form a more perfect union, etstabish justice, insure domestic tranquility, provide for the common defense, promote the general welfare, and secure the blessings of liberty, . . . " the people of the United States acting through their duly elected representatives ordained and established the Constitution of the United States of America as the fundamental and basic law of our land. This instrument is the oldest constitution of any country in the world. It established three separate branches of government: the legislative, the executive, and the judicial.

The legislative branch of the federal government is the Congress, composed of the House of Representatives and the Senate, which establishes the "written" law. The members of the House of Representatives are elected by the people of the various states based upon population. Two senators are elected from each state by the people of the state.

The executive branch is headed by the president, who is elected indirectly by the people and is charged with enforcing the law.

The judicial branch is composed of the Supreme Court and such inferior courts as Congress may from time to time establish. The chief justice and associate justices of the Supreme Court and all other federal judges are appointed by the president for life with the advice and consent of the senate.

Where nurses feel that there are laws affecting their profession, they have the right to petition the legislative body for a change. The various professional organizations are adept at providing guidance in this endeavor.

CHAPTER 44 PROFESSIONAL STATUS OF NURSING

■ It has frequently been stated that the right of an individual to engage in any lawful employment is guaranteed to our citizens under the provisions of the Constitution of the United States and the constitutions as adopted by the several states. However, the state retains the right to prohibit occupations and professions that affect the public health, morals, safety, or welfare, or restrict membership in such occupations to those persons who have met prescribed qualifications. This is particularly true even among the more learned professions if the good of the community requires that the public be protected from ignorance, incompetence, and fraud in the practice of such occupation.

Under the police powers of the state those who desire to engage in a particular occupation or profession, such as nursing, may be required to take and pass a suitable examination covering scientific or technical knowledge after they have given proof of possessing the physical, educational, and moral qualifications designated by the state. These regulations are established to protect the public, not to protect members of a particular profession. There is no doubt, however, that the licensing statutes tend to reduce the number of persons engaged in the profession and aid the profession by eliminating insofar as possible those persons who do not meet the moral, ethical, and educational standards required of qualified practitioners.

Boards are established in each of the states as agencies of the executive branch of government for the purpose of administering the licensure laws with respect to the various professions. The lack of uniformity found among the various state licensure regulations is due to the fact that the federal government delegates this responsibility to the states. In the case of nursing boards, board members are usually appointed from both the nursing and medical professions by the governor of the state. Some of the nursing boards operate in conjunction with the state health department. Frequently, after appointment to the board the board members elect officers from their own number and an executive director who is not a member of the board. The executive director normally has the duty and responsibility of carrying out the instructions of the board and acts as its secretary and treasurer.

In most states for an examination leading to certification and licensure as a registered nurse the applicant must be of good moral character, be a high school graduate, and have completed a course of study and graduated from an educational unit or school that has in turn been accredited by the board or a similar board or an accrediting agency of another state. For examination leading to certification and licensure as a licensed practical nurse or vocational nurse the applicant must be of good moral character, have completed the ninth grade of high school or its equivalent, and have completed a course of study and graduated from a program of practical nurse education accredited by the state board or one accredited by the legal accrediting agency of another state. Therefore it is a duty of the board of nursing to establish the classroom and clinical standards of the various nursing programs and to establish the method for determining the moral fitness of the applicant.

The board also has the responsibility of establishing the procedures for renewal of licenses and the enforcement of proper practice standards and disciplinary procedures for those in the profession.

The board of nursing may, without examination, issue by endorsement or reciprocity a certificate and a license to practice as a registered nurse or as a practical nurse to applicants who have previously been licensed under the laws of other states. However, the boards of the various states may require such an applicant to prove her competency and qualifications if in the opinion of the board there is a question concerning her competency.

RELATIONSHIP OF MEDICAL AND NURSING PRACTICE ACTS

The individual states establish the definition of the practice of medicine and the practice of nursing as well as the requirements of those persons who shall engage in such professions. It may well be that a registered nurse, a licensed practical nurse, and the physician can perform the same service. It could be possible under a given set of statutory and regulatory provisions for the nurse or the physician to administer drugs, anesthetics, or treatments.

As examples the practice of medicine has been defined by the New York legislature as follows:

A person practices medicine within the meaning of this article, except as hereinafter stated, who holds himself out as being able to diagnose, treat, operate or prescribe for any human disease, pain, injury, deformity or physical condition, and who either shall offer or undertake, by any means or method, to diagnose, treat, operate or prescribe for any human disease, pain, injury, deformity or physical condition.*

Medical practice is defined by statute in North Carolina as follows:

Any person shall be regarded as practicing medicine or surgery within the meaning of this Article who shall diagnose or attempt to diagnose, treat or attempt to treat, operate or attempt to operate on, or prescribe for or administer to, or profess to treat any human ailment, physical or mental, or any physical injury to or deformity of another person.†

New York law, again, defines nursing practice as follows:

a. A person practices nursing as a registered professional nurse within the meaning of this atricle who for compensation or personal profit performs any professional service requiring the application of principles of nursing based on biological, physical and social sciences, such as responsible supervision of a patient requiring skill in observance of symptoms and reactions and the accurate recording of the facts, and carrying out of treatments and medications as prescribed by a licensed physician or by a licensed dentist and the application of such nursing procedures as involves understanding of cause and effect in order to safeguard life and health of the patient and others.

b. A person practices nursing as a licensed practical nurse who for compensation or personal profit performs such duties as are required in the physical care of a patient and in carrying out of medical orders as prescribed by a licensed physician or by a licensed dentist requiring an understanding of nursing but not requiring the professional service as outlined in paragraph a.‡

The North Carolina legislature has defined nursing as follows:

a. Nursing by Registered Nurse.—The practice of nursing by registered nurse means the performance for compensation of any act in the observation, care, and counsel of persons who are ill, injured, or experiencing alterations in normal health processes, and/or in the supervision and teaching of others who are or will

*New York Education Law §6501, par. 4.
†North Carolina General Statute No. 90-18.
‡New York Education Law §6901, par. 2.

be involved in nursing care; and/or the administration of medications and treatments as prescribed by a licensed physician or dentist. Nursing by registered nurse requires specialized knowledge, judgment, and skill, but does not require nor permit medical diagnosis or medical prescription of therapeutic or corrective measures. The use of skill and judgment is based upon an understanding of principles from the biological, social, and physical sciences. Nursing by registered nurse requires use of skills in modifying methods of nursing care and supervision as the patient's needs change.

b. Nursing by Licensed Practical Nurse.—The practice of practical nursing means the performance for compensation of selected acts in the care of persons who are ill, injured, or experiencing alterations in normal health processes. Such performance requires a knowledge of and skill in simple nursing procedures, gained through prescribed preparation, but does not require the specialized knowledge, judgment, and skill essential for nursing by registered nurse. Practical nursing is performed under orders of a licensed physician or a licensed dentist, and/or under directions issued by a registered nurse.*

MONOPOLY AND CRIMINAL PENALTIES

Those who are licensed as physicians, registered nurses, and licensed practical nurses usually have the exclusive right to hold themselves out as practitioners within their respective professions. However, the

*North Carolina General Statute No. 90-158, subsection 3.

courts emphasize that the right to hold oneself out as a practitioner of a particular profession is reserved to any who meet the qualifications and obtain the proper license, rather than for the establishment of a monopoly by those already within the profession. However, each of the states that has adopted a nursing practice act has also provided that any unlicensed person who practices or offers to practice nursing or uses any title or abbreviation to indicate that such person is a licensed practitioner within such profession shall be guilty of a misdemeanor. A misdemeanor is a relatively minor crime as distinguished from a felony, which is usually defined as any criminal activity for which conviction may be punished by imprisonment.

Because of the increased complexity within the practice of medicine and the various nursing fields, many nursing organizations are promulgating and legislatures adopting more comprehensive statutes. Also, the medical profession, for its own protection, is seeking to upgrade the nursing profession's requirements for licensure.

With the advent of the medical assistant programs and the use of nurses as paramedical practitioners to relieve the shortage of medical doctors, the scope of the professional nurse is constantly expanding. New definitions and educational requirements are being studied by various medical societies, nursing organizations, and legislative committees.

CHAPTER 45 CONTRACTS

■ The term "contracts" is difficult to define succinctly, since the word arises in so many different circumstances. However, for our purposes a contract may be defined as an agreement supported by sufficient consideration to do, or refrain from doing, a lawful thing for the breach of which the law gives a remedy upon its breach. Contracts are made and performed so often in our daily lives that we sometimes fail to recognize them. This is true with respect to nurses in both their professional and nonprofessional lives.

People, including nurses and physicians, usually think that contracts must be in writing. However, the vast majority of contracts are oral, but there are some contracts that must be in writing to be valid. It is, of course, much better to reduce a contract to writing in order to prevent misunderstanding and disagreement brought about by imperfect memory or lack of comprehension.

Most states have adopted a statute, sometimes called "a statute for the prevention of frauds and perjuries," which normally provides that agreements in consideration of marriage; agreements not to be performed within a year; promises to answer for the debt, default, or miscarriage of another; contracts with respect to estates and interests in land; and sale of certain goods, wares, and merchandise must be in writing and signed by the person charged with the breach. These are sometimes called unenforceable contracts if oral.

Briefly, the necessary elements of a contract are (1) competent parties, (2) an offer and an acceptance of that offer, (3) definiteness and certainty as to the terms and requirements, and (4) consideration.

CAPACITY TO CONTRACT

It is a fundamental principle of law that the parties to a contract must be competent, that is, capable of understanding and agreeing to its terms.

Although ancient law provided that married women were incompetent to contract, this has been for all practical purposes abrogated in all states. Persons under 18 years of age in some states and 21 years of age in other states may contract, but the minor has the right to rescind or avoid his contract at any time except for necessities. A person is not incompetent to contract, however, because of advanced age or physical disabilities unless the advanced state or physical disabilities impair him mentally to the extent that he is unable to protect himself and his property.

OFFER AND ACCEPTANCE

An offer and acceptance is frequently referred to as a meeting of the minds. There must be a mutual agreement between the parties to the contract terms. An acceptance of an offer must be of the exact offer that was made for there to be a contract. A qualified acceptance or an acceptance that differs from the offer is referred to as a counter-offer, which may be accepted and become a contract.

For example, the merchant displays his wares and price. This is an offer. When the shopper selects an item from the merchant's display and presents payment, a sales contract has been entered into. However, if the customer attempts to "dicker" on the price, he makes a counter-offer, which the merchant may accept or reject. If the merchant accepts, a sales contract has been consummated. If the merchant rejects the counter-offer, there is no contract.

Whenever a physician opens his office for the practice of medicine, he makes himself available for employment by prospective patients. Legally he is not making an offer; he is inviting offers from those who seek his services. He does not agree to treat any particular patient or to accept the offer of all who may present themselves to him for his services. The same is true in the case of the nurse. She may pick and choose from among those who may seek her services. Once she accepts the offer made to her by a prospective patient, she has entered into a contract with the patient.

As a practical matter in many communities a nurse places her name on a roster maintained by either a nursing organization or a hospital, indicating her availability on terms that are standard with respect to the type of nursing service required. In many instances the nurse is given the option of accepting or rejecting the employment, but acceptance of such terms by the nurse makes the contract.

The whole offer must be accepted; anything else is a rejection. The offer cannot be accepted in part and rejected in part, although this may be considered as a counter-offer that may be accepted or rejected by the patient.

It should be noted, however, that the nurse and the patient need not, themselves, meet face-to-face to establish a contract relationship. Either the nurse or the patient or both may act through agents. The patient's physician, a nursing registry, or a member of the patient's family acting as the agent of the patient may make the initial contract with the nurse. The employment contract of a nurse with an institution is usually, if not aways, negotiated by an agent of the hospital.

There may be implied conditions based upon local custom that are never mentioned but that affect the totality of the contract. In private duty nursing the length of the workday or the furnishing of meals or other privileges may be so customary that they become a part of the contract. Of course, it is a better practice to discuss such conditions for better public relations and to prevent misunderstanding, but such may not be necessary.

It is implied in every nursing contract, as well as in every other professional contract, that the services will be performed within the existing professional standards and ethics. This implied condition is of utmost importance. Although the courts formerly held that the nurse in a particular community must furnish that standard of care which was prevalent in the community, the more recent decisions have extended the scope of the community to include the whole of the nursing profession throughout the country. The rationalization behind the extension of the boundary lines of the community is based on the improvements in communications and transportation that make it possible for the nurse to be exposed to the latest techniques and procedures.

An offer may be withdrawn at any time before it has been accepted. However, once an offer has been made, it must be accepted within a reasonable time under the circumstances or a rejection will be presumed. An offer transmitted to a nurse for immediate postoperative care must be accepted immediately or it will be presumed rejected. However, an offer made to a nurse for her employment in connection with elective surgery scheduled for a month in the future can be considered more leisurely, and a reasonable time might well be governed by extrinsic facts such as the availability of competent nurses in the community.

As was mentioned previously, nursing services are frequently contracted for the patient by someone acting on behalf of the patient. It is important to know whether the person acting for the patient has the authority of act for him. If the apparent agent does not have the authority to act and bind the patient, difficulties may arise with respect to payment for services. If the patient is incapable or incompetent to appoint an agent to enter into a contract, it may be necessary to contract with some responsible member of his family. If the responsible member of the family contracts to pay for the services, and if credit is extended to this responsible member of the family and not to the patient, the contract can be oral. However, if the person with whom the nurse contracts says he will pay for the nursing services if the patient does not, under the statute of most states the guarantee would be unenforceable unless it was in writing and signed by the contracting party.

LEGALITY OF THE ACT CONTRACTED

Before a contract is valid, the act to be done or not to be done must be legal. A contract to commit a crime or to do any other act that is against "public policy" is void and unenforceable. It is impossible to define in exact terms the meaning of the words "public policy" because it is variable and differs from state to state. However, agreements having a tendency to obstruct or interfere with the courts or the administration of justice, contracts based on illicit or immoral conduct, agreements to commit a crime or to reward someone else for the commission of a crime, agreements to defraud some other person, gambling contracts, and contracts prohibiting marriage have been generally held to be against public

policy. Therefore contracts whereby the nurse would be required to participate in illegal abortions, misuse of drugs, deviation from a proper standard of care, and services beyond the scope of her license would be against public policy.

CONSIDERATION

Consideration is an essential element of a contract; it is something within the contemplation of the parties given in exchange for the promise to do or not to do a particular legal act. It may be of benefit to the promisor or a detriment to the promises. It is some profit or benefit moving toward one party or a detriment, loss, or responsibility suffered or undertaken by the other party. The nurse may agree to go to the home of a patient daily to administer a prescribed drug, but if the patient has not agreed to pay or do anything in return, there is no contract because there is no consideration. If after a contract has been entered into between the nurse and her patient and the nurse agrees to render services beyond the scope of her original employment without the payment of additional consideration on the part of the patient, there is no contract for the additional services. An example of this would be the situation in which the licensed practical nurse is employed to render her nursing services in the home for the new mother and her baby for a stipulated fee, and, after the contract has been entered into, the licensed practical nurse agrees to cook the family's meals and wash the family's clothes without additional fees for her services. There is no contract with respect to the cooking and laundry services since there was no consideration to support the new agreement. Consideration is the "price" paid for a service.

BREACH

Once a contract has been entered into, each party has the option of either performing or not performing the contract on his part. The party who elects not to perform the contract is said to have breached the contract unless he has a legal excuse that prevents him from carrying out the terms of the contract.

When completion of the contract is prevented by the improper conduct of one of the parties, the other party may be excused. The party to the contract who makes performance impossible is the one who is said to have breached the contract. Impliedly, when a patient employs a nurse, he agrees that he will do nothing, willfully, to prevent the nurse from performing her services in a professional manner. When the patient, deliberately, becomes obstructive, he has breached the employment contract, and, if the improper conduct substantially prevents the nurse from rendering proper nursing services to the patient, the nurse may terminate the employment. However, the nurse should give the patient a reasonable opportunity to obtain the services of some other nurse. However, the courts generally hold that the nurse must be able to show that she was ready, willing and able to carry out her part of the employment contract.

Once a contract has been entered into for future nursing services, and before any services are rendered to the patient, if either party elects not to go through with the terms of the contract, it is said that he has repudiated the contract. Frequently a nurse repudiates a contract because it becomes inconvenient for her to render the services contracted for at the time and place required. The fact that it becomes inconvenient for a nurse to perform her professional services after she has contracted to do so is no excuse for repudiating the contract or for failing to do that which she has contracted to do. The nurse who fails to perform properly because it would be inconvenient for her to do so, breaches the contract and may be held liable for any damages that the patient may suffer. Her abandonment of the patient under such circumstances would be a breach of the contract and subjects the nurse to tort liability as well.

Where the failure to carry out the terms of the contract is beyond the control of the defaulting party because of an unforeseeable event, performance may be excused. If the nurse is prevented by an act of God from attending her patient, she may be excused from the performance while such condition exists. If she has partially performed her services and is prevented from completing them, she may recover her personal services already rendered. Some courts hold that recovery may be had for the value of services actually rendered when the completion of the entire contract is prevented by sickness or death. However, if this sickness is foreseeable, recovery is frequently denied. A particular limitation on the rule adopted by some courts is that sickness which should be anticipated is no excuse for nonperformance, such as where a pregnant nurse entered into a contract for her services and is prevented from completion of those services and is disabled for a period of time by confinement incident to childbirth unless this is contemplated by the parties at the time the contract is entered into. Of course, death terminates the nursing contract whether anticipated or not, and the nurse or her estate would be entitled to recover for her services up to the date of death.

Another defense to a breach of contract is a material misrepresentation on the part of either party. The nurse who is employed to care for a patient who is represented as being only slightly ill or only requiring minimal care, and who accepts employment relying upon such statements, will be excused from performance if the true facts reveal that the patient is seriously or critically ill and requires constant, specialized nursing services. Whenever a nurse holds herself out as having a particular type of license, education, or experience, she would be guilty of a material misrepresentation if the possession of such license, background, or education is important to the employer and such claim or claims are untrue. In this situation there would be no contract between the nurse and the employer because of the lack of understanding of the offer and acceptance.

REMEDIES

Basically the legal remedies for the breach of a contract are money damages or specific performance or both. Generally, when there has been a breach of a contract, damages are assessed in dollar amounts. However, in some situations where the damage is irreparable in terms of money, the court may enjoin the guilty party from refusing to carry out the terms of the contract. However, the nurse cannot be ordered to specifically perform her contract regarding her personal services because this might amount to slavery, which is prohibited by our constitution. A money judgment for the actual dam-

ages is the usual remedy. However, in extreme cases the court can award punitive or exemplary damages in addition to the actual monetary loss to punish the guilty party for his willful, deliberate, or capricious conduct.

There is a time limitation on bringing civil actions based on contracts. Uusually this limitation is three years, but some states have a longer period.

In conclusion it should be noted that contracts cover a wide range of situations with respect to the nursing profession and that the courts of the various states are not in agreement. Because of the variation in statute and judicial interpretation in the various states, the nurse should consult her attorney before entering into a contract while she still has the opportunity or election to accept, reject, or make a counter-offer.

CHAPTER 46 INDEPENDENT CONTRACTOR AND EMPLOYEE

■ In the law for all practical purposes the terms "master" and "servant" and "employer" and "employee" are the same. The employer is the master, and the employee is the servant. In this relationship the employer is entitled to exercise the right to control the manner in which the prescribed work is to be performed. There are four classic elements that are considered in determining whether the relation of employer and employee exists, to wit: the selection of the employee, the payment of wages, the right to dismiss, and the authority to control the employee's conduct, but the crucial element is the right to control. Usually the institutional nurse, the public health nurse, and the office nurse are employees of the institution, governmental unit, or doctor. If the nurse is an employee and negligently injures or causes damage to some third party, the nurse is liable to the injured party for damages, but her employer is liable or responsible for the actions of his employee.

Frequently, however, the nurse is engaged by the patient or his family to render nursing services of a private duty nature. In this situation she becomes an independent contractor. If the nurse is engaged as an independent contractor, she, alone, would be held responsible for her own negligent acts or improper conduct.

Therefore, insofar as the patient is concerned, the relationship of independent contractor or employer-employee is of great practical importance in as much as the patient would be more likely to recover damages from the employer than from a nurse, since nurses may have limited assets. However, the relationship may or may not be of importance to the nurse, since the employer has a right to require the employee to reimburse it or him for any monies the employer may have had to expend by virtue of the negligence of the employee.

RESERVATION OF CONTROL

The most important or decisive element or factor of those listed is the reservation of control or right to control over the activities of the employee. Where it appears that a nurse is employed to care for a patient or even several patients using her own procedure and without being subject to a detailed method by which she is to perform such services but is to be judged by the final result, she usually will not be held to be an employee but will be found to be an independent contractor.

When a patient employs a physician, the physician is usually an independent contractor who determines the diagnostic procedures to be followed. If the physician diagnoses his patient as having a surgical condition and refers the patient to a surgeon, the surgeon is an independent contractor who determines the proper operative procedure. The patient does not, normally, direct the surgeon in the selection of the operative site, length of incision, or in any other detail. In nearly all instances the private duty nurse is an independent contractor employed to care for the patient and to carry out the orders of the physician.

The staff nurse in a hospital is normally an employee since she does not retain control as to whom her services may be made available. Institutional or hospital nursing implies that the hospital as the employer will control the nurse as to which services shall be rendered, when, and to whom. Usually which services, and how they will be performed, will be dictated by superiors or by staff physicians.

Not infrequently a staff nurse of an institution is under the direct supervision of one or more physicians and surgeons in the hospital. This situation frequently arises where there is one nurse who scrubs only for one surgeon or in one surgical specialty field. This is called the "loaned or borrowed servant" doctrine. The nurse is employed by the hospital, who is her principal or usual employer. When the nurse is in the operating room, the surgeon becomes a special or temporary principal or master while the nurse acts under his direction and control. Although there is some confusion among the cases, it is generally held in the courts that the surgeon is responsible for the damage arising out of any negligent act on the part of the nurse while a loaned servant, and the hospital is normally released from liability except where it assigned a known incompetent nurse to the surgeon.

SKILL REQUIRED

In addition to the four classic elements above listed the courts occasionally consider the skill required to perform a particular task as indicative of the status of the person performing the task. If a task is within the grasp of almost anybody and only requires a minimal level of capacity, ability, and training to perform, the person performing the task would normally be considered to be an employee. Thus the courts usually find the private duty nurse to be an independent contractor because the performance of her services as a nurse requires professional judgment.

PAYMENT OF WAGES

Another of the classic elements of the employment contract is the method or manner of payment. When a person is employed at a stated wage per week or month with provision for overtime as provided by the Fair Labor Standards Act, the employee status is indicated. Independent contractors such as lawyers, doctors, nurses, or garagemen may determine his charges on a time basis, but the recipient of his services usually pays by the job. The method of charging a client or a patient is one thing, and the method of payment is something else entirely.

INSTRUMENTALITIES

In determining the relationship of employer and employee or independent contractor the courts frequently consider to some degree who supplies the instrumentalities, tools, and facilities to perform the work; however, this is only one factor to be considered.

SCOPE OF BUSINESS

Another question that arises in addition to the four classic elements is whether the services rendered were a part of the normal business of the employer. Hospitals normally furnish nursing services for the patients. However, hospitals do not normally provide private duty nurses for specific patients, and the providing of private duty nurses would not normally be within the scope of the business of the hospital. If the patient or his family requests the hospital to obtain a nurse and the nurse is paid by the patient or his family, the hospital would be acting as the agent of the patient or merely extending a courtesy for the patient. The private duty nurse would be an independent contractor to the patient and would have no relationship with the hospital. Taking it one step further, when the hospital obtains a private duty nurse upon the request of the patient and his family, pays the nurse, and bills the patient accordingly, a borderline situation may arise in which the courts may well determine that the hospital may be engaged in the business of obtaining laboratory tests and billing the patient for the special service.

INTENT

When all else fails, it may be that the intent of the parties involved in the contractual relationship must be determined. Merely calling or referring to the other as an independent contractor is not sufficient.

A painter may learn that an owner wants his house painted and agrees to paint the owner's house for a stipulated price with the owner furnishing paint, brushes, and ladders. The owner then tells the painter how he wants the house to look after it is painted and when the job is to be completed. The owner may then tell a friend, "I employed a painter to paint my house." Obviously the painter is an independent contractor regardless of the fact that the owner used the word "employed." The words will not change the relationship since the owner did not retain the right to indicate the manner or method by which the painter would perform the task. The manner of payment was to be for the completed job. The painter by approaching the owner held himself out as having the skill required to perform the task, even though the instrumentalities were to be furnished by the owner.

EMPLOYEE'S DUTY TO EMPLOYER

The law implies various obligations on the part of an employee toward the employer whether they are specifically included in the employment contract or not. By accepting employment the nurse implies possession of the skills and knowledge necessary to perform the services for which the nurse is employed; that all reasonable rules, orders, and instructions of the employer will be carried out; that the nurse will deport herself in such a manner as not to injure the employer; that the nurse will be ethical in dealings with others; and that the nurse will be loyal to her employer.

The employer, in turn, impliedly owes certain duties to the employee such as a reasonably safe place to work, suitable and safe tools or instrumentalities with which to work, and not to add new obligations, dangers, or inconveniences that were not contemplated by the nurse at the time of employment. In addition, the employer impliedly agrees not to require the nurse to perform services beyond the scope of the license.

Although the employer of an independent contractor is not normally liable for the negligence of the dependent contractor, if an injury is caused by the employer's own negligence, such as by the selection of an incompetent independent contractor, interference with the work of the independent contractor, or failing to prevent foreseeable improper conduct on the part of the independent contractor, the employer will be liable for such damages as may be caused thereby.

CHAPTER 47 TORTS

■ A tort is a legal breach of a legal duty directed and committed against another person or his property for which damages may be recovered in a civil action other than by reason of a contract. If civil actions are divided into two classifications, one would be contracts and the other would be torts.

A civil action is an action brought by one who claims to have been injured, called a *plaintiff*, against the party who he claims has injured him, called the *defendant*. It is usually instituted in a court by the filing of a complaint or petition and the issuance of a written notification called a *summons* or *citation* directing the defendant to appear and answer the complaint filed by the plaintiff within a designated period of time or suffer the consequences. After the summons and complaint have been served on the defendant and after the defendant has filed his answer admitting those facts that he contends are true and denying those facts that he contends are false, questions of fact arise called *issues*. In most jurisdictions there are procedures available to the parties to discover what evidence is in the hands of the other party. After all preliminary procedures have been completed, witnesses are directed by subpoena to appear in court to testify. Failure of the witness to appear will subject him to punishment for contempt and possibly other punishment. It is the duty of every citizen including nurses to appear and testify, truthfully, when required to do so. The trial may be before a jury or it may be before the judge depending upon the type of case or agreement between the parties. Where there is conflicting evidence, the jury (or the judge if the case is being tried without a jury) must decide where the truth lies and answer the questions or issues raised by the pleadings.

TORTS OTHER THAN PROFESSIONAL NEGLIGENCE OR MALPRACTICE

There are many, many different types of torts. A recital of all the torts other than negligence or professional malpractice would be difficult, however, we will examine a few.

Assault and battery

Often we hear the words assault and battery used together as though they had one meaning. An *assault* is the threat to unlawfully touch another with the apparent ability to carry it out. A *battery* is the unlawful touching of another. It includes every willful, deliberate, angry, violent, or negligent touching of another person's body, clothes, or anything connected or held by him without his consent.

The lack of consent or privilege is most important, but if the touching goes beyond that consented to or the privilege granted by law, the touching would still remain unlawful.

A parent or one other than a parent who has been given the right to exercise parental authority is privileged to use reasonable force by way of punishment. However, the parent or person standing in his place could and should be liable for excessive force that might inflict lasting injuries. This privilege extends to teachers and in many instances to nurses in the care of children. In determining whether a nurse has overstepped her privileges the courts will be interested in the act on the part of the child that brought about the punishment, the physical and mental condition of the child, and the resulting effect of the punishment on the child.

Nurses should be, and probably are, concerned with the consent of the patient to any touching. In recent years, more and more law suits have been instituted against nurses, physicians, and hospitals based upon an alleged lack of consent to an assault. Theoretically it is the surgeon's duty to adequately inform the patient concerning the aspects of any surgical procedure. The courts have gone far in defining the patient's right to know not only the benefits that can be derived from the surgical procedure but also the possibility of a bad result. Preferably the nurse or physician should present the consent form to the patient; this should not be delegated to ward secretaries or aides. The consent must be voluntary and when the patient's ability to make an intelligent decision has not been clouded by medications. The consent of a married woman's husband is not sufficient. However, if the procedure could affect the sexual functions of a married person, the consent should be signed, if possible, by the spouse as well as the patient. Even though consent can be given orally, written consent is highly desirable and should be required by all hospitals. Without a valid consent any surgical procedure or injection is a battery.

Consent may be implied if immediate surgery is necessary in an emergency situation to save the patient's life where an expressed consent cannot be obtained. However, there can be no implied consent to unnecessary or elective surgery or treatment.

If the patient is an unemancipated minor, consent for surgery must be obtained from the parent or guardian with whom the child resides.

If the proper consents are not obtained,

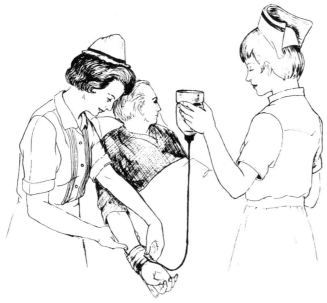

The laws governing the nurse's role in certain medical procedures, such as starting an intravenous infusion, vary from state to state.

all the nurses, physicians, and even the hospital could be held liable for the unlawful touching.

The nurse should realize that a patient has the right to decline treatment. The patient has the absolute right to refuse to be touched. When the nurse attempts to give a patient medication or treatment against his will, the nurse is liable to him for a battery, at least.

The patient has the right to withdraw any consent that he may have previously given. After he has withdrawn his consent, the nurse has no right to touch the patient. The patient has the right, unless he has been committed to the hospital by a court of competent jurisdiction, to leave the hospial, and any touching of the patient by a nurse to prevent him from leaving would be a battery, and the patient could bring a lawsuit against the nurse and her employer for his damages. In most jurisdictions there are damages that are called *punitive damages, exemplary damages,* or *vindictive damages* and that are sometimes referred to as "smart money." These are allowed, frequently, where the assault or battery is committed deliberately and without regard to the right of the person assaulted.

False imprisonment

False imprisonment is the unlawful restraint or unjustifiable detention of a person by another. As an example, to confine a patient by locking him in a room or placing him in restraint without medical justification is false imprisonment. Restraining a patient from leaving the hospital without first paying his bill is false imprisonment. A nurse may in some instances peacefully detain a patient for a few minutes to check on whether he has paid his bill, but she may not lawfully detain such a patient from leaving the hospital for his failure to pay his account. For example, a doctor had signed for the discharge of a patient from a small community hospital. The patient's husband, a farmer, went to the business office to make arrangements for the payment of the bill. He offered to pay a portion in cash and to sign a promissory note for the balance to become due in the fall when he would sell his crop. The business office refused to go along with this arrangement, and the nursing staff refused to allow the patient to leave upon being advised by the business office that she was to be detained until the bill was paid in full. The farmer made the remark as he left the hospital that his wife would not be much good to him until she fully recovered, anyway. Two weeks later the hospital sent the patient home by taxicab and sent the farmer a bill including the final two weeks. In the fall when the farmer sold his crop, he paid the hospital the amount of the bill up to the date the doctor discharged his wife. However, he refused to pay for the final two weeks, and the hospital sued him and his wife for the balance of their bill. The farmer and his wife counter-claimed for false imprisonment and successfully defended themselves and recovered damages from the hospital and the nursing staff for the false imprisonment.

Restraint of freedom of movement of a patient frequently involves the safety of the patient, but it also involves false imprisonment. The use of bed rails for a postoperative patient or in the case of the patient who is disoriented would be justified, and it might be negligent on the part of the nursing staff not to use bed rails under these circumstances. Mechanical restraints on irrational and violent patients is a common procedure and usually justified. However, the necessity for the use of such restraints has been greatly diminished with the advent of tranquilizing drugs. The nurse and the physician should be most careful in the decision as to whether or not mechanical restraints are justified before any are used.

Invasion of privacy

A person has a right to privacy. An invasion of this right of privacy may constitute a legal wrong for which a patient can recover damages. Some 40 years ago in a civil action in Georgia the parents of a deceased child were allowed to enjoin the publication of a picture of their child who had been born with his heart on the outside of his body and to recover damages for the invasion of their privacy by the hospital, a photographer, and the newspaper.

A patient has the unqualified right to privacy. The person guilty of permitting the invasion of this right is answerable at law. It is a nurse's duty to guard her patient against the invasion of his privacy. However, it is the nurse's duty to report cases of child abuse in most states, and the courts have made exceptions where the person or patient is a public figure. The safest course for a nurse to follow, however, is to allow the patient and the physician to make all decisions with respect to the patient and his public relations. All inquiries with respect to a patient should be referred to the physician or the proper hospital official regardless of the source of inquiry unless the inquiry is accompanied by an authorization signed by the patient himself. This includes inquiries from insurance adjustors, police officials, attorneys, newspaper reporters, and others.

Defamation

Defamation is the publishing of anything that is injurious to the good name or reputation of another or that might tend to bring the other person into disrepute. Defamation includes libel and slander. The distinction between the two terms is that *libel* is written and *slander* is oral. Libel can include written words, pictures, cartoons, or any other visual representation that might cause a person to be avoided, jeered at, ridiculed, or held in contempt either personally or in his occupation.

One requirement of both libel and slander is that it be published to a third person. That is, a nurse may make contemptuous uncalled-for remarks about a patient without being guilty of slander. A nurse may tell a doctor that he is a quack or otherwise incompetent without being guilty of slander. However, if she disseminates this information to a third person, she may be answerable in damages for defamation.

An unauthorized publication is defamatory *per se* when, standing alone, and stripped of any innuendo, it is susceptible to but one meaning, which would tend to disgrace and degrade the party or hold him up to public hatred, contempt, or ridicule, or cause him to be shunned or avoided, and it is not necessary that the words charge the commission of a crime or the violation of the law or impute immoral conduct. Where the injurious character of the words does not appear on its face as a matter of general acceptance, but only in consequence of extrinsic, explanatory facts showing its injurious effects, the plaintiff must be able to show some actual damage; none will be presumed in law.

As was previously stated, to form the basis of an action for libel or slander it is necessary that the defamatory matter be communicated to some person or persons other than the person defamed. Proof of the mere possibility that someone might have overheard the words is insufficient. But when a third person overhears the remarks, there is a publication, even though the person making the defamatory remarks could not see him and was unconscious of his presence.

There is a qualified privilege that extends to all communications made in good faith upon any subject matter in which the party uttering the statement has an interest or in reference to which he has some moral or legal duty to perform. In this situation the plaintiff must show malice. Therefore the nurse would be privileged to communicate otherwise defamatory matter to the treating physician concerning his patient when she does so in good faith and without malice. The falsity of the matter is not alone sufficient to establish malice.

There is an absolute privilege with respect to good faith testimony in court and comments made before legislative bodies.

MALPRACTICE OR PROFESSIONAL NEGLIGENCE

Until fairly recently it was rare for a nurse to be sued for malpractice or professional negligence because most nurses were not financially able to answer damages. The situation is now changing rapidly.

One by one the various states are taking away or disposing of the doctrine of charitable immunity. This doctrine was declared in 1876 when the Supreme Court of Massachusetts held that a charity patient, negligently injured by a student physician, could not hold the hospital responsible if due care had been used by its trustees in the selection of their inferior agents. The court held that the public and private donations that supported the charitable hospital constituted a trust fund that could not be used to pay damages.

Following the Massachusetts decision in 1876 other courts adopted the same charitable immunity rule upon several theories.

In relatively recent cases, 12 jurisdictions continued to recognize the charitable immunity doctrine but 31 others have either rejected it outright or have qualified the rule or doctrine to such a degree that for all practical purposes it has been abrogated. The state of Nevada has repudiated the rule by statute, and the other states have done it by court decree.

In a 1956 decision, abrogating the doctrine for the state of Pennsylvania, Justice Musmanno stated:

Thus, as a matter of integrity and nomenclature it must be stated that although the hospitals here under discussion are known as charitable hospitals, it does not follow that they offer their services through the operation of charity.*

In abrogating the doctrine for the state of North Carolina, Justice Susie Sharp stated:

Even though public hospitals are not operated for private gain, every effort is made to operate them

at a profit, which is put back into the facility. Nor are such hospitals principally supported by donations. Paying patients contribute largely to their support and maintenance—they provide the major share of defendant's operating funds. Furthermore, large payments in behalf of charity patients are made by governmental agencies from public funds. In short, today, some person or agency pays for the services a hospital renders. The hospital has lost its status as a charitable institution; a true charity requires no *quid pro quo* from its beneficiaries.*

The impact of these decisions on the hospital nursing staff is considerable. The patient who alleges that he was injured as the result of the negligence of the hospital nurse may now bring suit against the nurse and the hospital and expect to collect. The hospital may, in turn, seek reimbursement from the nurse for any damages that may be recovered by the injured patient since the nurse is the one who was actually negligent.

Under the generally accepted rule, tort liability for negligence rests on two factors: (1) the breach of a duty and (2) the resulting injury.

The nurse owes a duty to the patient. Exactly what that duty is may be debated. Until the early 1950's the cases generally held that the nurse owed the duty to the patient to provide the same standard of care as that generally exercised by reputable nurses in the same community. By the late 1950's the courts had begun showing their reluctance to rely, blindly, on the locality rule. By the middle 1960's it was possible to discern a trend away from the locality rule and for the courts to hold that the standard of care was to be that generally exercised by reputable nurses throughout a much broader area including the whole of the United States.

In 1966 the Wisconsin Supreme Court† seemed to base an opinion on the professional standards viewed in the light of

Flagiello v. Pennsylvania, 417 Pa. 486, 208 A2d 193 (1956).

Rabon v. Rowan Memorial Hospital, Inc., 269 NC1, 152 SE2d 485 (1967).
†*Carson v. City of Beloit,* 32 Wis. 2d 282, 145 NW2d 112 (1966).

public expectation. That is, the public expects nursing services to be of high caliber, and the court would hold the nurse to such expectation.

In another 1966 case tried in the Federal District Court in South Carolina,* a pathologist testified that periodic throat cultures on personnel assigned to a premature nursery was impractical and unusual in that locality. The testimony of a nonresidence specialist was to the effect that such practice was desirable as should be the usual practice in all areas. The court rejected the locality rule notwithstanding the general practice in the community.

In disregarding the locality rule the courts have generally referred to its historical background when travel and communication was difficult and the small town doctor and nurse had little opportunity to keep abreast with professional advances. With the advent of modern and rapid transportation and communication the courts are implying that there is little, if any, excuse for any professional not to keep abreast with his field of endeavor. In some instances the courts have implied that since the state requires the prospective nurse to meet a generally accepted standard for the whole of the state, the locality rule conflicts with the state licensure statute.

In addition the educational requirements of the nurse and the nurses' efforts to acquire for nursing the status of a "profession" have increased the public's expectation as to the quality of care to be expected from the nurse wherever the nurse may be. The locality rule has outlived its usefulness.

Negligence has been defined as the failure to do something that a reasonable person under the same or similar circumstances would do, or as doing something that a reasonable and prudent person under the same or similar circumstances would not do. Malpractice on the other hand includes not

only negligence but also all professional conduct that causes damage to a patient. It includes incompetence and immoral conduct that result in injury, unnecessary suffering, or death of the patient. It may come about as the result of ignorance, want of professional skill, recklessness, carelessness, or criminal act. Since the nurse is closely associated with the physician and is expected to understand the general and major problems arising in connection with the care and treatment of his patients, the sins of commission and ommission that give rise to suits against the physician may well entangle the nurse as either a defendant or witness. In other words, malpractice includes not only negligence but also deliberate acts causing damage to a patient.

Liability for negligence or malpractice

Everyone has the duty to handle himself so as to avoid injury to the person or property of others. If any person, including nurses and physicians, breaches the duty, he is answerable in damages to the injured party.

Common acts of negligence

ABANDONMENT. Once a private duty nurse accepts the responsibility of providing nursing care for a patient, she is liable if she abandons the patient without justifiable reason and without finding an acceptable replacement, just as the physician would be liable for any damages suffered by the patient if he abandoned the patient. Recently, on a Wednesday, Dr. A removed a tumor from the right breast of patient B. On the following day Dr. A walked into the patient's hospital room and told the patient he had reviewed her chart and had signed for permission for her to be discharged on Saturday. He further informed the patient that he was leaving that day for an extended vacation and advised her to seek another physician of her own choice to remove the stitches. He did not communicate with or consult any other physician in the com-

*Capuschinsky v. United States, 248 Fed. Supp 732 (1966).

munity with respect to the patient. He wrote no orders with respect to analgesics or other medication. The nursing staff of the hospital was most sympathetic but unable to administer anything to her for pain, and she was unable to locate a physician to take over her treatment while she was in the hospital. The community in which she lived was suffering from a severe shortage of physicians, and none could be found who was accepting new patients until Monday morning when a general practitioner relented because of her obvious distress. He rendered emergency treatment, administered analgesics, and referred her to a medical center where she subsequently had a mastectomy as the result of an untreated abscess. It was the opinion of the surgeon at the medical center that the second operation would not have been necessary had the first surgeon not abandoned the patient. The surgeon had not met the standard of care of surgeons, generally, by his abandonment of his patient.

If the illness of a patient is aggravated or extended by his being abandoned by the nurse, the nurse, herself, is liable in damages not only for the expense incurred but also for any additional suffering and loss of income on the part of the patient.

OPERATING ROOM. A significant number of law suits have been brought against nurses, along with the surgeons and the hospital, arising out of surgical procedures. The most frequent act of negligence on the part of the nurse in the operating room is concerned with her failure to account for sponges and instruments used during the procedure. Some courts have held that it is a nondelegable duty of the surgeon to see that all such foreign objects are removed. However, regardless of the stated reason, the courts generally hold that both the nurse and the doctor are responsible to the patient. Some few courts have relieved the surgeon from responsibility when he relied upon a nurse's sponge count, generally predicating the holding on the fact that the nurse was the employee of the hospital. However, these are old cases and should not be relied upon.

Recently the surgeon, anesthesiologist, nurses, and hospital were exonerated from damage for leaving a sponge in a patient when the surgeon closed the operative site on the direction of the anesthesiologist when the patient went into coronary arrest. The primary standard of care was and is to save the patient's life.

In any event the nurse can now expect to be made a party defendant in any such malpractice action whether or not the plaintiff enjoins the surgeon or the hospital or both.

SUPERVISION OF PATIENT. In the not too distant past the physician had the time to sit by his very ill patient's bed and give the patient close observation. At that time nurses were not expected to do much other than give the most basic attention to the patient. Now, with the advent of a higher quality of nursing education and with physicians having more patients and consequently less time to spend with each individual, it has become the duty of the nurse to provide close patient observation and supervision. If she holds herself out to be a professional nurse, she is expected to have sufficient training to recognize the need to communicate with the physician when certain signs appear or when the patient reacts abnormally to a prescribed treatment or deteriorates otherwise.

The failure of the nurse to act within the scope of her training and to render that standard of care which is expected of her would justify a finding that the nurse was guilty of malpractice. She cannot escape liability as a matter of law on the ground that she was merely carrying out the doctor's orders. Of course, the nurse is not authorized to make a medical diagnosis, but she should be able to observe and report symptoms and reactions when sound nursing judgment would require her to do so. The fact that the nurse knows that the particular physician does not appreciate being called after he has gone to bed at night does not relieve the nurse of her duty to communicate with him when the need arises. The patient is still the most important person in any hospital.

BURNS. Another source of malpractice litigation against nurses arises out of burns received by patients from improperly applied hot-water bottles or misuse of heat lamps and diathermy machines.

The negligence of the nurse in such situations is usually so obvious that the nurse and the doctor or hospital will be held liable without any other evidence with respect to proper procedure under such circumstances.

MEDICATION. Not long ago a nurse was expected to follow blindly the instructions of the physician with respect to the administration of drugs and other medications. She would only have been held liable if she had administered the medication contrary to the physician's oral or written instructions.

Because nurses now receive better education in the field of pharmacology, they are expected to use professional judgment in questioning an order with respect to dosage and route of administration and to seek further instructions from the physician. The nurse will be held liable for the administration of the wrong drug, or the right drug by the wrong route.

A professional nurse has the duty to her patient to refuse to administer a medication from which the order was obviously miswritten.

PATIENT'S PROPERTY. When a patient is carried to surgery, he is usually relieved of his jewelry and dentures. If these are taken from him by the nurse, she is responsible for seeing that they are redelivered to him. Every hospital has or should have a standard procedure for handling the personal property of the patient. This procedure should be followed. Whenever a person deposits personal property such as dentures, money, jewelry, or clothing, with another, a *bailment* is created. The depositer is called the bailor and the person receiving the property is called a bailee. The law says that a bailment is a contract and that failure to return the property at the time and place specified in the contract is a breach thereof, and the bailor may recover his damages for the loss of his property. The most usual situation outside of the hospital arises when clothes are delivered to a laundry or dry cleaners. The usual situation in the hospital arises when the nurse or hospital agrees to care for the property of the patient.

INFECTIONS. Nurses and physicians should know better than anyone else the problems that can arise from the lack of sterile or aseptic techniques. Most infections and cross-infections can be prevented by ordinary, clean techniques, and nurses are bound to use such care. The fact that a patient receives such a cross-infection to his damage while in the hospital may be sufficient in a particular case for a finding of negligence.

Exceeding licensure

As was previously discussed, the nurse is licensed to do a limited number of things. The nurse is not licensed to practice medicine, law, or pharmacy. The licensed practical nurse should not be expected or required to do those things reserved to the registered or professional nurse. The undertaking by a nurse to do or perform services that are beyond or outside the license or certificate held by the practioner and that damage a patient subjects the nurse to a legal claim for damages.

Professional liability insurance

Many nurses sincerely believe that they are covered and protected by the liability insurance policy of the hospital by whom they are employed. This is rarely the case. If the nurse is sued along with the hospital, and the hospital has to pay damages to the patient as the result of the nurse's negligence or malpractice, and if the hospital's liability insurance carrier pays the damages up to the limit on its policy, the insurance company or the hospital may take action against the nurse for the amount paid as the result of the nurse's negligence if there is no para-medical treatment. Even if the hospital does furnish negligence and malpractice coverage under its liability insurance policy, the nurse still needs to have a policy to cover those many situations when carrying out duties under the direction and assignment of a physician outside the scope of employment by the hospital. Although the physician or surgeon probably carries malpractice insurance that covers him, it might not cover the professional nurse. Nobody else's liability insurance would cover the nurse as an independent contractor.

There is one malpractice award against a hospital in the amount of $1,500,000, and a study indicates that the average award throughout the United States exceeds $85,000. Not many nurses could satisfy a judgment in any such amount without insurance.

CHAPTER 48 WILLS

■ A will can be defined as an instrument or legal declaration whereby a person disposes of his property. It takes effect on or after his death and is revocable during his lifetime. There are three general types of wills: (1) testamentary, (2) holographic, and (3) nuncupative.

A *testamentary will* is a written will executed in accordance with the necessary statutory requirements. Usually a testamentary will is witnessed by two or more subscribing witnesses, depending upon the state in which he lives and the state or states in which he owns real estate. A *holographic will* is a will written completely in the testator's own handwriting. To be valid in many states it must be deposited with another for safekeeping or be found among the decedent's valuable papers. A *nuncupative will* is recognized in some states and is usually defined as a deathbed declaration regarding the disposition of personal property, only.

TESTAMENTARY WILLS

The usual will is the formal, testamentary will. For such a will to be valid the requirements are (1) the person making the will must have testamentary capacity; that is, he (testator) or she (testatrix) must have sufficient mental capacity to know the general nature and extent of his property and the natural objects of his bounty (relatives). He must also have sufficient mental capacity to understand that he is executing a will and

understand the nature and effect of the will. (2) The testator or testatrix must declare that the instrument is his will to the witnesses. The witnesses do not need to know the provisions of the will. The only thing that the witnesses need to know about the instrument is that the testator has declared it to be his will. (3) In some states the testator or testatrix must sign the will in the presence of the witnesses, but in other states the testator or testatrix may acknowledge to the witnesses that he has signed the will. (4) A sufficient number of witnesses to the will must sign the instrument in the presence of the testator. The witnesses should not be beneficiaries under the will, since in many states they may be called upon to testify with respect to the execution and would be precluded thereby from receiving anything by virtue of the will.

The nurse should be particularly careful in dealing with a patient who wants his will prepared so that she may not be accused of practicing law. The practice of law is generally defined as performing any legal service for any other person, with or without compensation, specifically including the preparation or aiding in the preparation of wills. In some states there is a provision that allows someone other than a lawyer to prepare a will for another in an emergency when imminence of death leaves insufficient time to have the same drawn and its execution supervised by a licensed attorney at law.

It is a good practice on the part of the

nurse to note on the patient's chart when he sends for his attorney to prepare his will. Also, the nurse should note on the patient's chart when the lawyer returns with the prepared will and inform the lawyer of any medication or other condition that might cast doubt upon the patient's capacity to execute his will. This would particularly be true if the patient had been given narcotic or other mind-affecting drugs at periodic times or during the absence of the lawyer.

Wills may be challenged for three basic reasons: (1) lack of testamentary capacity on the part of the testator, (2) undue influence exerted upon the testator, and (3) the failure to meet the necessary legal requirements in connection with the execution of the will.

An example of undue influence exerted by others that takes away the testator's "free agency" would be a clergyman who tells the testator that he is going to hell unless he leaves his property to the clergyman or the church. Another example might be seen when a member of the family attempts to preclude other members of the family from visiting the testator and spends much time convincing the testator that the other members of the family do not care for him or where one member of the family convinces the testator that no one will care for him after he gets out of the hospital unless his will is prepared in a certain way.

There are two schools of thought in the nursing profession as to whether the nurse should be a witness to a will. One school of thought is that the nurse should not be a witness to a will because she might have to appear before some court at some time in the future and testify with respect to the execution of the will, which might cause her to lose some time and suffer some inconvenience. The other school of thought is that the nurse should witness the will, if requested, because it shows that she is concerned for her patient and is willing to be inconvenienced, if necessary. If the will is contested in court, all the doctors and nurses probably will be required to testify, anyway.

OTHER TYPES OF WILLS

If the patient knows he is dying and expresses a desire to dispose of his property in a certain way, the nurse should call several other competent persons to listen to the patient, carefully, so that his wishes may be carried out to the fullest extent of the law. If for no other reason, this should be done out of compassion for the patient. If the hospital procedures allow it, the directions and requests of the patient should be incorporated in the chart and signed by all the persons witnessing the statements or will. If the hospital procedures do not provide for such entries in the patient's chart, the witnesses should, immediately, record the wishes of the patient so that if and when they are called to testify, they can refresh their recollections and be accurate in their testimony. Some states have a special type of nuncupative will with respect to "soldiers and sailors." The requirements vary, but in those states that recognize these wills, an oral will can be perfectly valid to dispose of the entire estate of the decedent.

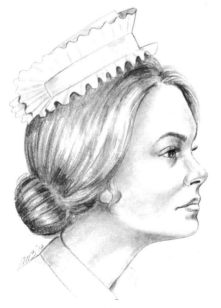

PHILADELPHIA GENERAL GRADUATE NURSE

INTESTACY

If a person dies without a will, his property will be disposed of in accordance with the statutory provisions. Often there is a substantial loss to the estate and the heirs arising from the different methods of administering the estate, administration expenses, taxes, and so on.

CHAPTER 49 CRIMES

■ We have discussed contracts and torts, which give rise to civil actions. These are private actions between the party wrongfully injured and the injuring person. Crimes are those violations of the law that the state can punish. Crimes are said to be "public wrongs." A criminal action is prosecuted in the name of the state or the people of the state, whereas a civil action is prosecuted in the name of the wrongfully injured plaintiff.

Criminal laws are constantly being changed and modified to meet the needs of society. The Congress of the United States passes laws that make certain conduct a violation of federal law, and the state legislatures pass laws making prohibited conduct a violation of the state law. The same act on the part of an individual may be both a state and a federal crime. Most of the states have adopted with modifications the Uniform Narcotic Drug Act making it illegal and a criminal offense for unauthorized persons to possess certain narcotics, hypnotics, and hallucinogens. Congress has made the possession of the same substances by unauthorized persons a federal criminal offense. An individual may be prosecuted, convicted, and punished in both the state and federal courts for possession of the same contraband substances.

WHAT CONSTITUTES A CRIME

As was previously stated, a crime requires the violation of a criminal law by the intentional commission of a criminal act.

The successful completion of the overt act is not necessary. The attempt to carry out the overt act is insufficent.

Intent alone is not sufficient. The intention to steal or kill or embezzle is not a crime until some overt effort is made to carry the intention into effect. The ultimate overt act need not correspond with the intention. As an example of this, H and his wife, W, had an agument that deteriorated into physical violence. H picked up a kerosene lamp and threw it at W. The lamp missed W and shattered against the wall spreading kerosene on the floor and igniting the flammable drapes. Before the fire could be extinguished, it had spread to the adjoining dwellings. The defendant intended the criminal act of assault and battery on his wife, but he was charged and convicted of arson, which is defined as the unlawful burning of the dwelling of another, and received a sentence of life imprisonment.

Another example is that of N. N takes from the drug cabinet a quantity of ergonovine maleate (Ergotrate) for the purpose of assisting a friend in an illegal abortion. The friend takes the ergonovine, hemorrhages, and dies. N's intention was to steal the drug and to participate in an illegal abortion, but she could be tried and convicted in most states of first-degree murder. The law presumes that the defendant intends the natural consequences of his act.

CLASSIFICATIONS OF CRIMES

All crimes are classified as either misdemeanors or felonies. Whether a crime is one or the other is usually determined by the seriousness with which it is regarded. If the crime is punishable by imprisonment in a state's prison, it is normally considered as a *felony*. Some states define a felony as one for which the convicted defendant can be imprisoned for longer than a designated period of time such as a year. All other crimes are classified as *misdemeanors*. Frequently the statute under which the defendant is being tried defines his crime as either a felony or as a misdemeanor.

In addition to the punishment pronounced by the court, the defendant convicted of a felony loses his citizenship, including his right to hold public office, right to vote, and the right to practice his profession.

SPECIFIC CRIMES
Homicide

The killing of another human being is a homicide. A homicide may be justifiable, excusable, or felonious. A *justifiable homicide* would include the slaying of an escaping felony prisoner by a law enforcement officer, among others. An *excusable homicide* includes the unintentional killing of another, such as where the patient died during legal surgery or in an unavoidable accident. *Felonious homicide* falls into two classifications: (1) murder and (2) manslaughter.

MURDER. A felonious homicide that shall be perpetrated by means of poison, lying in wait, imprisonment, starving, torture, or by any form of willful, deliberate, and premeditated killing is *murder in the first degree*. Some states include within this definition any unlawful or felonious homicide that shall be committed in the perpetration or attempt to perpetrate any arson, rape, robbery, burglary, or other felony.

Some states recognize a classification known as *second-degree murder,* which can be defined as the unlawful killing of a human

being with malice, but without evidence of premeditation and deliberation. As the law was brought to us from England, when the intentional killing by a deadly weapon was shown, the law presumed malice aforethought but does not presume premeditation and deliberation. The penalty for second-degree murder is less than that for first-degree murder.

MANSLAUGHTER. Manslaughter can be divided into two classifications: voluntary and involuntary. *Voluntary manslaughter* is an intentional homicide committed in a heat of passion caused by reasonable provocation. The classic example: the husband kills his wife or her boyfriend when he catches them together engaged in extramarital relations. *Involuntary manslaughter* is an unintentional homicide that is not excusable. It may arise as the result of a negligent act or while in the course of committing a misdemeanor. For example, an automobile driver operates his motor vehicle through a congested area at an unlawful rate of speed and strikes and kills a pedestrian. Another example would be the hunter who sees movement in a bush and fires, accidentally killing his hunting companion.

A second category of involuntary manslaughter arises from doing a lawful act in a grossly negligent manner. Many cases are on record in which physicians have been charged with manslaughter arising out of the deaths of their patients when the physician and surgeon operated while intoxicated or administered lethal overdoses of drugs.

A third type of involuntary manslaughter involves the failure to act when there is a duty to act. A good example of this is the death of a child brought about by parents who allow their child to starve to death or to suffocate in a closed automobile or who fail to provide medical attention when it is desperately needed.

Offenses against property

Larceny, robbery, embezzlement, false pretenses and cheats, obtaining property or services by false or fraudulant use of credit devices or other means, frauds, forgeries, and trespasses are crimes regarding property.

Larceny is the taking and carrying away of the property of another with the intention of depriving the owner or the person entitled to its possession of the use of the property. The crime is a highly technical one, since the courts of England were somewhat hesitant to invoke capital punishment for the larceny of small items. It was punishable by death in England for many, many years. Therefore the courts of England required strict proof before conviction.

Robbery is larceny with force. That is the taking of property from another by placing him in fear or through a threat of force.

If any person legally receives property for another and willfully misapplies or converts the property to his own use he can be guilty of a felony and is usually punished as in cases of larceny. The nurse is frequently entrusted with the valuables of her patient. She is obligated to keep these valuables for the patient and to return them to him. Not only may she be held liable, civilly, for her failure to return these valuables; but if she converts the property to her own use or does any act that would deprive the patient of his valuables, she can be guilty of embezzlement.

If the nurse obtains property under false pretense by a misrepresentation and then converts the property to her own use, she is also guilty of a criminal act. A patient who with the intent to defraud obtains hospital services with no intention of paying would, also, be guilty of obtaining property by false pretense.

Narcotics

The narcotic laws are probably the strictest and most dangerous laws that affect the nurse, directly. The narcotic laws covered in the Harrison Narcotic Act and the Uniform Narcotic Law are exceptions to the rule requiring intention. Nowhere in either of these two acts do the legislative bodies require that the violation be intentional. Several years ago a physician gave a patient three prescriptions for morphine: one dated the date of issuance, one dated two days later, and one dated four days later. The intention of the physician was to keep the patient from having too much morphine in her possession at any one time while he was on vacation. The pharmacist filled all three prescriptions on the date of original issuance. This was discovered by a narcotic agent during a check of the drug store's narcotic record, and the doctor was prosecuted for a violation of the Harrison Narcotic Act. The physician could have legally written one prescription for the total amount of morphine at one time. However, he was guilty of a violation of the federal law despite his good intentions.

The penalty for a violation of either the state or federal law with respect to narcotic drugs is severe.

CHAPTER 50 EVIDENCE

■ It would be ideal if we could always agree on all the facts and the law applicable thereto and act thereon accordingly, but as long as men differ, their disputes will always have to be decided by others. In our society the ultimate decision frequently has to be made in a court of law.

After all the pleadings have been filed and discovery has been completed, it is necessary to convince a judge or jury by the evidence of the facts in the case. The law of evidence is a system of rules and standards by which the admission of proof at a trial is regulated. Usually a trial is conducted in four stages:
1. The plaintiff's main case, or evidence submitted to support his claim.
2. The defendant's case or evidence in defense.
3. The plaintiff's rebuttal evidence.
4. The defendant's rejoinder.

In each part of the trial, witnesses are called by the party seeking their testimony, and examination of each witness may consist of (1) the direct examination conducted by the party calling it, (2) the cross-examination by his adversary, (3) redirect examination by the party calling the witness, and (4) recross-examination by the adversary. The party calling the witness implies that he vouches for the truth of what the witness says unless it becomes apparent that the witness has changed his testimony or is hostile to the party calling him.

Although the judge may in his discretion control the general form of the examination of a witness, he usually leaves it up to the trial lawyer as to whether he will ask specific questions or one question that will call for a free narrative of the events from the witness. The trial lawyer will usually make this decision based upon the intelligence of the witness and the ability of the witness to articulate what the witness knows in a vivid and accurate way. Ordinarily the judge will not allow the attorney calling a witness to ask questions that might lead the witness into a particular answer. The suggestion itself might plant the belief of its truth because it suggests to the witness the answer desired by the examiner. Also, usually, the lawyer will not be allowed over objection to ask a question that is argumentative. The policy of our system of proof is for the witness to testify to facts within his own personal knowledge and not based on what someone else may have told him. If a physician has examined an injured plaintiff, naturally he may describe what he has seen and give his expert opinion as to the cause or probable duration of the condition. The nurse in this situation could testify as to what she has seen, but she would not be entitled to give an expert opinion therefrom. However, she may be qualified as an expert in the field of nursing and give her opinion with respect to the standard of care of nursing or other aspects of the nursing care of the patient.

When the lawyer for the party calling her as a witness completes his examination, the opposing attorney has a right to cross-examine her. In England and in about one fifth of the states, the cross-examiner may question the witness about any subject relevent to any of the issues in the entire case. In the majority of the states, however, the cross-examination must be limited to the matters testified to on direct examination. One of the main functions of cross-examination is to bring out answers that will impeach the veracity, capacity to observe, impartiality, and consistency of the witness. It should be noted that if the witness has testified truthfully, he has nothing to fear from cross-examination.

PRIVILEGED COMMUNICATIONS

The privileged communications between husband and wife, attorney and client, physician and patient, and clergyman and parishioner are important enough to have separate treatments.

In common law, husband and wife are absolutely incompetent to testify in an action in which either was a party. Now, however, by statute in most states, husband and wife are both competent and compellable to testify either for or against each other in all civil actions. In some states there is a limitation surrounding testimony with respect to adultery of either party in order to prevent collusion in divorce actions. Also, in common law the husband or wife of the defendant in a criminal case was incompetent to testify either for the government or for the defense. This incompetency has been completely removed in most states by statute so far as testifying for the defendant is concerned, but it still exists, with specified exceptions, as to testimony against the defendant. A confidential communication between husband and wife is privileged, and neither may be compelled to disclose it when testifying as a witness. Only *confidential* communications are within the rule; hence a communication made in the known presence of a third party is not protected.

The law in North Carolina and in most states specifies that if a nurse is asked in

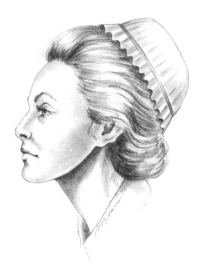

BELLEVUE HOSPITAL GRADUATE NURSE

court to answer a question concerning a privileged communication between herself and a patient, she should refuse to do so unless the judge specifically directs her to do so—in which case she must answer. If, however, she has received any information from the patient while specifically acting as agent for the physician, she may refuse to divulge such a communication.

The fact that a witness is the attorney for one of the parties does not necessarily render him incompetent to testify. A privilege exists, however, by virtue of which the attorney may not, without his client's consent, testify as to any confidential communication from the client to the attorney made on the faith of the relationship between them. The relation of attorney and client must have existed at the time of the disclosure. The communication must have been made in confidence. The communication must relate to the matter concerning which the attorney was employed or being professionally consulted. Although the attorney need not have been consulted with a view to actual litigation, the communication must have been made in the course of seeking legal advice for a proper purpose and not sought as an aid in the perpetration of a crime. The privilege is that of the client, and it may be waived by the client.

QUESTIONS AND STUDY PROJECTS FOR UNIT TWELVE

1. Discuss the purposes and duties of state boards of nursing.
2. What is the purpose of licensure for nurses?
3. Discuss the differences in the duties and responsibilities of the professional nurse and the licensed practical nurse.
4. What are the necessary elements of a contract? What is breach of contract? Why is the nurse concerned with contracts?
5. Define the following:

   a. Misdemeanor
   b. Felony
   c. Crime
   d. Tort
   e. Defamation
   f. False imprisonment

6. Define assault and battery. Give examples of hospital situations from which these charges might arise.
7. Explain the difference between negligence and malpractice. Give examples.
8. What is professional liability insurance? Does a nurse need this type of insurance? Explain your answer.
9. What is a will? Describe the three generally accepted types of wills. What is the nurse's role in regard to wills?
10. What is meant by "privileged communications," and what is the nurse's responsibility in this matter?

REFERENCES FOR UNIT TWELVE

American Jurisprudence, ed. 2, Rochester, N. Y., Jurisprudence Publishers, Inc.:
25 AmJur 2d, Drugs, narcotics, and poisons, section 4, 10-19, 52-73.
61 AmJur 2d, Physicians, surgeons, and other healers.
40 AmJur 2d, Hospitals and asylums.
American Law Reports, Rochester, N. Y., The Lawyer's Cooperative Publishing Co., Annotations:
Duty of physician or surgeon to warn or instruct nurse or attendant, 4 ALR 1527.
Liability of operating surgeon for negligence of nurse assisting him, 12 ALR 3d 1017. Malpractice in connection with intravenous or other forced or involuntary feeding of patient, 6 ALR 3d 668.
Nurse's liability for her own negligence or malpractice, 51 ALR 2d 970.
Applicability, in action against nurse in her professional capacity, of statute of limitations applicable to malpractice, 8 ALR 3d 1336.
Liability of private, noncharitable hospital or sanitarium for improper care or treatment of patients—failure to hire special nurse—failure of nurse to give constant attendance, 22 ALR 341, 345, 353, supplemented 39 ALR 1431, 1433, 1434, supplemented 124 ALR 186, 190.
Liability of surgeon leaving sponge or other foreign matter in incision—reliance on custom of nurse's count, 65 ALR 1023, 1026; 10 ALR 3d 9.
Libel and slander: privilege of statements by physician, surgeon, or nurse concerning patient, 73 ALR 2d 325.
Nurse as independent contractor or servant, 60 ALR 303.
Privilege of communications by or to nurse or attendant, 47 ALR 2d 742.
Admissibility of hospital chart or other hospital record, 75 ALR 378; 120 ALR 1124. Aspirin poisoning: liability for negligence in diagnosing or treating aspirin poisoning, 36 ALR 3d 1358. Hospital's liability for personal injury or death of doctor, nurse, or attendant, 1 ALR 3d 1036.
Liability of hospital for negligence of nurse assisting operating surgeon, 29 ALR 3d 1065.
Liability of physician for injury or death from blood transfusion, 59 ALR 2d 786. Liability of physician who adandons case, 57 ALR 2d 432. Liability of physician for lack of diligence in attending patient, 57 ALR 2d 379.

Proximate cause in malpractice cases, 13 ALR 2d 11.

Dressing patient: duty of physician or nurse to assist patient while dressing or undressing, 41 ALR 3d 1351.

Hypodermic injection: liability for injury allegedly resulting from negligence in making hypodermic injection, 45 ALR 3d 731.

Blackstone, Sir William: Blackstone's commentaries, ed. 3, Albany, N. Y., 1890, Banks & Brothers, Law Publishers.

Creighton, Helen: Law every nurse should know, Philadelphia, 1957, W. B. Saunders Co., chap. 1.

Culver, Vivian M., and Brownell, Kathryn O.: The practical nurse, ed. 7, Philadelphia, 1969, W. B. Saunders Co.

Hershey, Nathan: The law and the nurse. Minors and consent, American Journal of Nursing **68:** 2396, November, 1968.

Hershey, Nathan: You know what good practice is, American Journal of Nursing **68:**1057, May, 1968.

Kinkela, Gabrielle G., and Kinkela, Robert V.: Hospital nurses and tort liability, Cleveland-Marshall Law Review **18:**5369, January, 1969.

Pavalon, Eugene I., and Robin, Sidney: Damage suits based on nursing malpractice, Illinois Bar Journal **57:**282-298, December, 1968.

Sanner, Margaret: Trends and professional adjustments in nursing, Philadelphia, 1962, W. B. Saunders Co.

Sarner, Harvey: The nurse and the law, Philadelphia, 1968, W. B. Saunders Co.

Symposium on the nurse and the law, Nursing Clinics of North America, pp. 115-197, March, 1967.

INDEX